S. Suzuki · W.E. Hathaway
J. Bonnar · A.H. Sutor (Eds.)

Perinatal Thrombosis and Hemostasis

With 126 Figures

Springer-Verlag
Tokyo Berlin Heidelberg
New York London Paris
Hong Kong Barcelona

Professor SHIGENORI SUZUKI, M.D.
College of Medical Technology, Hokkaido University, Kita-ku, Sapporo 060, Japan

Professor WILLIAM E. HATHAWAY, M.D.
University of Colorado School of Medicine, Denver, CO 80262, USA

Professor JOHN BONNAR, M.D., FRCOG
University of Dublin, Trinity College, Department of Obstetrics and Gynaecology, St. James's Hospital, Dublin, Ireland

Professor ANTON H. SUTOR, M.D.
Universitäts-Kinderklinik, 7800 Freiburg, Federal Republic of Germany

ISBN 4-431-70055-2 Springer-Verlag Tokyo Berlin Heidelberg New York
ISBN 3-540-70055-2 Springer-Verlag Berlin Heidelberg New York Tokyo
ISBN 0-387-70055-2 Springer-Verlag New York Berlin Heidelberg Tokyo

Library of Congress Cataloging-in-Publication Data
Perinatal thrombosis and hemostasis / S. Suzuki . . . [et al.] (eds.)., p. cm. Includes bibliographical references. Includes index. ISBN 4-431-70055-2 : —ISBN 3-540-70055-2 : —ISBN 0-387-70055-2 : 1. Blood coagulation disorders in pregnancy. 2. Blood coagulation disorders in infants. 3. Thrombosis. 4. Hemostasis. I. Suzuki, Shigenori, 1936– . [DNLM: 1. Blood Coagulation Disorders—in infancy & childhood. 2. Blood Coagulation Disorders—in pregnancy. 3. Hemostasis. 4. Pregnancy Complications, Hematologic. 5. Thrombosis. WQ 252 P445]. RG580.B56P47 1990 618.3—dc20 DNLM/DLC for Library of Congress 90-10190

Typesetting: Asco Trade Typesetting Ltd., Hong Kong
Printing: Kowa Art Printing, Tokyo
Binding: Kubota Binding, Tokyo

Preface

Hemorrhage and thrombosis are major hazards for pregnant women and their newborn infants. This book is concerned with the developmental mechanisms, the diagnosis and treatment, as well as the prevention of these hemorrhagic and thrombotic disorders.

The topics discussed in this volume, (1) perinatal hemorrhage in mothers and their offspring; (2) coagulation disorders complicating pregnancy; (3) neonatal intracranial hemorrhage; and, (4) vitamin K deficiency in the neonate, will help bridge the gap between basic scientists and clinicians and between the pediatrician and the obstetrician. Hopefully, all those concerned with preventing these disorders will be stimulated by the information and questions raised in the following presentations.

Acknowledgements

We wish to thank Professors Takeshi Abe (Vice President, Teikyo University), Nobuyoshi Shinagawa (Hirosaki University), Hiroaki Soma (Tokyo Medical College), Tamotsu Miyazaki and Keisuke Sakurada (Hokkaido University) for their helpful advice.

SHIGENORI SUZUKI
WILLIAM E. HATHAWAY
JOHN BONNAR
ANTON H. SUTOR

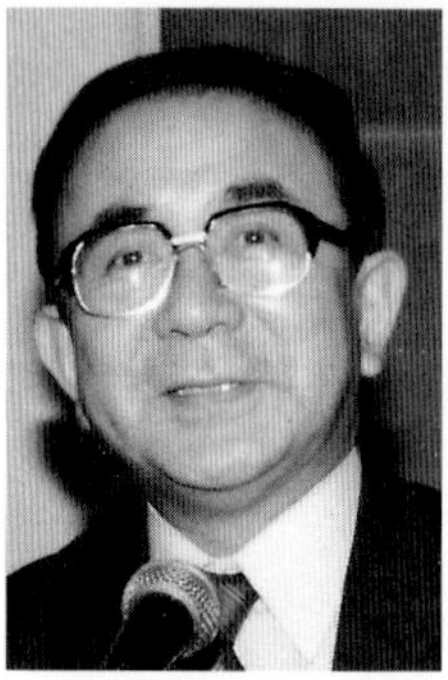

SHIGENORI SUZUKI. *1936 in Sapporo, Japan. M.D., University of Hokkaido, 1963. Lecturer, Hokkaido University, 1974. Alexander Humboldt-Foundation Scholarship, Free University of Berlin. University of Munich, 1974–1976. Former President, Japanese Society of Obstetrical, Gynecological, and Neonatal Hematology. President of International Symposium on Perinatal Thrombosis and Hemostasis (1989 Sapporo). Professor, College of Medical Technology affiliated with Hokkaido University since 1983.

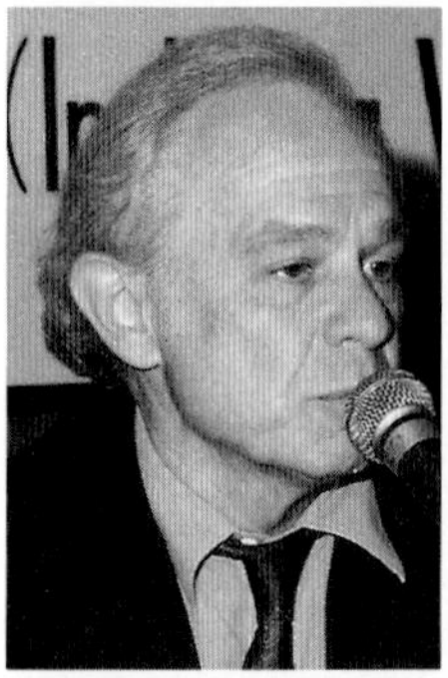

WILLIAM E. HATHAWAY. *1929 in Oklahoma, USA. M.D., University of Oklahoma, 1954. Fellow in Pediatric Hematology, University of Colorado School of Medicine, 1959. Head, Section of Pediatric Hematology-Oncology and Director of Special Coagulation Laboratory, University Hospital, 1973–1988. Professor of Pediatrics (1973–1988) and Professor Emeritus (since 1988), University of Colorado School of Medicine.

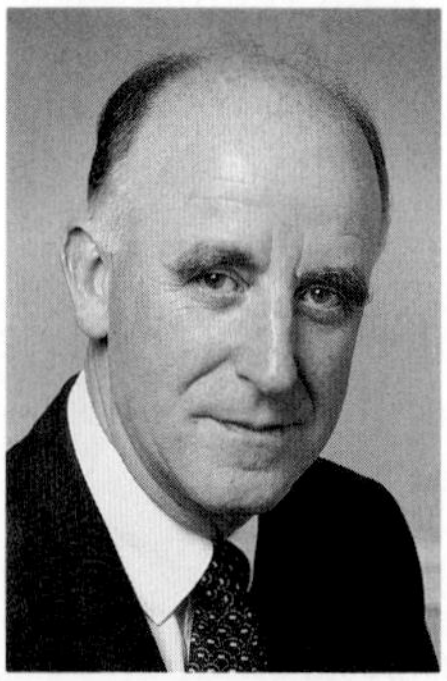

JOHN BONNAR. *1934 in Wishaw, Scotland. M.B., CH.B., University of Glasgow, 1958. M.D. with Honours, University of Glasgow, 1971. Elected to the Fellowship of the Royal College of Obstetricians and Gynaecologists, 1972. M.A., University of Dublin, 1976. Professor and Head, Department of Obstetrics and Gynaecology, Trinity College, University of Dublin since 1975.

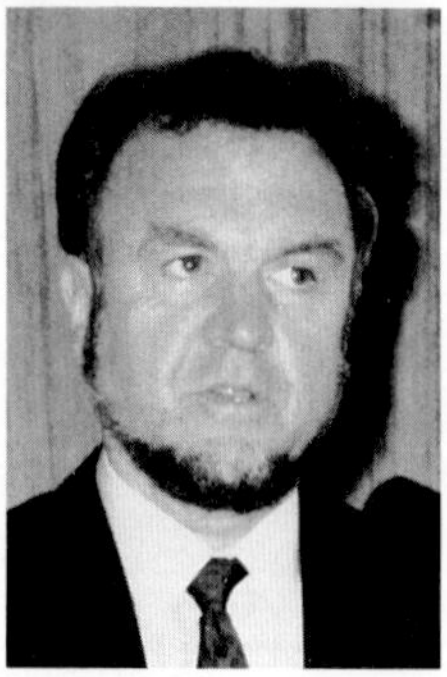

ANTON H. SUTOR. *1938 in Augsburg, Germany. M.D., Freiburg University, 1964. Fellow of Pediatric Hematology, Mayo Clinic (USA), 1969. Awarded the Goedecke Research Prize from Freiburg University, 1973 and the Alexander-Schmidt-Prize from the German Society of Haemostaseology, 1975. Professor of Pediatrics, Münster University since 1977. Head, Pediatric Hematology and Hemostaseology, University of Freiburg, Children's Hospital since 1982.

Contents

Part 1. Perinatal Hemorrhage in Mothers and Newborns (Diagnosis, Treatment, and Case Reports)

Diagnostic Value of Fibrin- and Fibrinogen Degradation Products in Perinatology

1.1 The Diagnostic Value of Fibrin- and Fibrinogen Degradation Products in Perinatology

REIMAR HAFTER and HENNER GRAEFF[1]

Introduction

Thromboembolic episodes and intravascular coagulation are more frequent during gestation and in certain groups of high-risk patients than in non-pregnant and healthy individuals. Hypercoagulability may be one of the underlying conditions. The so-called state of hypercoagulability is reflected in the levels of thrombin-mediated soluble fibrin monomer complexes (SFMC).

Fibrin monomer (des AA-fibrin) is generated from fibrinogen when fibrinopeptide A (FPA) is split off by thrombin. Fibrin monomer binds to fibrinogen to form soluble complexes (SFMC). Fibrin monomer and fibrinogen are in steady equilibrium with SFMC, fibrin (soluble polymerized fibrin monomer), and fibrinogen. When fibrin monomer is generated more abundantly, the equilibrium is shifted to favor SFMC and fibrin. Fibrin is taken out of equilibrium when it is cross-linked by factor XIIIa to form insoluble fibrin.

Activation of the coagulation system is linked to activation of the fibrinolytic enzyme system. One possible pathway is via factor XIIa and activation of prekallikrein to kallikrein. Kallikrein can activate plasminogen to plasmin directly or via plasminogen activator (scu-PA). As a result, concomitantly with the increase in SFMC, fibrin degradation products (FDP) arise. Elevated levels of SFMC are accompanied by elevated levels of FDP.

Application of Gel Filtration Chromatography

The soluble fibrin monomer complexes can be semiquantitated by gel filtration chromatography [1]. We adapted a method [2] by which a beta-alanine precipitated plasma sample is applied on a 4% agarose gel column, and SFMCs are separated according to their higher molecular weights as a shoulder in front of

[1]Frauenklinik der Technischen Universität München, Ismaninger Strasse 22, D-8000 München 80, Federal Republic of Germany

Table 1. Amounts of soluble fibrin monomer complexes (SFMC) in normal patients and in patients with hypercoagulability

Range of values	SFMC (%)
Normal (healthy young males/females, 18–30 years)	2.6–2.9
Hypercoagulability	3.8–8.0
Pregnancy (weeks 21 to 40)	3.6–4.9
During delivery	4.3–5.3
Early puerperium	6.0
Postoperatively (2 h)	4.0
In cases of intravascular coagulation (DIC)	8.0–25

the fibrinogen peak. The percentage of SFMCs in relation to the fibrinogen content can be planimetrically estimated [2]. This technique tends, according to the procedure involved, to result in what is probably a too-high estimation if the shoulder prior to the fibrinogen peak is very small. Therefore, the level of 2.6–2.9% SFMC for normal plasma could be slightly overestimated (Table 1).

In patients with hypercoagulability, values between 3% and 8% SFMC—or up to 5% above normal values—are found. During pregnancy a steady increase of SFMC from 2.6% to 4.9% was observed [3,4]. These data were confirmed by McKillop et al. [5], who applied the same procedure; and by van Royen and Ten Cate [6], who observed elevated levels of fibrinopeptide A (FPA) during pregnancy. During delivery a further increase of SFMC was measured (4.3% to 5.3%) which was statistically significant [7,8]. In addition, we could show [7] that the increase of SFMC was independent of the kind of delivery. Whether the delivery occurred spontaneously, was vaginal operative, or by section there was no difference in the increase in SFMC. This finding was in accordance with observations that the thromboembolic rate in postpartum patients was not dependent on the kind of delivery.

The highest values of SFMC were observed in the early puerperium [9]. The high levels (6%–7% SFMC) reflect the high incidence of thromboembolic episodes during the puerperium—20 times greater than in pregnancy. These data on hypercoagulability are in agreement with the increased risk for thromboembolism in certain groups of patients. Yet, in our limited experience, thrombosis or pulmonary embolism could not be monitored in any single patient by estimation of SFMC and by the finding of dramatically elevated levels of SFMC.

Elution Patterns in Patients with DIC

A different elution pattern by gel filtration is observed if the method of measuring SFMC is applied to beta-alanine precipitated plasma samples from patients with signs of disseminated intravascular coagulation (DIC). In Fig. 1 (*upper curve*), the pattern of a patient with amniotic fluid embolism accompanied by severe DIC is shown [9,10]. In comparison, the pattern from a patient in puerperium (hypercoagulability) is shown in the *lower curve*. The fibrinogen peak is diminished (*upper curve*) because of the decrease of clottable fibrinogen. The

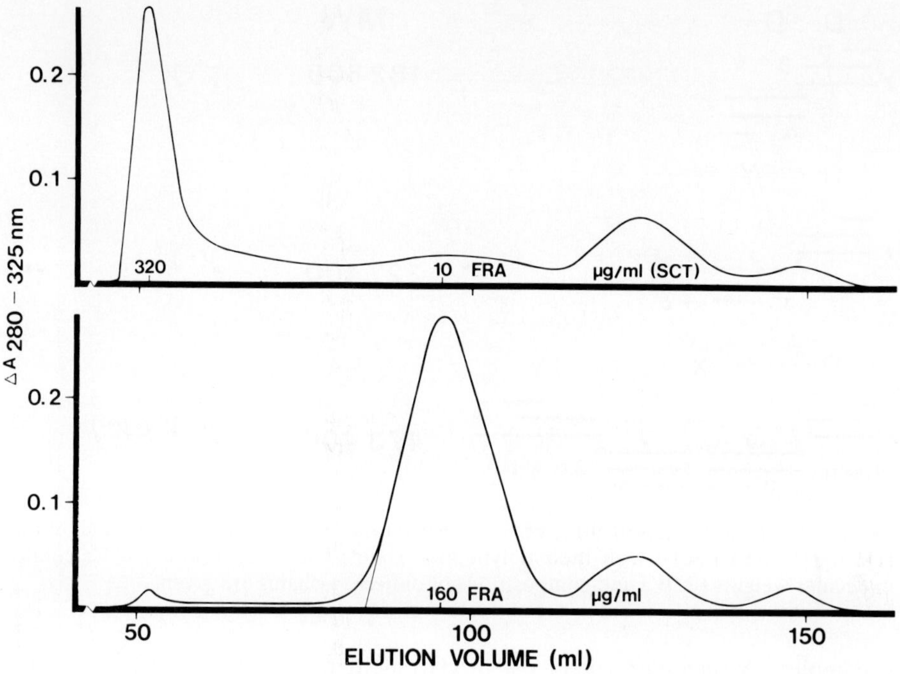

Fig. 1. Elution profile after 4% gel filtration of a beta-alanine precipitated plasma sample from a patient with amniotic fluid embolism (*upper profile*). Cross-linked fibrin oligomers are eluted with the void volume (at 50 ml of the elution volume) and the shoulder between void volume and fibrinogen peak (approx. 50–80 ml). The *lower profile* corresponds to one normally obtained in the early puerperium. Fibrinogen-related antigen (*FRA*) was estimated by the staphylococcal-clumping test (*SCT*)

fibrinogen is consumed via clotting to fibrin and degradation by plasmin to split products. When the split products are analyzed by SDS-polyacryamide gel electrophoresis, characteristic high molecular weight cross-linked fibrin derivatives can be demonstrated, which indicates that these products are derived from fibrin by the combined action of thrombin, factor XIIIa, and plasmin on fibrinogen [9,10].

In vitro investigations have provided detailed descriptions of these derivatives [10–16]. Figure 2 schematically depicts the formation of three derivatives (*DD*, *DY*, *DXY*) from their corresponding polypeptide subunit remnants. The first cross-linked fibrin derivative to be identified [17], D-dimer (DD), primarily occurs as DD/E complex in plasma [18]. It is the only fragment containing a dimeric gamma-chain shortened on both ends ($\gamma^1 - \gamma^1$). Fragment DY is the next higher homologous fragment [19]. Quantitatively, it is as prominent in biological fluids as DD [20]. Finally, fragment DXY is an example of the higher molecular weight derivatives, which, as early degradation products, still contain fragment X and are therefore also called "X-oligomers." Analogous to the DD/

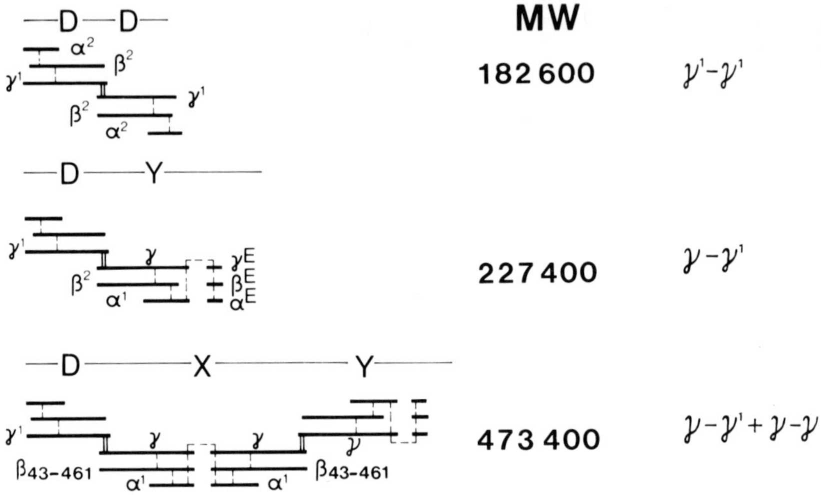

Fig. 2. Structural models of three characteristic cross-linked fibrin derivatives (D-dimer (*DD*), *DY*, and *DXY*) with their polypeptide chains and chain remnants. Calculated molecular weights (*MW*) and compositions of dimeric γ-chains are given

E complex, X-oligomers also exist in vivo as high molecular weight comlexes which are held together by hydrogen bonds [12,13].

The cross-linked high molecular weight fibrin derivatives (XDP) can be measured quantitatively by ELISA technique using monoclonal antibodies specifically directed against epitops in the cross-linking site. The method is known as the D-dimer test [21,22].

During a 7-year interval, severe DIC during pregnancy, with high levels of XDP, was demonstrated in our clinic [10]: five cases of abruptio placentae, seven cases of amniotic fluid embolism, five cases of endotoxin shock following septic abortion, two cases of endotoxin shock following pyelonephrites, two cases of dead fetus syndrome, and two cases of eclampsia (Table 2). In one case of abruptio placentae, XDP levels as high as 390 μg per ml were measured. The normal value in healthy subjects is less than 300 ng per ml.

Table 2. Demonstration of circulating cross-linked fibrin from obstetric patients with intravascular coagulation

	No. of Cases ($n = 23$)
Abruptio Placentae	5
Amniotic fluid embolism	7
Endotoxin shock following	
Septic abortion	5
Pyelonephrites	2
Dead fetus syndrome	2
Eclampsia	2

Thromboembolic disease can also be monitored by the D-dimer test. In young non-pregnant patients with deep vein thrombosis ($n = 6$) and pulmonary embolism ($n = 1$), elevated levels (808 ± 430 ng/ml) and a high level (4950 ng/ml) of XDP were measured [23].

The XDP are also elevated in the postoperative phase due to the wound healing process. In nine patients, (average age 44 ± 10 years) operated on electively because of benign gynecological disorders plasma samples were investigated from the 1st and 2nd postoperative day. The mean XDP concentration was 1280 ± 580 ng/ml. In a matched control group ($n = 20$), the mean XDP concentration was 197 ± 52 ng/ml [23]. If XDP is measured to monitor a thromboembolic event in the postoperative phase, this interference has to be considered.

The D-dimer test is so sensitive that even XDP which are generated during pregnancy and puerperium in the hypercoagulable state, caused through activation of coagulative and fibrinolytic systems, can be monitored. In a study of 23 subjects [23], we demonstrated that the plasma level of XDP increased distinctively during pregnancy. The highest values of 586 ± 57 ng/ml were noticed between the third trimenon and delivery, compared to 168 ± 87 ng/ml in matched controls ($n = 20$). A further marked increase up to about 2000 ng/ml was observed in the puerperium (1525 ± 630 ng/ml). These findings confirm very nicely that activation of the coagulation system responds to activation of the fibrinolytic system.

It is of particular clinical interest to distinguish between fibrinogenolysis and fibrinolysis, i.e., whether a fragment resulting from plasmin action is detectable before (fibrinogen derivative) or after (fibrin derivative) thrombin and factor XIII have acted on fibrinogen. This distinction is made possible with the help of appropriate monoclonal antibodies made available recently (reviewed in [24]). The antibodies can be used in ELISA technique to measure fibrin specifically in plasma samples [25] or, in another approach [26] to measure either fibrinogen degradation products or fibrin degradation products. The last two tests are already commercially available (Fg-DP and Fb-DP tests). Studies with these tests so far have shown that both kinds of degradation products are found at hypercoagulable states and in DIC, but fibrin degradation products are formed to a distinctively higher degree.

Summary. Hypercoagulability in obstetric patients and in the newborn reflects not only normal physiological changes often caused by hormonal stimulation, but also slight disorders caused by various dysfunctions. The biochemical correlates are the so-called soluble fibrin monomer complexes (SFMC). It has been shown that during pregnancy there is a constant rise in SFMC, which cumulates during birth and in puerperium. Elevated levels of SFMC are also observed in the asphyctic newborn. In obstetrical disorders accompanied by disseminated intravascular coagulation (DIC), an additional rise of fibrin degradation products occurs with the presence of cross-linked fibrin degradation products. These products can be monitored by gel filtration and further identified by SDS-PAGE. The characteristic fibrin degradation products are D-dimer. DY, and so-called X-oligomers. A more concise and specific method of measuring these products is achieved by ELISA technique using monoclonal antibodies which point out the cross-linking site. D-dimer proved to be a very sensitive parameter not only for DIC but also for local incidents of intravascular coagulation. This could be confirmed in patients with DIC following abruptio placenta, amniotic fluid embolism, etc. and in patients with thrombosis. Additional information concerning fibrinogen metabolism was obtained by ELISA using other specific monoclonal antibodies directed against fibrin-and/or fibrinogen degradation products.

References

1. Alkjaersig N, Fletcher AP, Burstein R (1971) Thromboembolism and oral contraceptive medication. Thromb Diathesis Haemorrh (Suppl) 49: 125–129
2. Hafter R, Graeff H (1976) Estimation of soluble fibrin monomer complexes by agarose gel filtration. In: Davidson JF, Samama MM, Desnoyers PC (eds) Progress in chemical fibrinolysis and thrombolysis, vol 2. Raven, New York, pp 137–149
3. Hafter R, Schneebauer T, Tafel K, Ernst E, Graeff H (1975) Bestimmung von löslichen Fibrinmonomerkomplexen zur Erfassung der Hyperkoagulabilität in der Schwangerschaft und unter der Geburt. Geburtsh u Frauenheilk 35: 518–525
4. Graeff H, Von Hugo R, Hafter R (1980) Hypercoagulability and intravascular coagulation in obstetrics and gynaecology. In: Coccheri S (ed) Vth International Congress on Thromboembolism, Bologna May 29-June 2, 1978. Proceedings, Quaderni della Coagulazine, pp 449–451
5. McKillop C, Forbes CD, Howie PW, Prentice CRM (1976) Soluble fibrin monomer complexes in preeclampsia. Lancet I: 56–58
6. Van Royen EA, Ten Cate JW (1976) Generation of a thrombinlike activity in late pregnancy. Thromb Res 8: 487–492
7. Graeff H, Hafter R, Von Hugo R (1976) Hyperkoagulabilität und Thromboseneigung in Schwangerschaft und Wochenbett. In: Ludwig H, Kurz H (eds) Die Beckenvenen. Schattauer, Stuttgart, pp 223–230
8. Graeff H, Wiemann A, Von Hugo R, Hafter R (1976) Amount and distribution pattern of soluble fibrin monomer complexes during the early puerperium. Am J Obstet Gynecol 124: 21–24
9. Graeff H, Hafter R, Bachmann L (1979) Subunit and macromolecular structure of circulating fibrin from obstetric patients with intravascular coagulation. Thromb Res 16: 313–328
10. Graeff H, Hafter R (1982) Detection and relevance of crosslinked fibrin derivatives in blood. Semin Thromb Hemost 8: 57–68
11. Hafter H, Graeff H (1982) Homologues of fibrin X oligomers. In: Henschen A, Graeff H, Lottspeich F (eds) Fibrinogen—recent biochemical and medical aspects. de Gruyter, Berlin, pp 291–305
12. Francis CW, Marder VJ (1982) A molecular model of plasmic degradation of crosslinked fibrin. Semin Thromb Hemost 8: 25–35
13. Marder VJ, Francis CW (1984) Plasmin degradation of cross-linked fibrin. Ann NY Acad Sci 408: 397–406
14. Gaffiney PJ (1982) Fibrin fragmentation by plasmin: molecular considerations and their relevance to DIC and thrombosis. In: Henschen A, Graeff H, Lottspeich F (eds) Fibrinogen—recent biochemical and medical aspects. de Gruyter, Berlin, pp 307–327
15. Gaffney PJ (1983) The occurrence and clinical relevance of fibrin fragments in blood. Ann NY Acad Sci 408: 407–423

16. Graeff H, Hafter R (1987) Clinical aspects of fibrinolysis. In: Bloom AL, Thomas DP (eds) Haemostasis and thrombosis. Churchill Livingstone, Edinburgh, pp 245–254
17. Kopec M, Teisseyre E, Dudek-Wojciechowska G, Kloczewiak M, Pankiewicz A, Latallo CS (1973) Studies on the double D fragment from stabilized bovine fibrin. Thromb Res 2: 283–292
18. Gaffney PJ, Lane DA, Kakkar VV, Brasher M (1975) Characterization of a soluble D-dimer-E complex in cross-linked fibrin digests. Thromb Res 7: 89–99
19. Whitaker AN, Rowe EA, Masci PP, Gaffney PJ (1980) Identification of a D-dimer-E complex in disseminated intravascular coagulation. Thromb Res 19: 381–391
20. Hafter R, Klaubert W, Gollwitzer R, Von Hugo R, Graeff H (1984) Cross-linked fibrin derivatives and fibronectin in ascitic fluid from patients with ovarian cancer compared to ascitic fluid in liver cirrhosis. Thromb Res 35: 53–64
21. Elms MJ, Bunce IH, Bundesen PG, Rylatt DB, Webber AJ, Masci PP, Whitaker AN (1983) Measurement of cross-linked fibrin degradation products—an immunoassay using monoclonal antibodies. Thromb Haemost 50 (2): 591–594
22. Hafter R, Schröck R, Von Hugo R, Graeff H (1985) Measurement of cross-linked fibrin derivatives in plasma and ascitic fluid with monoclonal antibodies against D-dimer using EIA and Latex test. Scand J Clin Lab Invest 45 (Suppl) 178: 137–144
23. Hafter R, Schröck R, Von Hugo R, Graeff H (1986) Clinical aspects of fibrin formation and fibrinolysis measured with monoclonal antibodies against D-dimer. In: Lane DA, Henschen A, Jasani MK (eds) Fibrinogen—fibrin formation and fibrinolysis. de Gruyter, Berlin, pp 303–312
24. Nieuwenhuizen W (1987) Plasma assays of fibrinogen/fibrin degradation products and their clinical relevance. In: Lowe GDO, Douglas JT, Forbes CD, Henschen A (eds) Fibrinogen—biochemistry, physiology and clinical relevance. Elsevier, Amsterdam, pp 173–180
25. Scheefers-Borchel U, Müller-Berghaus G, Fuhge P, Eberle R, Heimburger N (1985) Discrimination between fibrin and fibrinogen by a monoclonal antibody against a synthetic peptide. Proc Natl Acad Sci USA 82: 7091–7095
26. Koppert PW, Kuipers W, Hoegee-de Nobel, Brommer EJP, Koopman J, Nieuwenhuizen W (1987) A quantitative enzyme immunoassay for primary fibrinogenolysis products in plasma. Thromb Haemost 57 (1): 25–28

1.2 Bedside Diagnosis of Acute Obstetrical DIC

MASAHIRO MAKI[1]

Introduction

Obstetrical DIC is an acute or hyperacute serious complication associated with abruptio placentae, amniotic fluid embolism, severe hemorrhage, etc. In this situation, complicated and time-consuming tests are no help in making the diagnosis of DIC. This paper describes bedside diagnosis of acute obstetrical DIC.

Underlying Diseases of Obstetrical DIC

Each case of DIC always has its underlying disease. Therefore, when there is an underlying disease which is often accompanied by DIC, complication of DIC should be kept in mind. We experienced 185 cases of DIC in obstetrics. The underlying diseases found are shown in Table 1.

Table 1. Underlying diseases of obstetrical DIC

Underlying diseases	No. of cases (%)
Abruptio placentae	94 (51)
DIC type postpartum hemorrhage	45 (24)
Septic infection	17 (9)
Postcesarean DIC	7 (4)
Eclampsia	6 (3)
Amniotic fluid embolism	5 (3)
Dead fetus syndrome	2 (1)
Others	9 (5)
Total	185 (100)

[1] Department of Obstetrics and Gynecology, Akita University School of Medicine, 1-1-1 Hondo, Akita, 010 Japan

Clinical Signs

Clinical signs and vital signs are of course most important in the diagnosis of DIC. The DIC patient is usually in serious condition or in shock. Blood lost through the wound or drawn out from a blood vessel is often noncoagulable, or clot formation is weak, soft, and small. Subcutaneous bleeding, especially in injection or puncture sites is a common sign of hemorrhagic diathesis. Gangrene is also a rare complication in obstetrical DIC. An edematous appearance is often observed in serious DIC. In such cases, the plasma bradykinin content is very high—reading several hundred compared with the normal range of 20–40 pg/ml plasma.

Laboratory Tests

Laboratory tests for obstetrical DIC can be classified into 2 groups: group 1 for diagnosis of underlying disease and group 2 for diagnosis of DIC. Only the group 2 category will be discussed here.

Coagulation, fibrinolysis, and kinin formation are proteolytic processes. DIC is an intravascular proteolytic state of these enzymes resulting in consumption of terminal substrates (fibrinogen in coagulation, kininogen in kallikrein) and zymogens, their enzyme inhibitors, and increases in enzymeinhibitor complexes and proteolytic split products, including activation peptides. Platelets are consumed, thereby platelet factors are released from α-granule. From these events in DIC, various laboratory tests have been presented as shown in Tables 2 and 3. These tests give us useful information on the clinical and pathological states of DIC. In particular, newly developed techniques for detecting enzyme-inhibitor complexes are very sensitive and give us more detailed information on coagulation and fibrinolysis, which is important in understanding the basic mechanisms of DIC. Even in normal pregnancy, the levels are elevated (Table 4) indicat-

Table 2. Tests for coagulation system

Increase of coagulation time
Prolonged whole blood clotting time
Prolonged prothrombin time
Prolonged activated partial thromboplastin time
Increases in r and K, decrease in ma in thrombelastography
Decreases in fibrinogen, prothrombin, and other almost all coagulation factors
Decrease of coagulation inhibitor
Decreases in antithrombin III, including protein C and protein S
Increases in enzyme-inhibitor complexes
Increase in thrombin-antithrombin III complex
Increases in proteolytic split products
Increases in fibrinopeptides A and B
Increase in soluble fibrin monomer complex
Increases in activation peptides

Table 3. Tests for fibrinolysis and kinin-forming systems and platelet

Fibrinolytic system
Decreases in plasminogen and α_2-antiplasmin
Increase in enzyme inhibitor complex (plasmin-α_2 antiplasmin complex)
Increases in proteolytic split products
FDP (fibrin, fibrinogen degradation products)
D-D dimer (fibrin specific FDP)
Kinin-forming system
Decreases in prekallikrein, HMW Kininogen,
Factor XII and C_1 esterase inhibitor
Increase in split products (bradykinin)
Platelet
Decreased platelet count
Prolonged bleeding time
Increases in β-thromboglobulin and platelet factor 4

ing that a pregnancy is a state of latent DIC. Unfortunately, these are time-consuming tests to perform and, therefore, not helpful in making a prompt diagnosis of acute obstetrical DIC.

Diagnosis of DIC by Scoring

Obstetricians not rarely encounter acute typical and life threatening DIC as in abruptio placentae. In this situation, both prompt diagnosis and prompt initiation of therapy are required.

DIC Score by the Ministry of Health and Welfare (MHW)

In Japan, a diagnostic score for DIC presented by the DIC research group of the Ministry of Health and Welfare (MHW) is widely used (Table 5). In this scoring system, higher points are given to the laboratory tests rather than such clinical items as underlying diseases, hemorrhagic symptoms and organ failure. In acute emergency DIC, even simple tests like FDP, platelet, fibrinogen and prothrombin time are no help in making prompt diagnosis of DIC.

In 1988, the DIC research group of the MHW proposed the following 7 items [1]:

1. Abnormal D-D dimer level
2. Positive soluble fibrin monomer complex
3. Abnormal level of thrombin-antithrombin III complex
4. Abnormal fibrinopeptide A level
5. Abnormal level of plasmin-α_2 antiplasmin complex
6. Serial increase in DIC score, rapid decreases in platelet and fibrinogen, and rapid increase in FDP within a few days
7. Improvement by anticoagulant therapy

Table 4. Concentrations of thrombin-antithrombin III complex (TAT) and plasmin-α_2 antiplasmin complex (PAP) during pregnancy and labor

Test	Nonpregnant	1st trimester	2nd trimester	3rd trimester	Intrapartum	Postpartum[a]
TAT (ng/ml)	1.07 ± 0.77 (15)			4.22 ± 1.26 (42)	8.99 ± 9.83 (9)	12.0 ± 9.82 (8)
PAP (μg/ml)	0.37 ± 0.26 (13)	0.22 ± 0.35 (12)	0.34 ± 0.37 (29)	0.43 ± 0.37 (48)	0.49 ± 0.34 (21)	0.75 ± 0.35 (21)

* Statistically significant
[a] Immediately after delivery.
Figures in parentheses are number of cases tested.

Table 5. DIC score in Japan by a research group of the Ministry of Health and Welfare

	Point			
	3	2	1	0
Underlying diseases			present	none
Hemorrhagic tendency			present	none
Organ failure			present	none
Laboratory tests				
FDP (μg/ml)	≧40	20 ~ 40	10 ~ 20	< 10
Platelet ($10^3/\mu$l)	≦50	50 ~ 80	80 ~ 120	>120
Fibrinogen (mg/dl)		≦100	100 ~ 150	>150
Prothrombin time (PT,s) or		≧ 20	15 ~ 20	< 15
Patient PT (s)/control PT (s) ratio		≧1.67	1.25 ~ 1.67	<1.25

Criteria: 7≦, DIC; 6, suspicious; 5≧, DIC(−)
If there are two or more of the following items, the diagnose can be DIC. High concentrations of (1) soluble fibrin monomer, (2) D-D dimer, (3) thrombin-antithrombin III complex, (4) plasmin-$\alpha_2$antiplasmin complex, (5) rapid decrease in platelet or fibrinogen in a few days, or (6) improvement of DIC by anticoagulant therapy.

Obstetrical DIC Score

We provided a new obstetrics-specific DIC scoring system, in which higher points were given for clinical items rather than laboratory tests. The scoring system consists of 3 parts: (1) underlying diseases, (2) clinical symptoms, and (3) laboratory tests (Table 6) [2]

Taking the example of abruptio placentae as an underlying disease, when there was stiffening of the uterus with a dead fetus, 5 points were given. Taking the example of acute renal failure as of one of the clinical symptoms, when there was anuria, 4 points were given. In contrast to the high points given for underlying diseases and clinical symptoms, only 1 point was given to each abnormal item found in the laboratory tests. The DIC score was counted as the sum of points for all items.

In spite of the different scoring systems, there was a close relationship between the MHW and the obstetrical score results (Fig. 1). When obstetrical DIC score reached 8 points or more, the parameters of AT III, fibrinogen, platelet, FDP, prothrombin time, and erythrocyte sedimentation rate were mainly out of the normal range by a large percentage (Fig. 2). It was decided that when the obstetrical DIC score reaches 8 points or more, it is time to start therapy for DIC.

Significance of Erythrocyte Sedimentation Rate (ESR) in Diagnosis of Acute Obstetrical DIC

Various factors such as macromolecular plasma proteins like fibrinogen and glycoproteins and the erythrocyte count influence ESR. Of these, the plasma fibrinogen concentration has a key effect. ESR and fibrinogen concentration

Table 6. DIC diagnostic criteria in obstetrics and gynecology

Criteria	Score
Underlying diseases	
Abruptio placentae	
Stiffening of the uterus, death of the fetus	5
Stiffening of the uterus, survival of the fetus	4
Confirmatory diagnosis of abruptio placentae by ultrasonic tomographic findings and CTG findings	1
Amniotic fluid embolism	
Acute cor pulmonale	4
Artificial ventilation	3
Assisted respiration	2
Oxygen flux alone	1
DIC type postpartum hemorrhage	
Blood from the uterus has low coagulability	4
Hemorrhage of ≧ 2 000 ml (within 24 h after the start of hemorrhage)	3
Hemorrhage of ≧ 1 000 ml, but not exceeding 2 000 ml (within 24 h after the start of hemorrhage)	1
Eclampsia	
Eclamptic attack	4
Severe infection	
Fever accompanied by shock, bacteremia, and endotoxemia	4
Continued or remittent fever	1
Other underlying diseases	1
Clinical symptoms	
Acute renal failure	
Anuria (≦ 5 ml/h)	4
Oliguria (5 ~ 20 ml/h)	3
Acute respiratory failure (amniotic fluid embolism excluded)	
Artificial ventilation or occasional assisted respiration	4
Oxygen flux alone	1
Organ failure	
Heart (rales or foamy sputum)	4
Liver (visible jaundice)	4
Brain (clouding of consciousness, convulsion)	4
Digestive tract (necrotic enteritis)	4
Other severe organ failure	4
Hemorrhage diathesis	
Macroscopic hematuria and melena, purpura, hemorrhage from the mucous membrane, gingival bleeding, and/or bleeding at the site of injection	4
Shock symptoms	
Pulse rate ≧ 100/min	1
Blood pressure ≦ 90 mmHg (systolic) or blood pressure reduction of ≧ 40%	1
Cold sweat	1
Pallor	1
Laboratory findings	
Serum FDP ≧ 10 μg/ml	1
Platelet count ≦ $10 \times 10^4/mm^3$	1
Fibrinogen ≦ 150 mg/dl	1
PT ≧ 15 (s) (≦ 50%) or hepaplastin test ≦ 50%	1
Erthrocyte sedimentation rate ≦ 4 mm/15 min or ≦ 15 mm/h	1

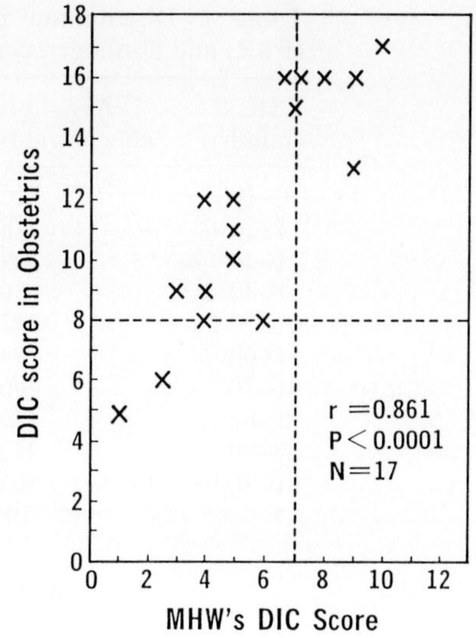

Fig. 1. Correlation between the Ministry of Health and Welfare's (*MHW's*) DIC score and the DIC score in obstetrics

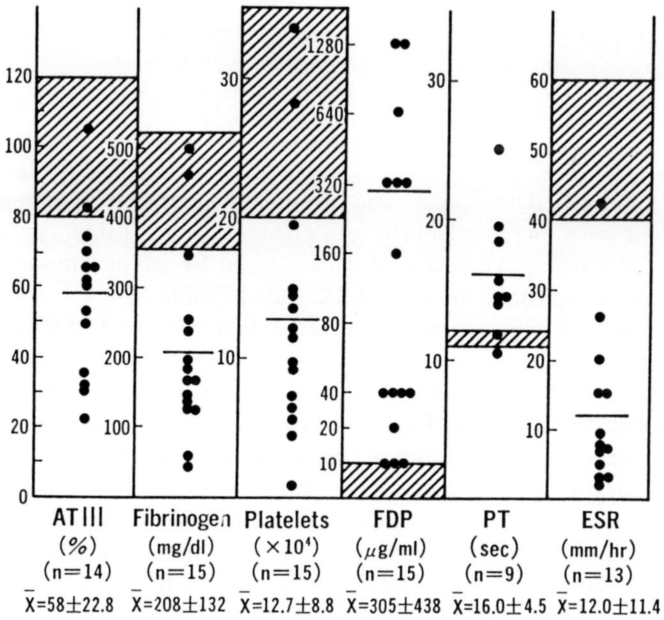

Fig. 2. Coagulation test findings at more than 8 points by DIC score in obstetrics. *PT*, prothrombin time; *ESR*, erythrocyte sedimentation rate

Table 7. Distribution of erythrocyte sedimentation rate (ESR) and fibrinogen concentration

ESR (mm/h)	Avg. fibrinogen concentration (mg/dl)	No. of cases studied
0–10	226	15
11–20	278	21
21–30	309	21
31–40	356	23
41–50	392	32
51–60	394	23
61–70	406	29
71–80	433	21
81–90	442	18
91–100	507	9

Table 8. Effect of fibrinogenolysis induced by streptokinase (SK) on erythrocyte sedimentation rate (ESR)

SK added (units)	ESR (mm/h)
0 (control)	75
6.25	50
12.5	38
25	36
50	29
100	22
200	17
400	11

were simultaneously determined. The results indicated that an increase in ESR was observed with increased fibrinogen concentration (Table 7). When fibrinogenolysis in citrated whole blood was induced by streptokinase (SK), ESR decreased according to the amount of SK added (Table 8).

During pregnancy, fibrinogen concentration increases, and ESR also increases with the advance of gestational age. The average ESR value was approximately 50 mm/h at the end of pregnancy. In acute obstetrical DIC, ESR is below 15 mm/h or below 4 mm/15 min (Fig. 3). In two cases of amniotic fluid embolism, ESR rapidly decreased after onset of the symptoms (Fig. 4).

Determination of ESR is very simple, economic, and reliable. When plasma fibrinogen concentration in obstetrical DIC patients was lower than 120 mg/dl, ESR always remained within 15 mm/h or 4 mm/15 min. However, delayed ESR is observed in about 1 % of normal late pregnancies. It is therefore very important to observe concomitantly clinical symptoms of DIC to avoid misunderstanding. ESR is not a direct expression of fibrinogen concentration. Indication by ESR change is available not only for obstetrical DIC but also for DIC associated with infection and advanced malignancy. In these conditions, fibrinogen concentration increases and ESR accelerates, unless DIC is accompanied.

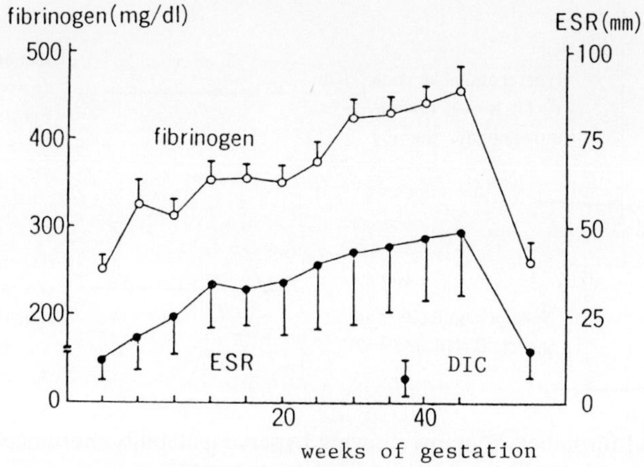

Fig. 3. Fibrinogen concentration (○—○) and erthrocyte sedimentation rate (*ESR*) (mm/h) (●—●) during pregnancy and in DIC

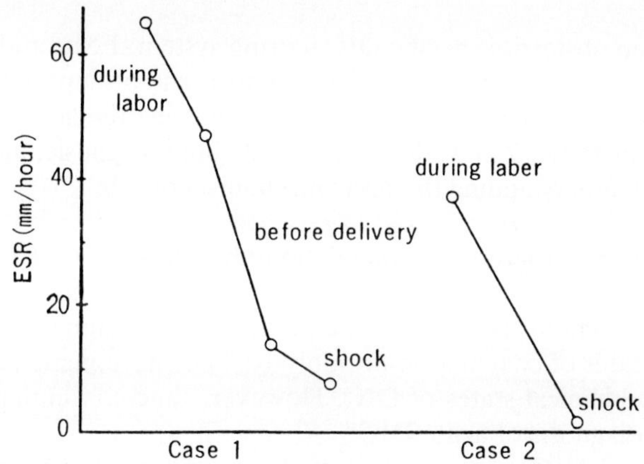

Fig. 4. Rapid change of erythrocyte sedimentation rate (*ESR*) in cases of amniotic fluid embolism. *Case 1:* 27-year-old, *gravida* 3, *para* 2. Labor was induced with oxytocin. The patient delivered a 3400 g male 2 h after the induction. Immediately after delivery, she fell into severe shock with dyspnea, convulsion, and massive bleeding. In spite of intensive care, she died 2 h after delivery. ESR: 48 mm before induction, 14 mm after delivery. *Case 2:* 22-year-old, *gravida* 3, *para* 1. The patient delivered a 3300 g male uneventfully. After delivery she suddenly developed severe shock with dyspnea and cyanosis. She recovered from shock 4 h later by heparin and antishock therapy. Laboratory tests showed findings typical of DIC. ESR: 34 mm during labor, 0 mm in shock state

Thrombelastography (TEG)

TEG gives global information on coagulation and fibrinolysis including platelet function and also provides orientation as to how to manage coagulation defect (Fig. 5). We include this instrument among our delivery room equipment.

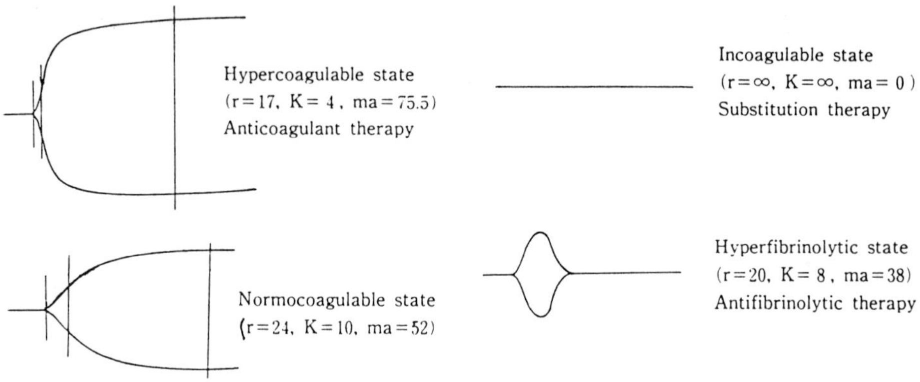

Fig. 5. Typical thrombelastograms showing hypercoagulability, normocoagulability, incoagulability, and hyperfibrinolysis and their management

Discussion

I recommend an obstetrics-specific DIC scoring system, ESR, and TEG as bedside tests. These are important for quick diagnosis and prompt initiation of therapy. However, I never neglect, rather would like stress the necessity of detailed tests as shown in Tables 2 and 3 for making a definite diagnosis, judging effect of treatment, and understanding the basic mechanism of DIC.

Summary. Recent progress in coagulation-fibrinolysis research has brought various new tests for diagnosis of DIC. The enzyme-inhibitor complexes, e.g., thrombin-antithrombin III complex and plasmin-antiplasmin complex, are good indicators of states of coagulation-fibrinolysis. They have made possible the explanation of subclinical states of DIC. However, time-consuming tests are not useful for the diagnosis of acute DIC.

The obstetrical DIC score in which high scores are given to underlying diseases and clinical signs, but not to laboratory tests, correlates well with the DIC score of the Ministry of Health and Welfare in which high scores are given to laboratory tests, but not to clinical states. Erythrocyte sedimentation rate and thromboelastography are recommended as bedside tests in acute obstetrical DIC.

References

1. Hasegawa A (1989) Diagnostic criteria of DIC in 1988 (MHW). In: Annual review of hematology (in Japanese). Chugai Igakusha, Tokyo, pp 224–228
2. Maki M, Terao T, Ikenoue T, Takemura T, Sekiba K, Shirakawa K, Soma H (1987) Clinical evaluation of antithrombin III concentrate (BI 6.013) for disseminated intravascular coagulation in obstetrics. Gynecol Obstet Invest 23: 230–350

1.3 Analysis of γ-γ Dimer and Factor XIII (Fibrin Stabilizing Factor, FSF) During Pregnancy and Labor

SHIGENORI SUZUKI[1], HENNER GRAEFF[2], and REIMAR HAFTER[2]

Introduction

It is well known that the final stage of pregnancy is characterized by a state of hypercoagulability in which the levels of all coagulation factors, with the exception of factor XIII, increase. When fibrin and fibrinogen polymerize to form the matrix of the blood coagulation-fibrinolytic system, factor XIII, which acts like an adhesive, is the only coagulating factor that decreases. This perhaps suggests that the structure of the fibrin clot is weakened and that fibrinolysis increases.

In the final stage of blood coagulation, thrombin, which converts fibrinogen to fibrin, is formed. This covers the wound in vessels and also induces fibrinolysis by plasmin which dissolves fibrin and fibrinogen to form degradation products (FDP). The degradation products of fibrinogen which are formed during hyperfibrinolysis impair blood coagulation.

These mechanisms are sufficient under normal conditions as well as during delivery and puerperium. Changes in this sensitive balance cause considerable difficulties leading to abnormal hemorrhage or thrombosis at the time of delivery.

Because of uterine contractions, the blood loss in normal deliveries is only approximately 200–300 ml. However, this is true only when fibrin, the final reaction product of blood coagulation, is not degraded by the fibrinolytic system. Thus blood coagulation and fibrinolysis both participate in hemostasis around delivery. The stability of clots against fibrinolysis is dependent on the action of factor XIII, the fibrin stabilizing factor (FSF), which was first described in 1948 by Laki and Lorand [1]. However, up to now, its role in the perinatal period has scarcely been investigated. The changes in factor XIII during the late stages of

[1]College of Medical Technology, Hokkaido University, Kita 12-jo, Nishi 5-chome, Kita-ku, Sapporo 060, Japan

[2]Frauenklinik der Technischen Universität München, Ismaninger Straße 22, D-8000 München 80, Federal Republic of Germany

pregnancy and during delivery, with special reference to fibrinolysis, are hereby reported in this paper.

Materials and Methods

Samples: Thirty normal female adults in the vesicular ovarian follicle period, 51 cases of normal pregnancy and normal delivery, 15 cases of premature separation of placenta, 16 cases of placenta previa, and 16 cases of atonic bleeding were examined. In order to evaluate the effects of estrogen and progesterone, changes to FSF brought about by administration of oral contraceptives (pill) (21 cases) were also examined.

Blood samples were taken from the cubital vein, nine parts blood to one part of 3.8% sodium citrate. Immediately after withdrawal, o.1ml of trasylol 1000 KIE units was added and the sample was centrifuged at 3000 r.p.m. for 20 min.

Factor XIII Determination

Anti-factor XIII Subunit A serum (Behringwerke, Marburg, West Germany) was used. The antiserum was diluted as indicated by the manufacturer (Fig. 1). Into each of the eleven test tubes, 0.1 ml of one of the various anti-factor XIII serum dilutions and 0.2 ml of patient plasma were pipetted, mixed, and allowed to stand for 30 min at room temperature (20°–25°C). Then 0.1 ml thrombin/calcium chloride solution was added to each test tube and mixed well. For clot formation and stabilization the tubes were left standing for 60 minutes at room temperature (20°–25°C). Three ml of 1% monochloroacetic acid solution was pipetted into each of the test tubes and the tubes were sealed with rubber stoppers. They were left standing at room temperature and cautiously tilted 10 times every 10 min in order to obtain through rinsing by the monochloroacetic acid. At 90 min, the highest dilution of anti-factor XIII serum in which the clot had been dissolved was noted, and the factor XIII content of the sample calculated as percent of norm according to the package insert [2].

FDP and Fibrinogen

Tanned red cell hemagglutination inhibition immune assay (TRCHII, Teikokuhormone, Tokyo, Japan) was used as indicated by the manufacturer. Fibrinogen was detected by the method of Blomback [3]. The resulting fibrinogen content had to be corrected for anticoagulant dilution and hematocrit. According to Seligsohn [4] the following formula can be used:

$$\text{mg fibrinogen corr./dl} = \text{mg fg/dl} \times \frac{100 - \text{hematocrit}}{(100 - \text{hematocrit}) - 10}$$

SFMC

Purification Procedure. Fibrinogen and its derivatives were precipitated from plasma with β-alanine. A 40% aqueous solution of β-alanine was added at 0°C to

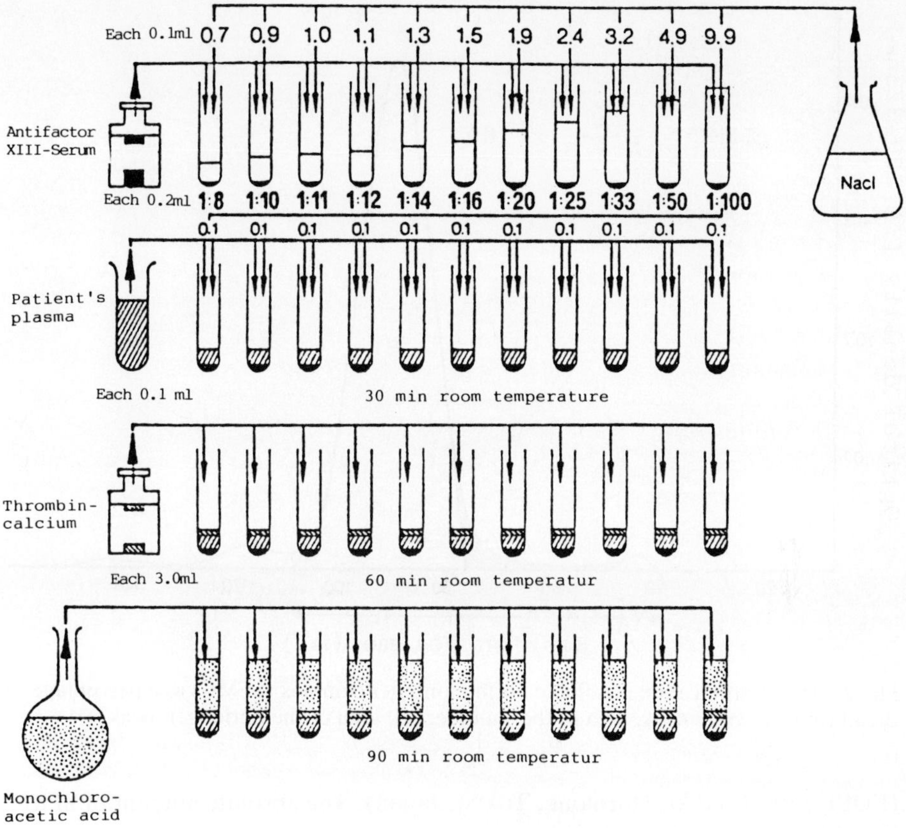

Fig. 1. Qualification of factor XIII

the plasma specimen (2.5 ml) up to a final concentration of 2.5 m, and the precipitate was dissolved in 2 ml TESCL-citrate buffer (pH 7.6) containing 100 KIU Trasylol per milliliter.

Quantitative Agarose Gel Filtration. A 4% agarose gel filtration was performed using Biogel A-15 m spherical agarose, 100–200 mesh (Bio-Rad Laboratories, Munich, West Germany). A 2 ml sample containing 6 mg protein was applied to a 1.5 × 95 cm column and eluted with Tris-Cl-citrate buffer, pH 7.5 (0.05 M Tris, 0.116 M NaCl, 0.0129 M trisodium citrate, 0.025 Mϵ-aminocapronic acid (EACA), 0.025% sodium azide). The flow rate was kept at 12 ml/h. The optical density was measured at 280 and 325 nm with a Hitachi 181 spectrophotometer (Tokyo, Japan) and the elution profile plotted on millimeter paper.

The quantification of Soluble Fibrin Monomer Complex (SFMC) as a percentage of the fibrinogen content was achieved by planimetric evaluation of the elution pattern (area of the shoulder between void volume and ascending part of the fibrinogen peak versus fibrinogen peak). SFMC percentage = A × 100/(A + B), where *A* is the area of the shoulder and *B* the area of the fibrinogen peak (Fig. 2). The presence of FR-antigen material in the eluted fraction of the shoulder of the peak was confirmed in certain cases by use of the Latex-test

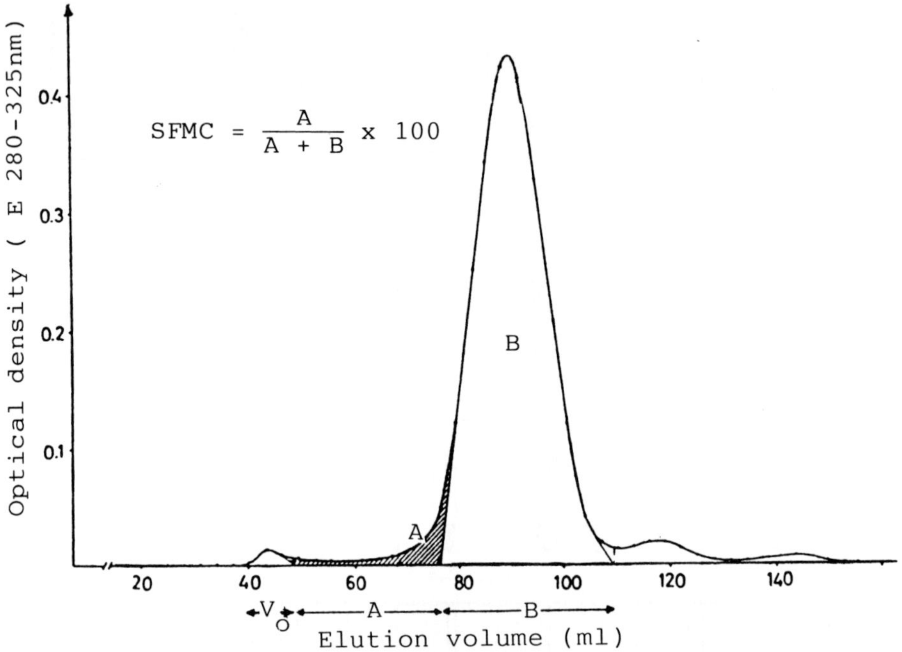

Fig. 2. The quantification of soluble fibrin monomer complex (SFMC) as a percentage of the fibrinogen content. *A*, area of the shoulder; *B*, area of the fibrinogen peak

(FDPL-test, Teikoku-Hormone, Tokyo, Japan). The absolute amount of SFMC in milligrams per 100 ml of plasma was calculated by relating the relative amount of SFMC to the fibrinogen concentration in the respective plasma sample.

Polyacrylamide Gel Electrophoresis. Gel electrophoresis was performed with 7.5% or 5% gels; in 7.5% or 5% separating gels (6 × 60 mm) with 0.1 M phosphate buffer, pH 7.0, containing 6 M urea and 0.1% sodiumdodecylsulfate (SDS). Reduction was performed by incubating the samples at 37°C for 2 h in the presence of 1% (v/v) 2-mercaptoethanol, 0.2% (w/v) SDS and 6 M urea, after dialysing the samples against 0.1 M phosphate buffer, pH 7.0. Staining was done with coomassie brilliant blue.

γ-γ Dimer

γ-γ dimer was tested by RAPIDA-D dimer (A latex agglutination test for detection of cross-linked fibrin derivatives).

Results

Changes in Factor XIII in the Latter Half of Pregnancy

While normal values were 85.4 ± 12.8% without any significant differences up to the 6th month of pregnancy, FSF hovered around the lower limit of normal

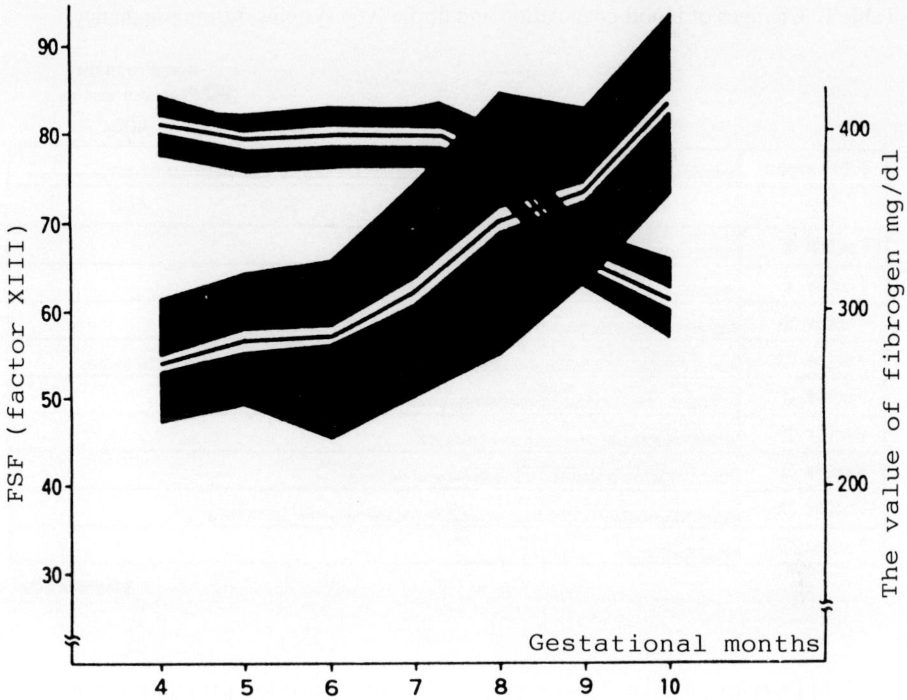

GM / items	4	5	6	7	8	9	10
factor XIII (FSF)	82.0±6.8	80.6±7.4	78.6±5.4	75.4±7.2	74.2±6.6	65.4±6.8	58.7±9.0
Fibrinogen	276±30	282±29	285±59	314±68	359±78	371±41	416±51

Fig. 3. Changes in fibrinogen and fibrin stabilizing factor (FSF) during pregnancy

values from about the 28th week of pregnancy. The 8th and 9th months of pregnancy showed values of 74.2 ± 6.6% and 65.4 ± 6.8% respectively, which became even lower, down to 58.7 ± 8.9%, in the 10th month. At the commencement of delivery, the values were 55.6 ± 6.4%; immediately after delivery the values were 54.8 ± 3.9% while they showed a marked lowering, to 50.2 ± 4.1% on the 2nd day of puerperium. However, on the 7th day of puerperium, the values rose to 65.4 ± 5.1%, and they returned to normal (78.6 ± 4.9%) one month after delivery (Fig. 3).

Changes in Fibrinogen and other Coagulating Factors

When the changes in fibrinogen and other factors were noted at the end of pregnancy, so-called Vitamin K dependent factors II, VII, IX, and X, showed a rise of approximately 1.2–1.8 times their values during the non-pregnant period. Factor V especially showed a 1.5 fold increase while factor VIII showed an almost threefold increase. As seen in Fig. 5, *fibrinogen showed a remarkable increase from around the 28th week of pregnancy, and had an approximately

Table 1. Changes of blood-coagulation and fibrinolytic systems during pregnancy

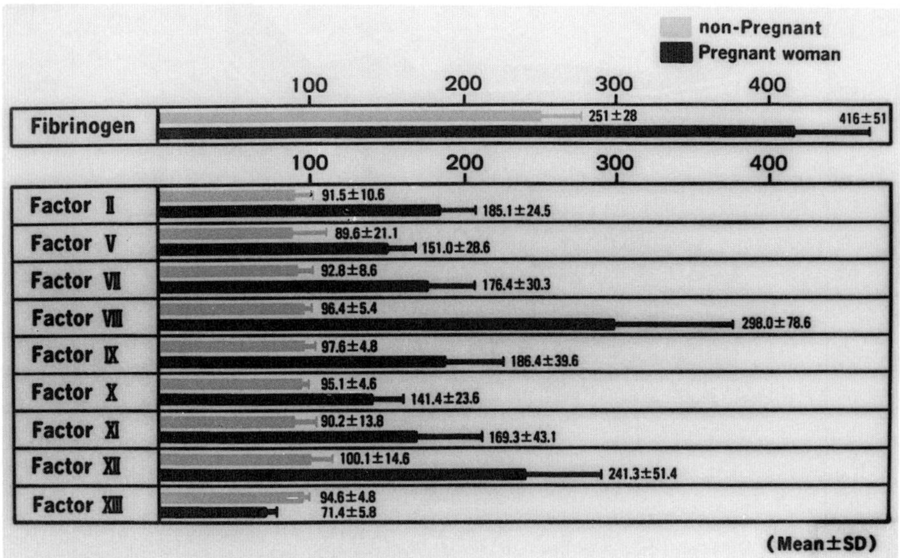

twofold increase, of 41.6 ± 5.1 mg/dl, in the later period of pregnancy compared with the non-pregnant period* (Table 1).

Results of the Quantification of Soluble Fibrin Monomer Complex (SFMC) by Agarose Gel Filtration

As may seen seen in Fig. 4, rises similar to those in fibrinogen were present during the course of pregnancy. In addition, from the first period of pregnancy until delivery (second period) and up to around the 2nd day of puerperium, an additional remarkable rise was recognized. In DIC cases, portion A (Fig. 2) occupies 10% or more; this can be calculated by the formula:

$$\text{SFMC} = \frac{\text{A}}{\text{A} + \text{B}} \times 100$$

The normal adult value in the present method was 2.1 ± 0.6%. After delivery, the return to a normal range required about 2 months.

Changes of FSF Brought About by Administration of Oral Contraceptives

Quantification of fibrinogen, SFMC and factor XIII was carried out on 21 subjects who had had the oral contraceptive Ovulen (Böhringer, West Germany) administered to them for at least one year. Resulting SFMC values of 3.79 ± 0.8% with a risk ratio of 0.1% compared with the control value of

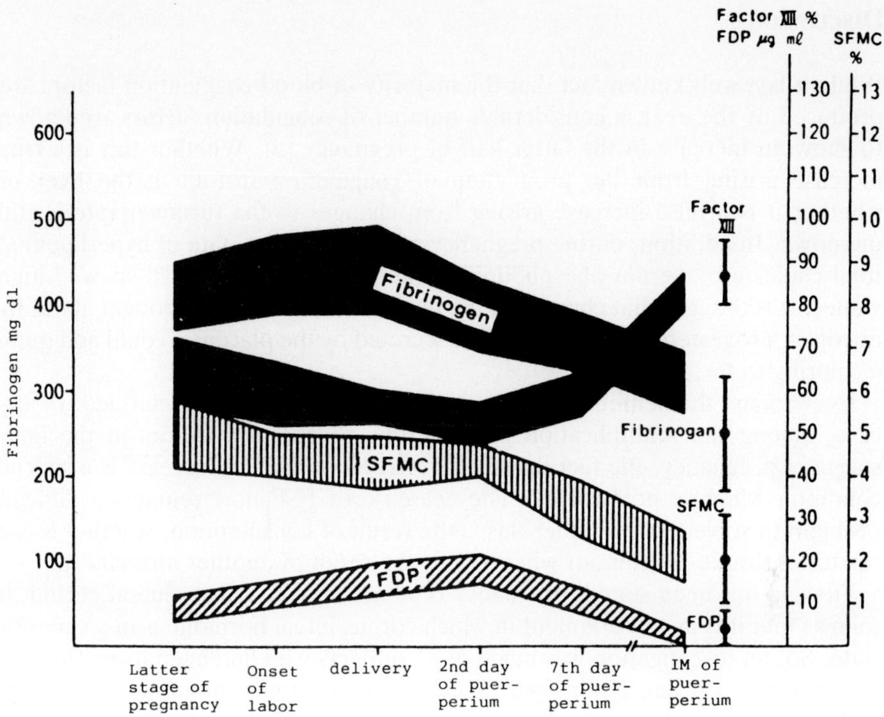

Fig. 4. Increase of fibrinogen, FDP, SFMC and reduction of factor XIII around delivery

2.87 ± 0.5%. Fibrinogen showed a value of 263 ± 41 mg/dl compared with the control value of 224 ± 45 mg/dl, a significant increase, with a risk ratio of 0.5%. However, for values of factor XIII no significant differences were observed between the administered group and the non-administered group (Table 2).

Table 2. The activity of factor XIII and the amounts of fibrinogen and SFMC in plasma of controls and of Ovulen users

items		(Mean ± SD)	
Examination	Control (31)	Ovulen users (21)	Statistical evaluation
Factor XIII (%) (FSF)	94.1 ± 16.5	85.6 ± 19.4	P > 0.05
SFMC (%) (percent of fibrinogen content)	2.87 ± 0.51	3.79 ± 0.75	P < 0.001
SFMC (mg/dl)	6.46 ± 1.78	9.92 ± 2.27	P < 0.001
Fibrinogen (mg/dl)	224 ± 45	263 ± 41	P < 0.005

Discussion

While it is a well-known fact that the majority of blood coagulation factors are produced by the liver, a considerable number of coagulation factors are known to show an increase in the latter half of pregnancy [5]. Whether this is a true increase arising from the production of coagulation factors in the liver or whether it is a false increase arising from changes in the turnover rate is still unknown. In addition, during pregnancy as well as in the state of hyperlipemia, total cholesterol, serum phospholipids, and serum triglyceride all showed high values. It is thought that changes in the hormone environment brought about by estrogen, progesterone, etc., which are secreted by the placenta, could add quite a coloring to the above.

Even today, the definition of hypercoagulability has not been clarified. In any case, among the multiplication of numerous coagulation factors in the later stages of pregnancy, the fact that factor XIII alone fails to increase is a special condition which is noteworthy. The decrease of FSF now remains a difficult problem to solve; i.e., whether this is the result of consumption, whether it is a matter of simple dilution, or whether it is the result of another mechanism.

First, as has been stated, pregnancy is an accentuaed corpus luteal period; it follows that it is an environment in which corpus luteal hormone is in a superior state. So, an investigation was made of 21 subjects who had been using the oral contraceptive Ovulen (Böhringer, West Germany) for a minimum of $1\frac{1}{2}$ years and a maximum of 5 years. Results obtained showed that, as was the case in the pregnant subjects, no decrease in FSF was observed, while an increase in Fibrinogen and SFMC was seen (Table 2). Firstly it may be said that FSF shows a special change which does not depend on the hormonal environment accompanying pregnancy or on the state of hyperlipemia.

Secondly, if the behavior which is different from the other coagulating system is caused by changes in circulating behavior arising from pregnancy, in other words, if the cause may be attributed to the increase of the plasma volume during pregnancy, the following assumptions may be tentatively advanced. Namely, it is generally accepted that a maximal circulating plasma volumn is seen at the eighth month of pregnancy; it is known that this total plasma volume is 4,000 ml (Fig. 5). When this is compared with 2,500 ml in the non-pregnant state, the dilution rate should be 62.5%. The normal value of FSF in the non-pregnant state is 70%–100% and if this is extrapolated, a 45%–63% change in the FSF values should be obtained. However, the actual measured value is 75%. In this respect, the actual measured value per unit ml is higher than the theoretical value, and it may therefore not be said that the values show a decrease. We, however, can state here that, as may be seen with the other coagulating factors, a remarkable rise was not seen. There is a report [6] available on this point which postulates a connection with fibrinolysis which appears in the latter period of pregnancy.

Based on the results of in vitro experiments, Coopland et al. [5] confirmed that the higher the concentration of urokinase registered, the lower the cross-linking ability of factor XIII became. This suggests the influence of fibrinolysis

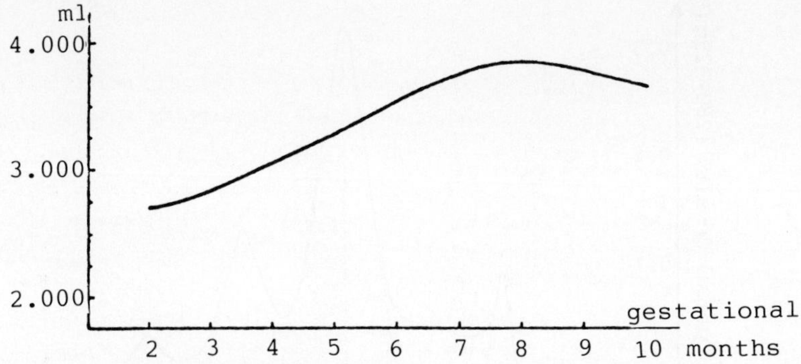

Fig. 5. Change of total plasma-volume during pregnancy. Comparison of total plasma-volume (8 months). Non pregnant 2500 ml factor XIII (FSF) 90%. Eight months 4000 ml factor XIII (FSF) 75%. Theoretical value 56.3%. (90 × 0.625).

Ratio of dilution $\frac{2500}{4000} \times 100 = 62.5$ (%)

on the lowering of FSF activity. By analogical influence based on this fact, a slight rise of FDP would be seen in the latter period of pregnancy, especially in the last half of the 9th month of pregnancy; this can be seen even in a normal pregnant woman. This seems to provide solid evidence for the results of Coopland et al. [6]. At the onset of labor, the coagulating fibrinolytic system of blood has a completely different aspect from that in pregnancy, as previously reported by the authors [7]. In other words, FDP shows a rise in the latter period of pregnancy and at the onset of labor, the elongating tendency of Euglobulin lysis time is shortened.

The changes in values of factor XIII were therefore scrutinized, focussing attention on the time of delivery. At the onset of labor, namely at the beginning of delivery, the value was 58.7 ± 8.9%. It decreased to 54.8 ± 3.9% immediately after delivery of the fetus. On the 2nd day of puerperium, a remarkably low value of FSF, down to 50.2 ± 4.1%, was seen. In relation to the above, during the course of delivery levels of fibrinogen, FDP and SFMC rose, and eventually returned to their former levels during puerperium.

However, in early separation of the placenta, in which separation of the placenta occurs prior to the onset of labor, this tendency is more pronounced, especially in cases accompanied by DIC [8]. In these cases, high values of 40–640 μg/ml in FDP and over 10% in SFMC were seen. These events can probably be interpreted as follows: the high rise of split products indicates that coagulation followed by reactive fibrinolysis has taken place. Perhaps the changes of factor XIII activity which have a completely different kinetic from the other blood coagulating factors during pregnancy-delivery-puerperium are due to consumption, because factor XIII is very thrombin sensitive as has been shown by Triantaphyllopoulos [9]. The pathophysiology, with special regard to thrombosis in the puerperium also seems to be very important in solving this question [10]. Based on the present data, it can only be speculated that both the lowering

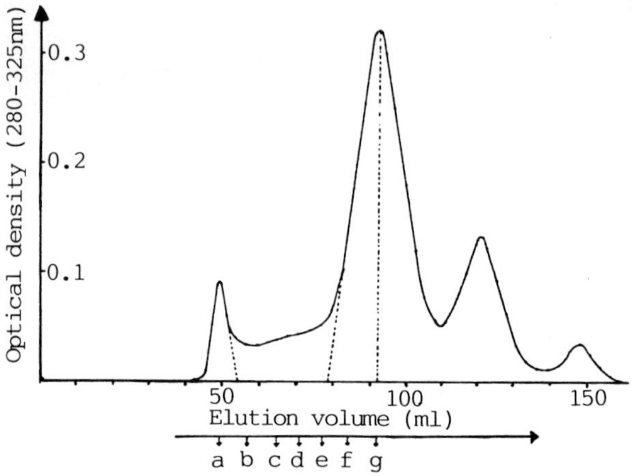

Fig. 6. Cases of DIC

of factor XIII and the increase of fibrinolytic activity seem to be reasonable mechanisms for the prevention of thrombus formation arising from hypercoagulability which is due to a rise in the other coagulation factors. Thus, the lowering of factor XIII together with an increase in fibrinolysis would contribute to counterbalancing coagulation.

It would be worth mentioning that a portion of SFMC quantified by agarose gel filtration (Figs. 2, 6) and a fraction thereof were investigated by PAA gel electrophoresis. This showed weakened α-chains and the appearance of γ-γ dimer in the DIC cases (Fig. 7). In such cases, this is probably because activated FSF has a value as low as 20%, which we may reasonably consider to be the result of consumption by secondary fibrinolysis which has arisen from DIC (Fig. 7). Conversely, a conjecture may be made that FSF, even with such a low level of activity, still retains a cross-linking function. While the lowering of FSF is also seen in placenta previa and atonic bleeding, the frequency of γ-γ dimer appearance is extremely low in such cases (Table 3). In the cases of premature separation of the placenta, the incidence of γ-γ dimer appearance is much higher than that of placenta previa (Fig. 8).

This is a study in which differences in the image of the disease have been clarified; it is also a matter of great interest. It is strongly suggested that the

Table 3. Values and percentage of Factor XIII, SFMC, and γ-γ dimers

	Factor XIII (%)	SFMC (%)	Incidenees of γ-γ dimers (%)	Decreases of α-chains (%)
Normal delivery	54.8 ± 8.9	5.6 ± 2.8	0 (0/51)	80.3
Premature separation of placenta	23.6 ± 10.4	10.4 ± 3.8	86.7 (13/15)	100
Placenta previa	37.6 ± 9.6	7.6 ± 2.9	6.3 (1/16)	100
Atonic bleeding	48.6 ± 7.8	6.8 ± 4.3	6.3 (1/16)	100

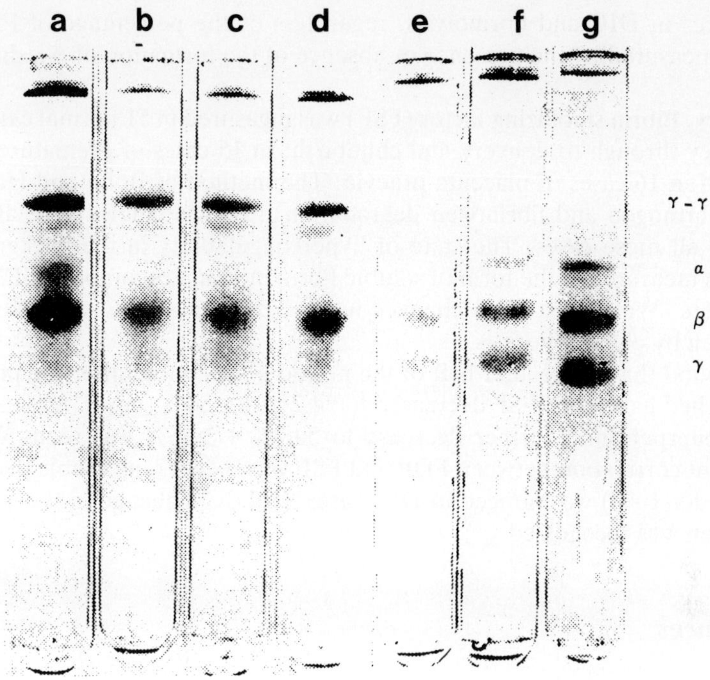

Fig. 7. Electrophoresis of areas **a–g** as seen in Fig. 6.

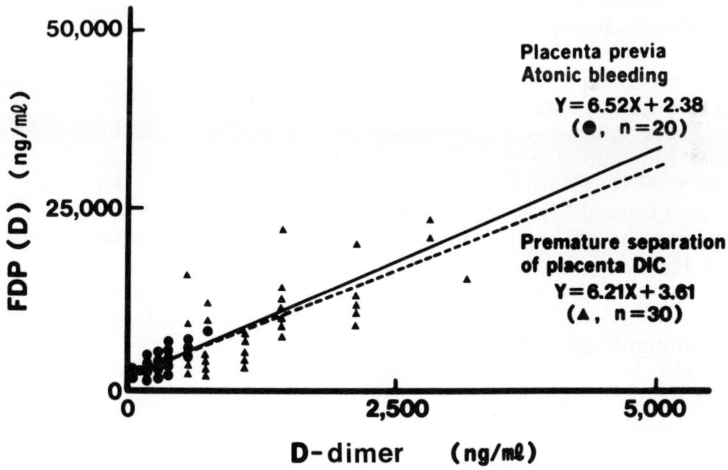

Fig. 8. Concentration of γ-γ dimers appearing in the cases of premature separation of the placenta and placenta previa

differences in DIC and fibrinolysis, regardless of the percentage of FSF, may well be measured by the presence or absence of the formation of γ-γ dimer.

Summary. Fibrin stabilizing factor (FSF) was measured in 51 normal cases, from pregnancy through to delivery and childbirth; in 15 cases of premature separation; and in 16 cases of placenta praevia. The method of Bohn and Haupt was used. Fibrinogen and fibrinogen degradation products (FDP) were also measured in all these cases. The state of hypercoagulability in the background of DIC was measured in the form of soluble fibrin monomers complex (SFMC) and γ-γ-dimers. We also studied changes in the respective α, β, and γ chains of fibrinogen by electrophoresis.

We found that in the later half of the period of gestation, after the pregnancy had reached half term, FSF decreased to 74.2% ± 6.50% (norm. 80% − 120%). In the puerperium a further decrease to 50.2% + 2.05% was seen. While no significant correlation between FDP and FSF was seen a remarkable decrease in FSF (under 10%) was noticed in DIC cases. In DIC a change in the γ chain of fibrinogen was recognized.

References

1. Laki K, Lorand L (1948) On the solubility of fibrin clots. Science 108: 280
2. Bohn H, Haupt H (1968) Eine quantitative Bestimmunge von Faktor XIII mit Anti-Faktor XIII-Serum. Thrombos Diathes Haemorrh (Stuttg) 9: 509
3. Blomback BM (1956) Purification of human and bovine fibrinogen. Arkiv Kemi 10: 415
4. Selingsohn U, Rapaport SJ, Kuefler PR (1972) Extra-adrenal effect of ACTH on fibrinogen synthesis. Am J Physiol 224: 1172
5. Ludwig H (1972) Thromboembolische Erkrankungen in der Schwanger schaft und unter Geburt. Z Geburtshilfe Perinatol 176, 3: 1169
6. Coopland A, Alkjaersig N, Fletcher A (1969) Reduction in plasma factor XIII (FSF) concentration during pregnancy. J Lab Clin Med 73, 1: 144
7. Suzuki S (1974) Consumption coagulopathy in obstetrics (in Japanese). Japanese Journal of Clinical Medicine 32, 5: 1077
8. Hafter K, Schneebaker T, Tafel K, Ernst E, Graef H (1971) Bestimmung von löslichen Fibrinmonomerkomplexen zur Erfassung der Hypercoagulabilität in der Schwangerschaft und unter der Geburt. Geburtshilfe Frauenheikd 35: 513
9. Triantaphyllopoulos DC (1973) The inactivation of factor XIII during blood coagulation. Thromb Res 3: 241
10. Graeff HA, Wiedermann R, Von Hugo R, Hafter R (1976) Amount and distribution pattern of soluble fibrin monomer complexes during the early puerperium. Am J Obst Gynecol Vol 124, 1: 21

1.4 Perinatal Emergencies in Sapporo Medical College

Emi Horimoto, Etsuji Satohisa, Takao Sano, and Masayoshi Hashimoto[1]

Introduction

Abnormal bleeding can occur quite suddenly during delivery, which can easily cause hypovolemic shock, thus threatening the maternal and neonatal lives. This paper presents some of our findings from perinatal emergencies in our clinic.

Material and Methods

During the years from 1979 to 1988, 5803 patients were admitted to our clinic. Of these, 114 patients were transferred from various hospitals and clinics throughout the Sapporo area. Among the transferred patients, we had 25 hemorrhage cases.

We investigated the frequency of transferred patients, the source of transfer, and the type of disease seen in the past 10 years. During this period we had 25 hemorrhage cases, which we will discuss in detail.

Results

Figure 1 shows the changing trend in the source of transfer. Patients were classified as coming from either a clinic with one obstetrician, more than one obstetrician, or transferring from another general hospital. You will notice that the number of patients transferring from other hospitals is increasing, while those from clinics are decreasing.

Figure 2 illustrates the distribution of cases according to the type of disease. Until 1988, toxemia of pregnancy was the leading disease among the transferred

[1]Department of Obstetrics and Gynecology, Sapporo Medical College, South 1 West 16 Chuou-ku, Sapporo, 060 Japan

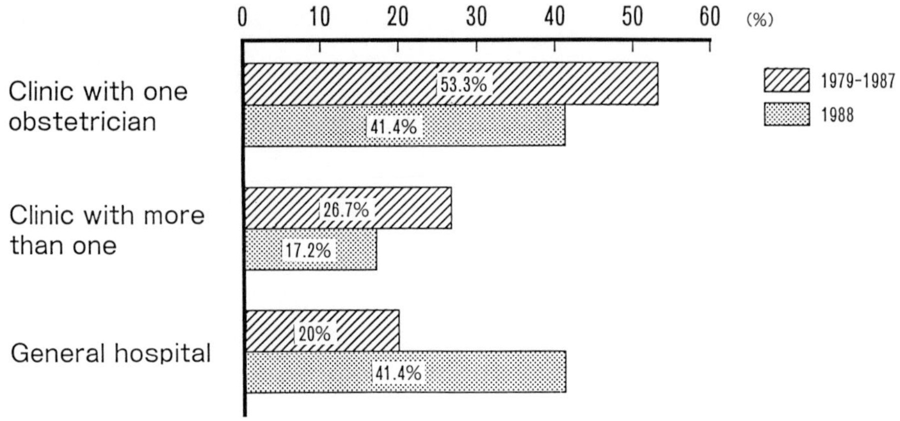

Fig. 1. Source of transferring patients

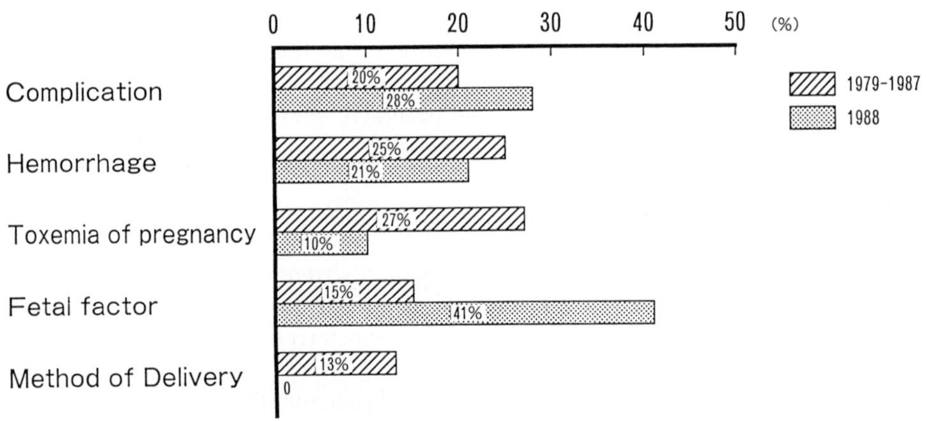

Fig. 2. Diagnosis of transferred patients

patients. Due to the recent development of the nonstress test (NST), ultrasound echogram, etc., fetal factor is now the leading disease. This was also reflected in the acute increase in the number of patients for 1988. On the other hand, the percentage of hemorrhage cases has been rather steady over the years, with a total of 25 patients being transferred.

The 25 hemorrhage patients treated were of various types (Fig. 3). Eight of these women developed hypovolemic shock with five of them further developing DIC. Table 1 provides a summary of the five DIC cases.

Case 1

The patient delivered by having vacuum extraction 3 times. The clinical record revealed that about 30 min after delivery, she complained of abdominal pains

Table 1. Summary of DIC cases 1–5

	1	2	3	4	5
Diagnosis	Uterine rupture	Atonic bleeding	Atonic bleeding, Ventricular fibrillation	Placental, abruption	Bleeding following C-section
Laboratory Data					
FDP	20			>40	
Fibrinogen				150	97
AT III				56	29
Platelet (10^3)	130	73		112	103
ESR (mm) (60 min)	1				
Japan Obstetrics DIC score	17	18	33	13	13
Blood transfer (cc)	4800	9000	5000	1200	8000
Operation	Hysterectomy	None	Supravaginal hyster-ectomy Direct counter shock 4x	Cesarean section	Hysterectomy
Drugs	Foy Inovan Miraclid	Inovan, Digitalis Meylon, Heparin Fibrinogen Hydrocortisone Xylocaine	Adrenalin Heparin Meylon, Noradrenaline Xylocaine, Foy Calcium	Transamin Inovan Meylon Foy	Foy Inovan Haptoglobin Globulin
Prognosis	Non-A, non-B hepatitis	Died	Died	Now pregnant	Graft versus host
Transfer time (min)	120	190	162	100	127

ESR, erythroeyte sedimentation rate

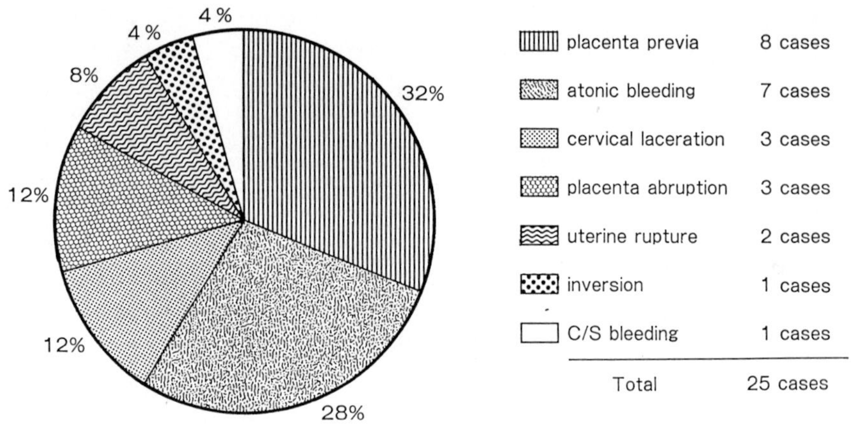

Fig. 3. Distribution of hemorrhage cases by disease. *C/S*, cesarean section

many times. Forty-five minutes later, the patient complained of nausea, vomiting, and gastric pain, but her blood pressure was normal. Approximately 30 min later, the patient suddenly went into shock. She arrived at our hospital only 15 min after that, and we operated immediately. The patient required two operations and a significant amount of blood.

Case 2

Shortly after delivery the patient went into shock. She arrived at our hospital 2.5 h after pre-shock was detected. Before arrival she had already entered a severe state of DIC. We gave her a large amount of blood; however, she continued to bleed throughout the body and died. We made a diagnosis of atonic bleeding of the uterus. Her family did not authorize an autopsy. However, since she had sudden dyspnea, cyanosis, and was in shock, we suspect that amniotic fluid embolism may have caused shock.

Case 3

This patient also required more than 2 h to be transferred. She had a large amount of bleeding, hypovolemic shock, DIC, and ventricular fibrillation upon arrival. We administered a blood transfusion, direct counter shock 4 times, and performed two operations. In spite of our effects she died. If the patient had been transferred earlier, we may have had a better chance to save her.

Case 4

There was a placental abruption and the patient had complained of bleeding. She was transferred fairly quickly after discovery of the bleeding and indication of fetal distress. We performed a cesarean section and although the fetus was stillborn, we were able to take protective measures to save the mother. It is interesting to note that the mother is pregnant again at this time.

Case 5

Fetal distress was recognized at another hospital and a cesarean section was performed. After the cesarean section bleeding continued. The attending doctor tried to treat the bleeding, but her condition worsened. She was then transferred to the emergency department about 2 h after the original bleeding had begun. Although it was not too late to save her life, she suffered DIC and required two operations.

Discussion

An important principle in the management of DIC is prompt diagnosis [3]. We usually use the Japan Obstetrics DIC score (J.O.S.) and start the DIC treatment if a patient scores more than 8 points [4]. It has been valuable to start DIC treatment as soon as possible. The evidence shows that for the two cases which resulted in death unusually long transfer times transpired. Of the other three cases, two of them took 2 h to be transferred, and both patients required hysterectomies and hemostatic operations.

The focus should be placed on the time elapsed between the discovery of a hemorrhage condition and arrival at (our hospital) a treatment center. Perhaps if these patients had arrived earlier, we could have avoided the hemostatic operations.

In conclusion, there are three points to consider:

1. Usually there is a relatively high percentage of hemorrhage cases which arrive in perinatal emergency.
2. The sooner a hemorrhage condition is diagnosed by a clinician and the patient is transferred, the better our chances are to save the patient.
3. An important consideration in the management of hypovolemic shock, DIC, and multiple organ failure (MOF) is a high index of suspicion or anticipatory attitude on the part of the clinician.

With respect to hemorrhage cases, the first priority is quick diagnosis and original treatment of the disease in order to prevent the need for a subsequent operation. Therefore, we stress the importance of reducing the time it takes to transfer emergency patients.

Summary. Abnormal bleeding can occur quite suddenly during delivery and can easily cause hypovolemic shock and be a threat to the maternal and neonatal lives. An important principle in the management of hypovolemic shock is a high index of suspicion or an anticipatory attitude on the part of the clinician.

There were 5653 patients admitted to our clinic for the years 1979–1988. Twenty-five transferred from various hospitals throughout Hokkaido Prefecture were treated for abnormal bleeding. Of the 25 treated, there are 8 patients with placenta previa (32%), 7 with atonic bleeding of the uterus (28%), 3 with cervical lacerations (12%), 3 with placental abruption (12%), 2 with uterine rupture (8%), 1 with inversion of the uterus (4%), and 1 with abnormal bleeding following cesarean section (4%). Eight of the patients developed hypovolemic shock with five of them further developing DIC. Of these five, three had atonic bleeding of the uterus, one was a cervical laceration, and one was a uterine rupture. The three cases of atonic bleeding required blood transfusions with two recoveries and one death. The patient with uterine rupture was saved with a blood transfusion and a hysterectomy. Direct current shock, transfusion, and operation were required for the cervical laceration, as her heart had stopped upon arrival at the hospital. However, she developed severe DIC and died. The diagnosis and the management of the five DIC cases are discussed.

References

1. O'Leary J L, O'Leary JA (1974) Uterine artery ligation for control of postcesarean section hemorrhage. Obstet Gynecol 43: 849
2. Hayashi RH (1986) Hemorrhagic shock in obstetrics. Clin Perinatol 13: 755
3. Suzuki S (1989) The treatment of abnormal bleeding during delivery. Sanfujinkachiryou 58: 179 (in Japanese)
4. Terao T (1989) Management of DIC. Sanfujinkachiryou 58: 185 (in Japanese)

1.5 Can We Predict Bleeding in Pregnancy? Computer Graphic Analysis of Obstetric Bleeding

SHIGENORI SUZUKI, TUKASA MURAMATU[1], and TOSHIHIKO TERAO[2]

Introduction

As is already well known, the amount of bleeding at childbirth greatly affects the prognosis for the mother and her baby. According to statistics compiled by the Japanese Welfare Ministry the major cause of maternal death has been gestosis; the second most important cause of maternal death has been bleeding. These facts show that bleeding at childbirth is an important factor in the mortality of pregnant women.

Many obstetric factors are involved in the process of childbirth. The importance of some of them, e.g., blood coagulation, fibrinogenolysis, the kallikrein kinin system, the possibility of gravidas, and the mother's physical and mental condition at the time of delivery, cannot always be clearly estimated.

The first aim of our study was to investigate which risk factors for gravidas were present before childbirth, and by applying the idea of multi-risk using the multiple logistic function method, to attempt to construct some guidelines that would help predict abnormal bleeding at childbirth.

The second aim of the study was to clarify how the physical condition of the mother was related to hemorrhagic diathesis in her newborn baby. Advances in prenatal medicine have increased opportunities for treating extremely premature infants. Therefore a more systematic approach to evaluating the numerous factors involved in the embryonal and newborn periods is needed. For example, in conditions such as asphyxia of the newborn, or intracranial hemorrhage (which involves intracranial hemorrhage in early infancy), the relation between maturation value of the liver function of affected infants and obstetric factors affecting their mothers during pregnancy and childbirth, has not been elucidated.

[1] College of Medical Technology, Hokkaido University, Kita 12-jo, Nishi 5-chome, Kita-ku, Sapporo 060, Japan

[2] Department of Gynecology & Obstetrics, Hamamatsu Medical University. Handa-cho. Mamamatsu, Japan

Computer graphic analysis is a useful tool for predicting intracranial hemorrhage and for making follow-up treatment plans. The period of life from newborn to juvenile infant, referred to as the "valley" by obstetricians and pediatricians, is particularly troublesome and calls for accurate judgment and evaluation of data. Screening by computer graphic analysis may provide valuable information otherwise overlooked during this critical period.

Materials and Methods

We collected data from 217 pregnant women who had been treated in the department of Obstetrics and Gynecology at Hokkaido University Hospital and Hamamatsu Medical College. Records of medical examinations and treatments were coded on file and stored in a computer. Blood samples were taken from the elbow vein during the first stage of labor.

We studied the patients who had an abnormal quantity of bleeding at childbirth (from period I to period IV of childbirth), and examined several factors as shown in Fig. 1. They were consisted of 26 factors. The items of determination was the haploid relation number. In the qualitative items, we analyzed the related number by X official approval (using direct way of probability at the same time) and investigated the main items.

A) Private factors (1. Age, 2. Use of health insurance, 3. Address, 4. Hospital used for delivery).
B) Case histories of pregnancy and delivery (5. Gravidity, 6. Parity, 7. Abnormal birth, 8. Cesarean section, 9. Gestosis, 10. Anemia of pregnancy).
C) Cases of abnormal childbirth (11. Perineum tear, 12. Injury of soft parturient canal, 13. Tear of cervical duct, 14. Abruptio placentae, 15. Extremely large fetus, 16. Opacity of amniotic fluid).
D) Obstetric treatment (17. Derivative childbirth, 18. Dilatation and curettage operations, 19. Cesarean section, 20. Episiotomies, 21. Cristerel fetal expression).
E) Measurements of mother (22. Weight, 23. Height, 24. Fundus of uterus, 25. Width of chest).
F) X-ray of the pelvis (26. Confugata, 27. Isthmian occipitofrontal diameter, 28. Diameter transversa of infant's head).
G) Data of delivery (29. Gestational days, 30. Delivery time, 31. Weight of placenta).
H) Measurements of neonate (32. Weight, 33. Length, 34. Size of head, 35. Small diameter tranversa, 36. Large diameter transversa).
I) Examination of gravidic blood (37. Fibrinogen, 38. Factor VIII, 39. Factor XI, 40. FDP, 41. Platelet aggregation, 42. Number of red blood cells, 43. Hemoglobin, 44. GOT).

Using the assay of multiple logistic functions,

$$P(X) = \frac{1}{1 + e^{-\lambda}} \qquad P(X) = \text{the incidence of abnormal bleeding.}$$

However, $\lambda = \alpha + \beta_1 X_1 + \beta_2 X_2 + \ldots\ldots\ldots + \beta n X n$

We analysed the comprehensive influence of multivariates on the quantity of bleeding, making the incidence of abnormal bleeding the purpose variable; each factor which was judged to be related to the amount of bleeding was used as an explanation variable.

Results

The relation between abnormal bleeding and the quantity of each unit double phased number of the 44 items was 0.75. (Fig. 1). We divided the cases into two groups: the disseminated intravuscular coagulation (DIC) group and the non-DIC group. In the non-DIC group, obstetric factors which were considered to have a high significant standard, i.e., delivery time, external conjugate and conjugata, were examined. In addition to these, the number of red blood cells and the fluctuation of factor XI were also taken into account. In the DIC group, fibrinogen plaque and Fibrin degradation products (FDP) were highly correlated (Fig. 2) (Table. 1).

Similarly, in the assay of multiple logistic function, the weight of the embryo was correlated with the highest risk of abnormal bleeding. Furthermore, judging from the estimated value, high risk factors such as gravidity and cesarean section were analyzed.

The Neonatal Hepaprastin test value is usually measured four days after birth as a screening of plasma prothrombin. We examined the relation between low values on this test and obstetric factors, and found that such low values are related to Base Excess, duration of labor, and caput succedaneum.

Considerations

The problem of maternal bleeding is of continuing concern to obstetricians, not only for maternal mortality but also for perinatal death. We considered that a bleeding amount of more than 500 ml at childbirth was abnormal and we called this atonic bleeding or third stage bleeding. As is generally known, spontaneous contractions of uterus muscle lead to biological ligation that causes the fine blood vessels of the uterus to contract. This natural process helps limit the amount of bleeding at childbirth to a level of 150–250 ml.

In our study of the non-DIC group, there was a significant correlation between duration of labor and external conjugate and conjugata as obstetric factors. However, a number of clinical problems remain to be elucidated. One of them concerns the duration of labor, one of the three critical organs involved in childbirth. It is not clear how the parturient canal is related to the gestation of the embryo or to the placenta, and it is not clear how it affects the quantity of bleeding at delivery.

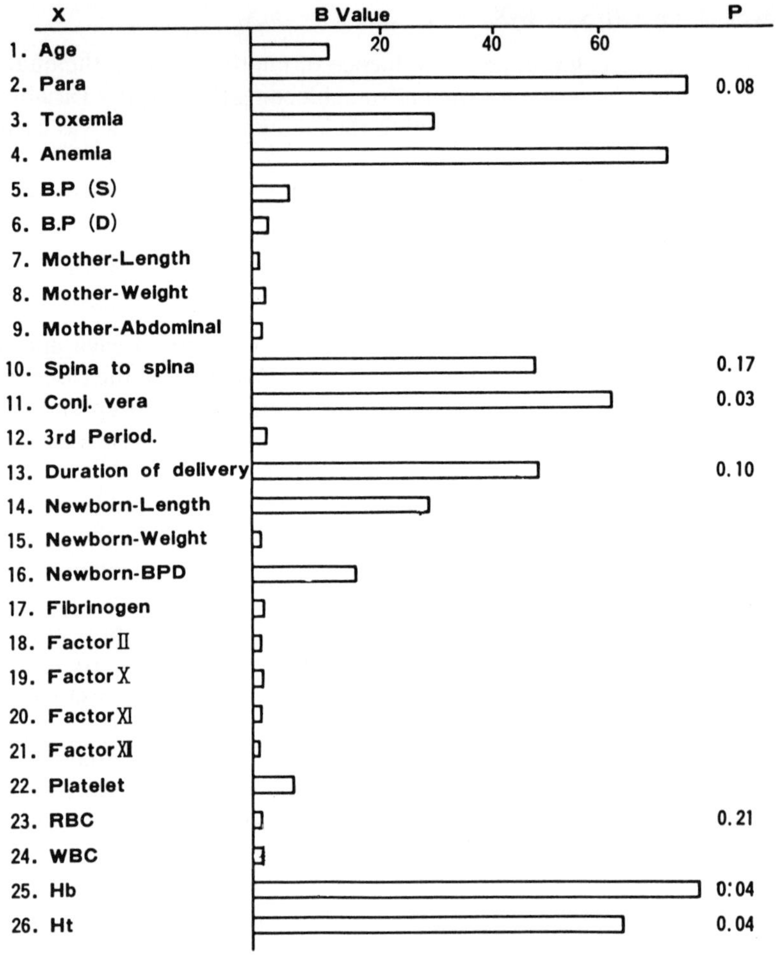

Fig. 1. Maximum R-square improvement for dependent variable bleeding
R-square = 0.77505708
Y (bleeding) = $a_1x_1 + a_2x_2 + \ldots\ldots + a_{26}x_{26}$.

The number of red blood cells and the Hb condition of pregnant women are related to the problem of pregnancy anemia. For examle, there is a tendency for anemia pregnant women are nursing mothers (Fig. 1) to bleed excessively, which could induce shock. The importance of good eating habits and the intake of extra doses of iron cannot be overemphasized in this regard.

We next considered if the quantity of bleeding at childbirth is related to the number of platelet and the blood coagulation factors. In the non-DIC group, which included cases of normal childbirth, no significant correlation was noted (Fig. 2). The only exception was factor XI, (Fig. 3). When examining values of 90%–180% for factor XI it can be seen that when factor XI shows a high value,

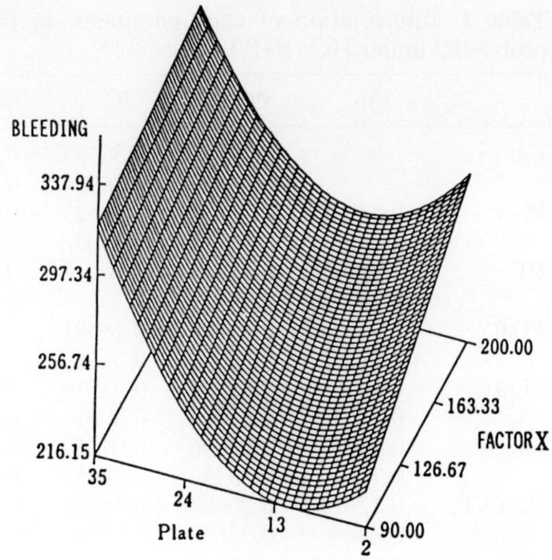

Fig. 2. Three-dimensional graph by computer graphics. Relationship between platelets and bleeding (non-DIC group)

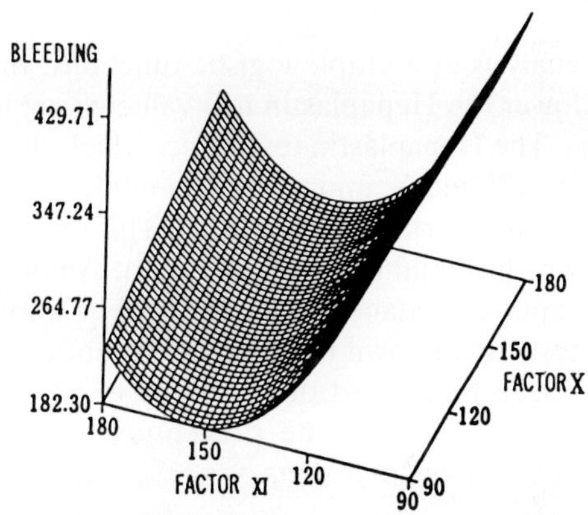

Fig. 3. Three-dimensional graph by computer graphics. Relationship between factor XI, bleeding, and factor X

the quantity of bleeding tends to increase. This suggests the activation of a contact factor. In the non-DIC group, the kinin and kinin-kallikrein system appeared to be related to abnormal bleeding.

In the DIC group, 15 cases, with one exception, demonstrated abruptio placentae. The number of platelet and the values of fibrinogen and FDP were considered to have a significant effect on this result (Table 1). We thus confirmed the DIC Index of the Japanese Welfare Ministry to be a useful score for the evaluation of abruptio placentae.

Prothrombin time is one of the factors also included in the DIC Index of the Japanese Welfare Ministry. However, this factor is important mainly in cases of chronic DIC such as liver disease. For the diagnosis of obsteric diseases considered to be related to acute DIC, only three items—the number of platelet, the values of fibrinogen, and the values of—FDP are needed.

Concerning the relation between the neonatal Hepaplastin test values (obtained the 4th day after birth) and the obstetric factors, it was proved, by the

Table 1. Interrelation of each parameter in the DIC cases. Correlation coefficients/ prob >!R! under HO: RHO = 0/ N = 15

	Fib	Plate	PT	FDP	SFMC	Fact V	Fact VII
Fib	*	0.54975 0.0338	0.30487 0.2692	−0.07431 0.7924	−0.60129 0.0177	0.43463 0.1055	0.12919 0.6463
Plate	0.54975 0.0338	*	0.38127 0.1609	−0.11804 0.6752	−0.18384 0.5119	−0.03856 0.8915	0.26669 0.3366
PT	0.30487 0.2692	0.38127 0.1609	*	−0.18091 0.5188	−0.23214 0.4051	0.07539 0.7895	0.16539 0.5558
FDP	−0.07431 0.7924	−0.11804 0.6752	−0.18091 0.5188	*	0.46009 0.0844	−0.09885 0.7260	0.21242 0.4472
SFMC	−0.60129 0.0177	−0.18384 0.5119	−0.23214 0.4051	0.46009 0.0844	*	−0.40929 0.1298	0.15332 0.5854
Fact V	0.43463 0.1055	−0.03856 0.8915	0.07539 0.7895	−0.09885 0.7260	−0.40929 0.1298	*	0.21258 0.4469
Fact VII	0.12919 0.6463	0.26669 0.3366	0.16539 0.5558	0.21242 0.4472	0.15332 0.5854	0.21258 0.4469	*

analysis of multiple logistic functions, that the longer the delivery time was, the lower the Hepaplastin test value was (Fig. 4).

The Hepaplastin test value, which shows the comprehensive activity of factors II, VII and X among the vitamin K dependent factors, may give low liver values on the fourth day after birth. This may be attributed to delayed delivery, a point which should be given attention. Among the haploid relation number especially caput succedaneum, etc. also has a important meaning to do with Hepaplastin-test. It is known that certain synoptic factors of the newborn infant may have a farreaching effect on its ability to adjust to life outside the womb. Considering this, we studied the prevention of vitamin K deficiency-induced intracranial hemorrhage in infants.

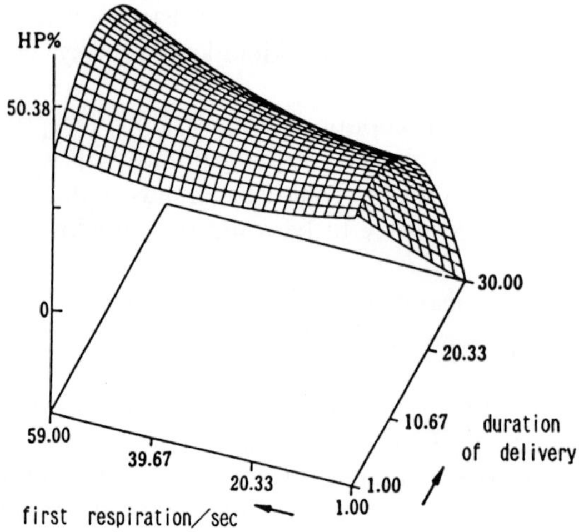

Fig. 4. Three-dimensional graph by computer graphics. Relationship between Hepaplastin test values, delivery time, and the first respiration per second

Summary. In order to detect risk factors which will cause abnormal bleeding during delivery, we tried to project abnormal bleeding using a multi-logic factor model. Fifteen DIC cases and 217 non-DIC cases were tested. As far as the correlation between abnormal bleeding and each obstetric factor is concerned, it should be clearly noted that in the non-DIC cases the duration of delivery, red cell count, and changes of factor XI, correlated highly with Fibrinogen, platelet counts and FDP. The high risk factors of abnormal bleeding during labor consisted of fetal-birth weight, duration of delivery, Conj. vera, and so on. Among the various hematologic factors, RBC and Hb exert a very important influence. In the non-DIC cases, no significant correlations between bleeding and many coagulation-factors, including platelet counts, were proved.

The total volume of the bleeding was apt to increase as the value of factor XI increased. This fact strongly suggests that the Kinin-kallikrein system is closely connected with contractions of the uterus and with activating the contraction factors.

References

1. Haller UB, Frielingsdorf M, Litschgi M (1986) Perinatal gynecological information system. Arch Gynecol 239: 278–282.
2. Baumann H, Huch R, Huch A (1987) Geburtshilflich-perinatologische Datenerfassung mit dem Personal Computer. Geburtshilfe Frauenheilkd 47: 401–405
3. Anderson HF (1985) Developing a perinatal database on a microcomputer. Am J Perinatol 2: 148–149
4. Houlton MJ, Austin D, Jenkins GM, Turner DG, Wilkins (1984) A microcomputer in the delivery suite. Br J Obstet Gynaecol 91: 555–559

AT III

1.6 AT III in Pregnancy and Newborn Infants

HERMANN ERICH KARGES[1]

Introduction

Blood fluidity is determined by the balance between the components of the coagulation and fibrinolytic pathways. The balance is maintained by the activators and inhibitors of the respective proenzymes and enzymes (Fig. 1). Disturbances in either of these systems lead to thrombosis or bleeding.

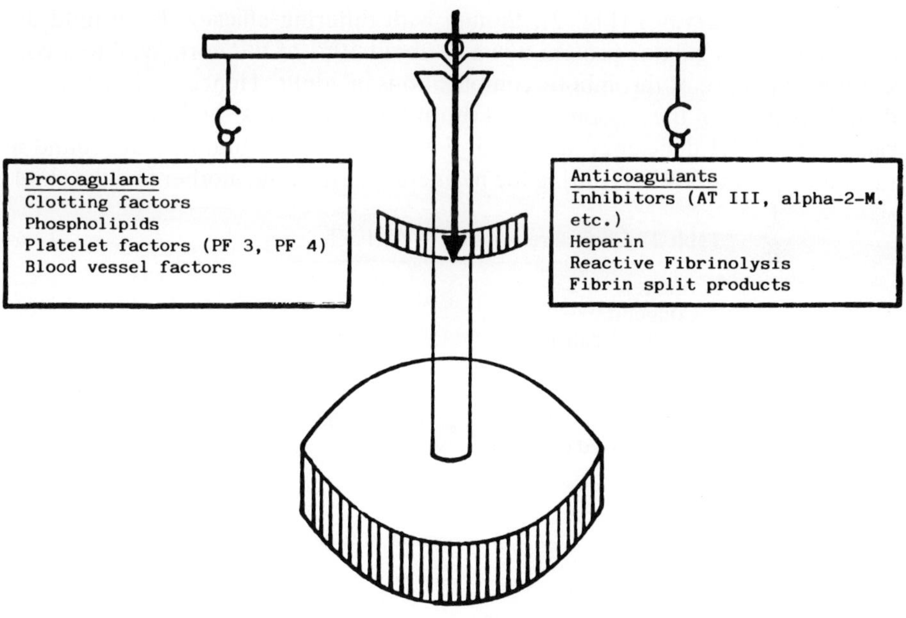

Fig. 1. Homoeostasis of the blood clotting system

[1]Research Laboratories of Behringwerke, Postfach 11 40, D-3550 Marburg 1, Federal Republic of Germany

Excessive activation of the blood clotting system results in thrombosis; however, counterbalanced by the fibrinolytic pathway, it may also lead to bleeding due to the consumption of the clotting factors. Both thrombosis and bleeding due to unbalanced enzymatic systems may occur in late pregnancy and the perinatal phase. Possible reasons for thrombosis are compiled in Table 1.

Table 1. Reasons for thrombosis

Increased coagulation due to
Increased level of procoagulants (F VIII, F IX, etc.)
Increased activation of clotting cascade (F III, tumor coagulant, etc.)
Reduced level of regulator proteins (AT III, PC, PS, HC II, etc.)
Dysproteinemia of regulator proteins (AT III, etc.)
Cellular events (platelets, granulocytes)
Vessel wall effects (thrombomodulin defects, etc.)
Reduced fibrinolysis due to
Plasminogen deficiency/dysplasminogenemia
Increased levels of α-2-PI
Plasminogen-activator deficiency (t-PA, u-PA, F XII)
Increased level of plasminogen-activator-inhibitor (PAI)
Increased level of HRG (carrier of plasminogen)

This contribution is restricted to the role of the main inhibitor of thrombin, the antithrombin III (AT III), which not only inhibits thrombin but also all the other clotting enzymes (Fig. 2), though with differing efficacy. Even mild decreases of this regulator protein down to about 50% of the norm lead to a considerable increase of thrombotic complications in adults. Hence, isolated AT III deficiency is often the reason behind thrombotic disorders. In Table 2 the main causes of AT III deficiency are listed. Several of these conditions are found in thrombotic complications during the perinatal phase in the mother and the child.

Table 2. Clinical reasons for AT III deficiency

Permanent
Congenital
AT III deficiency
AT III dysproteinemia
Acquired
Reduced synthesis (e.g., liver cirrhosis)
Increased excretion (e.g., nephrotic syndrome)
Transient
Consumption
DIC (infections, polytrauma, intoxication, burns)
Inflammation
Carcinoses
Heparin overdosage
Reduced synthesis
Transient liver damage
Oral contraceptives

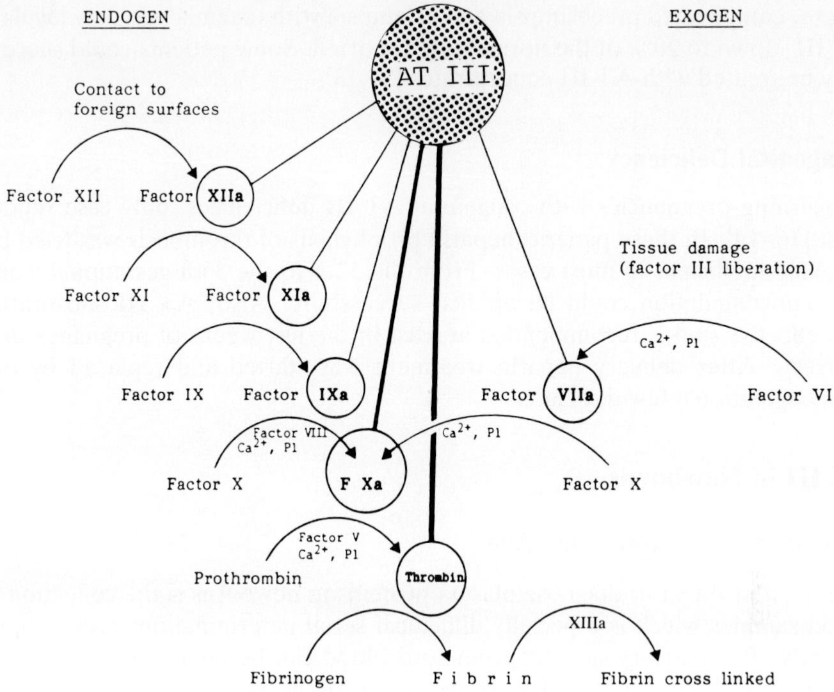

Fig. 2. Antithrombin III sites of action

AT III in Pregnancy

Normal Pregnancy

Reports on plasma AT III-levels in normal pregnancy are scarce and contradictory. While Gjønaess et al. [1] and Ambrus et al. [2] found decreased AT III levels during uncomplicated pregnancy in the third trimester, Weiner and Brand [3], Hellgren and Blombäck [4], and Weenink et al. [5] reported normal values during pregnancy and post partum. Nevertheless, thromboembolic complications during pregnancy between 0.27% to 1% and 1.8% to 4.3% in the puerperium are reported [6–10]. Thus, risks other than AT III deficiency must also be considered in these patients.

Preeclampsia, Hypertension, and Eclampsia

Often in patients with preeclampsia, hypertension, or eclampsia low levels of AT III were detected [11–15]. AT III levels in mild preeclampsia are often found in the lower normal range, about 80% of the norm, with a tendency of decrease. In the last days antepartum [15] the AT III activity decreased even further to 65% of the norm. After delivery the AT III values normalized within a few days. In severe, complicated preeclampsia and eclampsia with toxemia very low levels of AT III, down to 20% of the norm, were reported. Some patients could successfully be treated with AT III concentrates [11,13].

Congenital Deficiency

Concerning pregnancies with congenital AT III deficiencies, only case reports exist [16–19]. In these patients heparin prophylaxis of thrombosis was tried but revealed inefficient in most cases. From the 12th to the 36th gestational week, oral anticoagulation could be applied successfully. Also, AT III substitution was effective and is recommended at least in the last weeks of pregnancy until delivery. After delivery heparin treatment was started and replaced by oral anticoagulation a few days later.

AT III in Newborns

Dependence on Gestational Age

The main problem to diagnose plasma proteins in newborns is the collection of blood samples which is especially difficult if serial determinations are planned. Directly after delivery samples from cord blood can be obtained with an anticoagulant to blood ratio of 1:9. However, cord and venous blood samples resulted in different protein levels for most parameters (A.N. Blanco et al. 1984, personal communication). Even in plasma samples from umbilical vein and umbilical artery differences were seen [20]. The most convenient method of blood sampling in newborns seems to be heel puncture [21]. Though by this method capillary blood is obtained, no marked difference with venous blood samples could be detected. Micromethods were used for determination of different clotting and fibrinolytic factors. With these methods, it could be shown that the AT III levels in newborn plasma is dependent on the gestational age (Table 3) and increases until term to about 50% of the adult norm. At the same gestational age, the AT III content of plasma was found proportional to birth weight [22]. Due to the very low AT III levels, newborns small for gestational age have an additional risk of thrombosis; since the AT III pool of their plasma is small, they are prone to dysregulation in every consumption situation.

Plasma Protein levels and AT III Activity in Healthy, Full-term Neonates

In accordance with the necessary balance between procoagulant factors and the inhibitors, most clotting factor levels in newborns are also low: F II 48%, F IX 53%, F X 40%, F XI 38%, F XII 53%, Prekallikrein 37%, and HMW-Kininogen 54% [23]. The same is true for the fibrinolytic factors: plasminogen 58%. On the other hand, some protein levels are increased beyond the adult value: F VIII: vWF 153% fibrinogen 102%, and α_2-macroglobulin 139%. Also, the main inhibitor of fibrinolysis is relatively high with 85%; it exceeds the plasminogen level by 47% relatively. Up to now, the reason for the different levels

Table 3. Plasma AT III level of newborns dependent on gestational age

Week	AT III (*n*) (% of norm)	Parameter	Sample	Author
30	29 (M*)	activity	capillary	Peters et al. [37]
32	34 (M*)	activity	capillary	Peters et al. [37]
34	39 (M*)	activity	capillary	Peters et al. [37]
36	44 (M*)	activity	capillary	Peters et al. [37]
38	50 (M*)	activity	capillary	Peters et al. [37]
40	55 (M*)	activity	capillary	Peters et al. [37]
>37	45 (20)	activity	cord	Hadnagy et al. [38]
>37	40 (20)	activity	venous	Hadnagy et al. [38]
38–41	59 (16)	activity	capillary	Peters et al. [25]
38–41	70 (16)	antigen	capillary	Peters et al. [25]
28–35	35 (10)	activity	capillary	Peters et al. [25]
28–35	45 (10)	antigen	capillary	Peters et al. [25]
37–42	63 (58)	antigen	venous	Andrew et al. [23]
>36	57 (70)	activity	venous	v. Kries et al. [29]
>36	64 (70)	antigen	venous	v. Kries et al. [29]

*From curve Fig. 1 [37]

of plasma proteins in neonates, as compared to the adult norm, is not clear and further studies are needed to elucidate the physiological background.

To draw conclusions from the analytical data, it is not only important to know the amount of a plasma protein but also its activity. It is well known that different clotting factors are altered in newborns compared to the adult protein: Prothrombin complex factors are only partially γ-carboxylated due to viatamin K deficiency and hence have reduced activity; fibrinogen is differently glycosylated and shows altered clotting properties. With newborn AT III, contradictory results have been reported. McDonald et al. [24] did not find any functional difference in kinetic studies with isolated newborn AT III compared to adult AT III, whereas Peters et al. [25] reported a reduced activity/antigen ratio in newborn AT III down to 0.68 in preterm neonates with idiopathic respiratory distress syndrome (IRDS). They postulate an abnormal AT III molecule in newborns. Whether this really is the case has to be further clarified. It is possible that either the different protein pattern in newborns influenced the determination of AT III by Peters et al. [25] or Mc Donald et al. [24] only isolated the functionally active AT III molecules.

Protein Concentration in Newborns

A further aspect which has not been considered so far is the protein concentration in newborn plasma. In a few newborn plasma samples analyzed in our laboratory, we found not only a reduced AT III level but also a reduced protein content measured by the absorption difference at 280–320 nm. Correction of the AT III values according to the protein content of the plasma sample resulted in nearly normal AT III levels in newborns (Table 4). Since the number of plasma samples is too small to draw general conclusions, this aspect should be

Table 4. Protein- and AT III-levels in newborns

No.	Gestational age (weeks)	Length (cm)	Weight (g)	Protein (g/l)		AT III (% of norm)	
				m	c	m	c
1	35	47	2000	25	55	36	79
2	38	48	3460	31	55	31	55
3	40	51	3620	36	55	47	72
4	40	55	4100	44	55	55	69
5	41	54	4060	33	55	51	85
Mean value	38.8	51	3448	33.8	55	44	72

m, measured; c, corrected

further investigated. Furthermore, it has to be shown whether the absorption coefficient 10 at 280–320 nm = 1% protein, applicable for adult plasma, can also be used for newborn plasma. Nevertheless, it seems necessary to consider the plasma protein content of the sample when analyzing plasma samples; otherwise, wrong conclusions can be drawn from the analytical data. Our results are supported by the data of Schmidt et al. [26], who found in newborn rabbits and infants a good correlation ($r = 0.76$ and 0.79, respectively) between the albumin content of a sample and the AT III level.

AT III in Diseased Newborns

In newborns with IRDS or DIC, AT III is further drastically decreased below the level of age-matched, healthy infants [27–29]. Peters et al. [30] found the lowest levels in newborn infants who died. Also an acquired dysfunctional AT III was detected by immunological methods and AT III activity/antigen-ratio in premature sick infants [31]. Those especially in danger of developing thrombosis are newborns with the rare congenital AT III deficiency [32,33].

Treatment of Neonatal AT III Deficiency

Due to the low AT III level in diseased newborns, heparin is often inefficient [34]. After the availability of AT III concentrates, a substitution therapy has been used with good success. AT III was substituted either alone or combined with low doses of heparin [35].

Conclusions

AT III is an important parameter for the regulation of the blood clotting cascade in pregnancy and newborns as well. In normal pregnancies its level remains constant. The increase of thrombotic events during pregnancy seems to result from an activated clotting system in the early and late pregnancy period. If, however, further thrombotic risk factors like hypertension, preeclampsia, toxemia, septic conditions, or congenital AT III deficiency aggravate this latent thrombotic risk, pregnant patients are highly endangered to develop severe thromboses. Therapeutic measures have to be initiated in these cases to prevent life-threatening conditions. In addition to disease specific treatments, anticoagulation and AT III substitution are indicated.

Newborns, on the other hand, have physiologically low AT III levels of about 50% of the adult norm, which is in balance with the levels of most clotting factors. In premature infants, the AT III level is even lower and depends on the gestational age. These children are prone to coagulation disorders like IRDS and DIC—often with lethal outcome. Not just the small amount of AT III in these neonates contributes to this dangerous situation, but also the lower level of plasminogen together with relatively high levels of α_2-antiplasmin. Even a slight consumption of plasminogen leads to conditions in which fibrin clots deposited in the microvasculature cannot be removed by the reactive fibrinolysis. Under this aspect, the results of the IRDS prophylaxis study in premature infants by substituting plasminogen merits consideration [36]. The authors found a considerable reduction of IRDS in the plasminogen treated group, though the substituted plasminogen doses were extremely low. It seems resonable to regulate clotting disorders in newborns with non-activated proteins like AT III without heparin or plasminogen without activators of fibrinolysis to support the physiological regulation systems. To take the right therapeutic measures, exact analyses have to be performed to define the clinical status of the patients. Under this aspect, the determination of the protein content of a sample could be additionally helpful.

Summary. AT III is the main inhibitor of the blood clotting cascade. Even mild decreases, down to about 50% of the norm, lead to a considerable increase of thrombotic complications in adults.

During normal pregnancy, the AT III level remains unchanged and also during labor and the postpartum phase. However, in eclampsia very low levels of AT III together with thrombotic complications have been reported. In the fetus, the AT III level increases with gestational age and reaches a level of about 50% of the adult norm in full-term infants. The adult AT III level is reached at an age of about 90 days. Activity/antigen relationship was reported by most authors to be near 1. Also, kinetic studies on inhibition of clotting factors revealed no difference between adult and newborn AT III. Hence, the decreased AT III level in newborns is not a qualitative but only a quantitative problem.

In our investigations we found not only low levels of AT III in newborns, but also low plasma protein levels. If the AT III levels of newborns are corrected according to the protein content of the plasma, normal values result. Nevertheless, if the clotting system of newborns is activated due to traumatic of septic complications, they are at high risk for thrombotic complications, and early substitution of AT III seems to be indicated.

References

1. Gjønnaes H, Fagerhol MK (1975) Studies on coagulation and fibrinolysis in pregnancy. Acta Obstet Gynecol Scand 54: 363–367
2. Ambrus JL, Ambrus CM, Lillie MA, Browne BJ, Hanson FW, Niswander K, Witul M, Jung DS, Bartfay-Szabo A (1976) Effects of various estrogen treatment schedules on antithrombin III levels. Commun Chemic Pathol Pharmacol 14: 543–549
3. Weiner CP, Brand Y (1980) Plasma antithrombin III activity in normal pregnancy. Obstet Gynecol 56: 603–610
4. Hellgren M, Blomäck M (1981) Studies on blood coagulation and fibrinolysis in pregnancy, during delivery and in the puerperium. Gynecol Obstet Invest 13: 141–154
5. Weenink GH, Treffers PE, Kahlé LH, ten Cate JW (1982) Antithrombin III in normal pregnancy. Thromb Res 26: 281–287
6. Villesanta U (1965) Thromboembolic disease in pregnancy. Am J Obstet Gynecol 93: 142–160
7. Husni EA, Pena LI, Engle-Lenhert A (1967) Thrombophlebitis in pregnancy. Am J Obstet Gynecol 97: 901–905
8. Aaro LA, Juergens JC (1971) Thrombophlebitis associated with pregnancy. Am J Obstet Gynecol 109: 1128–1136
9. Flessa HC, Glueck HI, Dritschilo A (1974) Thromboembolic disorders in pregnancy: pathophysiology, diagnosis, and treatment with emphasis on heparin. Clin Obstet Gynecol 17: 195–235
10. Hillesma V (1960) Occurrence and anticoagulant treatment of thromboembolism in gravidas, parturients and gynecologic patients. Acta Obstet Gynecol Scand (Suppl 2) 39: 5–76
11. Büller HR, Weenink AH, Treffers PE, Kahlé LH, Otten HA, ten Cate JW (1980) Severe antithrombin III deficiency in a patient with pre-eclampsia. Scand J Haematol 25: 81–86
12. Hellgren M, Nygards E-B, Robbe H (1982) Antithrombin III in late pregnancy. Acta Obstet Gynecol Scand 61: 187–189
13. Schregel W, Straub H, Wölk G, Schneider R (1984) Successful treatment of massive dissiminated intravascular coagulation in EPH gestosis with multiple organ insufficiency. Anasth Intensivther Notfallmed 19: 201–203
14. Goubran, F, Fareed A, Elian A, Abolouz S (1985) Antithrombin III and α_2-macroglobulin in normal pregnancy and preeclampsia. Thromb Haemost 54: 204
15. Friedman KD, Borok Z, Owen J (1986) Heparin cofactor activity and antithrombin III antigen levels in preeclampsia. Thromb Res 43: 409–416
16. Brandt P (1981) Observations during the treatment of antithrombin III deficient women with heparin and antithrombin concentrate during pregnancy, parturation and abortion. Thromb Res 22: 15–24
17. Handeland GF, Abildgaard U (1985) In vivo recovery of antithrombin concentrates. Thromb Res 39: 133–138
18. Schoch U, Zanetti E, von Felten A (1987) Prevention of thromboembolism during pregnancy in 3 sisters with congenital antithrombin III deficiency and decreased inducible fibrinolysis. Schweiz Med Wochenschr 117: 1807–1810
19. De Stefano V, Leone G, de Carolis S, Ferelli R, di Donfrancesco A, Moneta E, Bizzi B (1988) Management of pregnancy in women with antithrombin III congenital defect: Report of four cases. Thromb Haemost 59: 193–196
20. Jürgens H, Göbel U, Bokelmann J, von Voss H, Wahn V (1979) Coagulation studies on umbilical arterial and venous blood from normal newborn babies. Eur J Pediatr 131: 199–204
21. Peters M, Breederveld C, Kahlé LH, ten Cate JW (1982) Rapid microanalysis of coagulation parameters by automated chromogenic substrate methods—application in neonatal patients. Thromb Res 28: 773–781

22. Peters M, ten Cate JW, Koo LH, Breederveld C (1984) Persistent antithrombin III deficiency: Risk factor for thromboembolic complications in neonates small for gestational age. J Pediatr 105: 310–314
23. Andrew M, Pars B, Milner R, Johnston M, Mitchell L, Tollefsen DM, Powers P (1987) Development of the human coagulation system in the full-term infant. Blood 70: 165–172
24. McDonald MM, Hathaway WE, Reeve EB, Leonard BD (1982) Biochemical and functional study of antithrombin III in newborn infants. Thromb Haemost 47: 56–58
25. Peters M, Jansen E, ten Cate J, Kahlé LH, Ockelford P, Breederveld C (1984) Neonatal antithrombin III. Br J Haematol 58: 579–587
26. Schmidt BK, Muraji T, Zipursky A (1986) Low antithrombin III in neonatal shock: DIC or non-specific protein depletion? Eur J Pediatr 145: 500–503
27. Hathaway WE, Neumann LL, Borden CA, Jacobsen LJ (1978) Immunologic studies of antithrombin III heparin cofactor in the newborn. Thromb Haemost 39: 624–630
28. Henriksson P, Westström G, Hedner U (1979) Umbilical artery catheterization in newborns. Acta Paediatr Scand 68: 719–723
29. von Kries R, Schweickert M, Gunzelmann KH, Göbel U (1984) Antithrombin III activity and concentration in healthy and ill newborns. Lab Med 7: 353–357
30. Peters M, ten Cate JW, Breederveld C, de Leeuw R, Emeis J, Koppe J (1984) Low antithrombin III levels in neonates with idiopathic respiratory distress syndrome: Poor prognosis. Pediatr Res 18: 273–276
31. Andrew M, Massicotté-Nolan P, Mitchell L, Cassidy K (1985) Dysfunctional antithrombin III in sick premature infants. Pediatr Res 19: 237–239
32. Schander K, Niesen K, Rehm A, Budde U, Müller N (1980) Diagnosis and therapy of a congenital antithrombin III deficiency during the neonatal period. In: Deutsch E, Lechner K (eds) Fibrinolyse, Thrombose and Haemostase. Schattauer Verlag, Stuttgart, pp 483–486
33. Brenner B, Fishman A, Goldsher D, Schreibman D, Tavory S (1988) Cerebral thrombosis in a newborn with a congenital deficiency of antithrombin III. Am J Hematol 27: 209–221
34. Markarian M (1982) Heparin resistance in newborn infants. J Pediatr 103: 175
35. von Kries R, Stannigel H, Göbel U (1985) Anticoagulant therapy by continuous heparin-antithrombin III infusion in newborns with disseminated intravascular coagulation. Eur J Pediatr 144: 191–194
36. Ambrus CM, Choi TS, Cunnanan E, Eisenberg B, Staub HP, Weintraub H (1977) Prevention of hyaline membrane disease with plasminogen. A cooperative study. JAMA 237: 1837–1841
37. Peters M, ten Cate JW, Jansen E, Breederveld C (1985) Coagulation and fibrinolytic factors in the first week of life in healthy infants. J Pediatr 106: 292–295
38. Hadnagy J, Giertler U, Halvax L, Sulyok E, Ertl T, Csaba IF, Buchenan W (1983) The antithrombin III-activity in the newborn age. Dtsch Gesundh Wesen 38: 1719–1720

1.7 Thrombin-Antithrombin III Complex and D-Dimer in Neonates:

Signs of Thrombin Generation During Birth

W. MUNTEAN[1], M. DANDA[1], and H. ROSEGGER[2]

Introduction

In neonates, especially in sick neonates, signs of enhanced proteolysis are observed: (1) after birth the fibrinolytic activity is high, (2) fibrin/fibrinogen degradation products are elevated, and (3) fibrinogen is lower immediately after birth than after 3 days of life. Factor VIII activity is very high immediately after birth and activity of factor VIII is higher than factor VIII antigen suggesting activation of factor VIII [1–5].

The question is whether an enhanced proteolysis in the neonate predominately leads to hypocoagulability because of primary degradation of procoagulant proteins or whether limited proteolysis leads to activation of procoagulant proteins and induction of hypercoagulability. In sick neonates this hypercoagulability then may progress to DIC and secondary hypocoagulability.

Clinical experience favors the latter. Peters et al. [6] observed that low antithrombin III correlated significantly with poor prognosis in infants with idiopathic respiratory distress syndrome (IRDS). Mc Donald et al. [7] reported that coagulation profiles in infants with severe grades of intracranial hemorrhage were suggestive of an initial clotting activation resulting in consumptive coagulopathy. And, there are also the old reports about the increased risk of intracranial hemorrhage after the administration of prothrombin complex concentrates to newborns [8]. Obviously, whether a hypocoagulability in newborns is the result of an initial activation of the clotting system or not has important implications for the treatment regimens.

Two relatively new clotting tests may help to answer the question. Thrombin forms a complex with its most important inhibitor, antithrombin III. These thrombin-antithrombin III complexes (TAT) can be measured by means of two

[1]Department of Pediatrics and [2]Department of Gynecology and Obstetrics, University of Graz, Auenbruggerplatz, A-8036 Graz, Austria

antibodies and reflect intravascular thrombin generation. High TAT complexes are found in DIC and thrombotic states [9].

D-dimer is a fragment of cross-linked fibrin that can be measured by means of monoclonal antibodies. The advantage of the assay over other determinations of fibrin/fibrinogen degradation products is that the antibodies do not react with fibrinogen or its degradation products; therefore, elevated D-dimer is not only a sign of enhanced fibrinolysis but also of fibrin formation [10]. Since we have observed very high TAT and D-dimer values in nearly all sick newborns, we investigated what can be found after a normal birth in normal neonates.

Material and Methods

Thirty healthy term neonates were investigated. Each were spontaneous deliveries after an uncomplicated pregnancy and labor. Gestational age ranged from 38–42 weeks. All had a normal fetal heart rate pattern, Apgar values >8, and pH >7.20. All neonates were without any problems for the first 48 h of life. Blood samples were collected into 0.1 M sodium citrate from a peripheral vein by a clean puncture immediately after birth and 1 h, 10 h, and 24 h afer birth. All samples were assayed within 1 h. *Thrombin-antithrombin III complexes (TAT)* were determined by means of a commercially available enzyme-linked immunosorbent assay (ELISA) obtained from Behring Corp. (Enzygnost-TAT, Behring, FRG). *D-dimer* was determined by ELISA obtained from Boehringer Corp. (ELISA D-Dimer, Boehringer Mannheim, FRG). *Factors II, V, VIII* were determined by one stage assays (Behring Corp, FRG). *Fibrinogen* was determined according to Clauss.

Results

TAT levels were very high in all neonates immediately after birth. Some neonates showed extremely high values; in all neonates TAT was above the upper

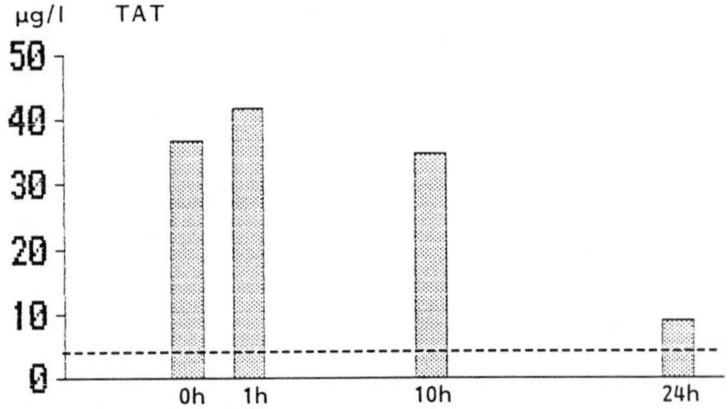

Fig. 1. Mean thrombin-antithrombin III complex values (*TAT*) in 30 neonates at 0, 1, 10, and 24 h after birth

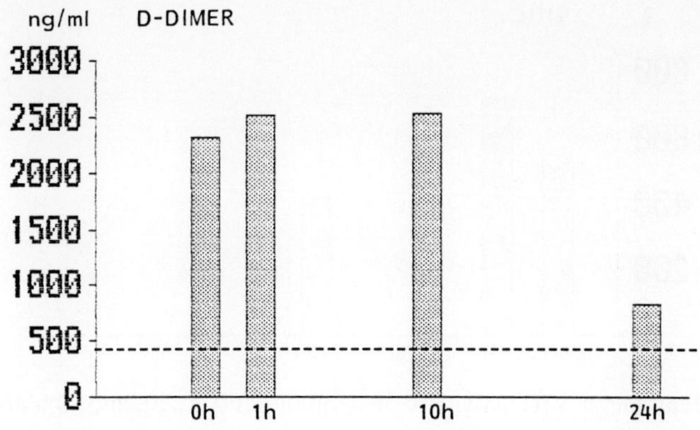

Fig. 2. Mean D-dimer values in 30 neonates at 0, 1, 10, and 24 h after birth

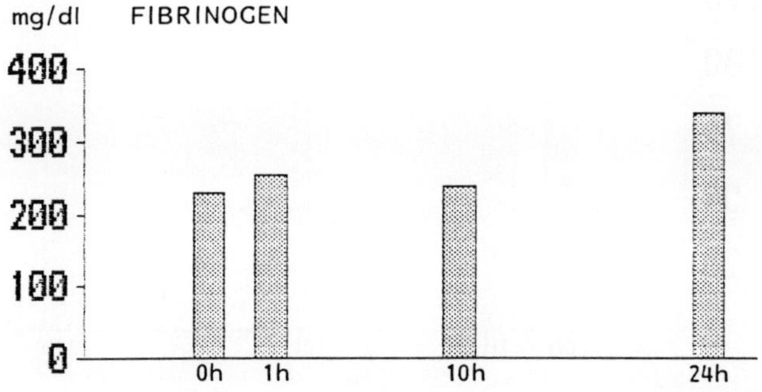

Fig. 3. Mean fibrinogen values in 30 neonates at 0, 1, 10, and 24 h after birth

limits of normal for adults. TAT remained elevated in all neonates for the first 10 h of life and decreased to near normal values for adults until 24 h after birth (Fig. 1).

D-dimer values also were very high immediately after birth, the values being above the upper limits of normal for adults in all neonates. Similar to TAT, D-dimer values were still high after 10 h and decreased to near normal values for adults until 24 h after birth (Fig. 2).

Fibrinogen was about the same at 0.1, and 10 h after birth and showed an increase after 24 hours (Fig. 3). In contrast, factor VIII activity was very high at 0 and 1 h after birth and then decreased (Fig. 4). Factor V showed a similar pattern, but activity was not that much elevated immediately after birth (Fig. 5). Factor II activity decreased slightly until 24 h after birth (Fig. 6).

Further analysis of the data showed a strict correlation between TAT and D-dimer values in neonates (Fig. 7). There was also a significant correlation of high TAT values with low fibrinogen values (Fig. 8). No correlation was observed between fibrinogen and D-dimer values (Fig. 9). High factor VIII activity correlated significantly with high TAT values (Fig. 10), but no such correlation was observed between D-dimer and factor VIII activity (Fig. 11). Similar to factor VIII activity, high factor V activity correlated significantly with high

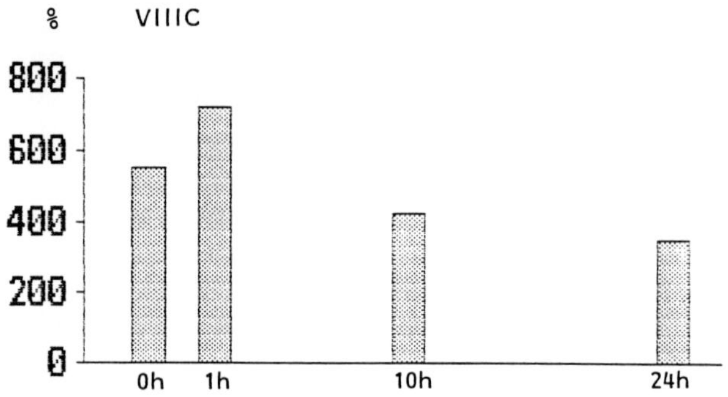

Fig. 4. Mean factor VIII activity in 30 neonates at 0, 1, 10, and 24 h after birth

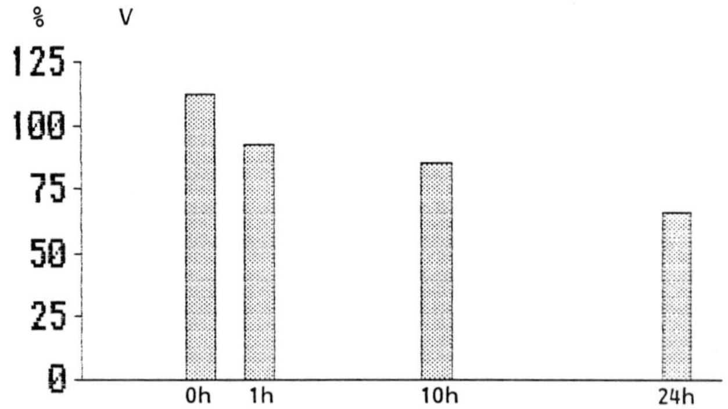

Fig. 5. Mean factor V activity in 30 neonates at 0, 1, 10, and 24 h after birth

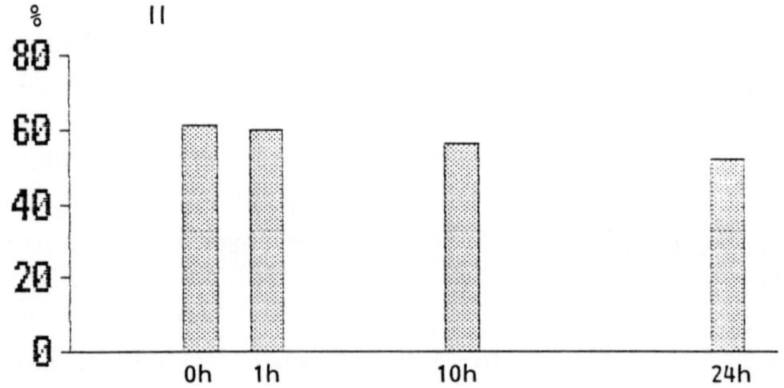

Fig. 6. Mean factor II activity in 30 neonates at 0, 1, 10, and 24 h after birth

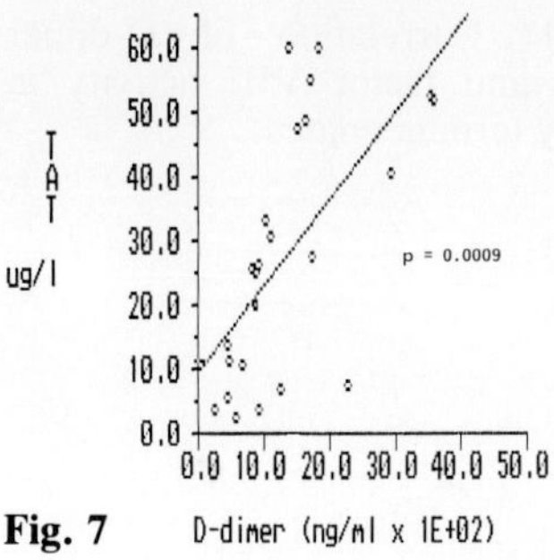

Fig. 7

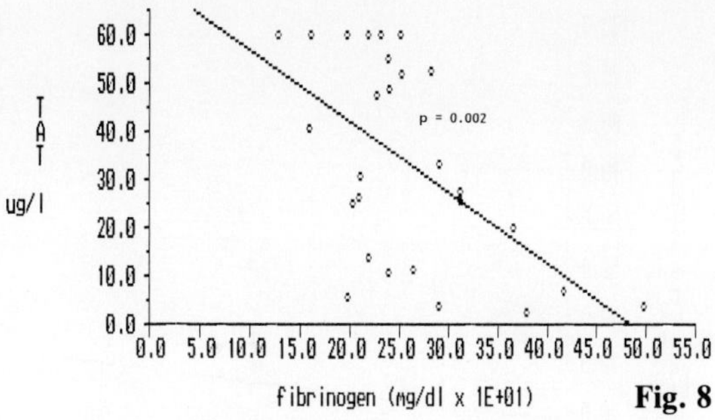

Fig. 8

Fig. 7. Correlation of thrombin-antithrombin III complex values (*TAT*) and D-dimer values in healthy neonates

Fig. 8. Correlation of thrombin-antithrombin III complex values (*TAT*) and fibrinogen values in healthy term neonates

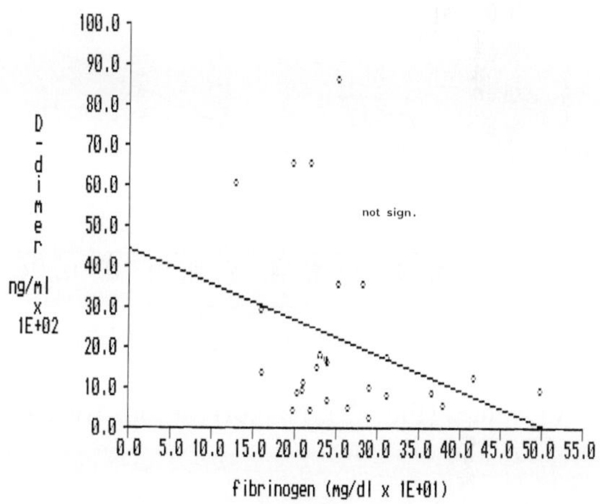

Fig. 9. Correlation of D-dimer and fibrinogen values in healthy term neonates

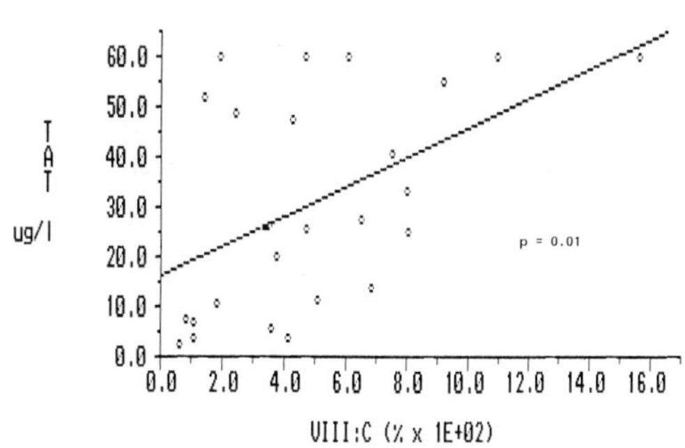

Fig. 10. Correlation of thrombin-antithrombin III complex (*TAT*) and factor VIII activity in healthy term neonates

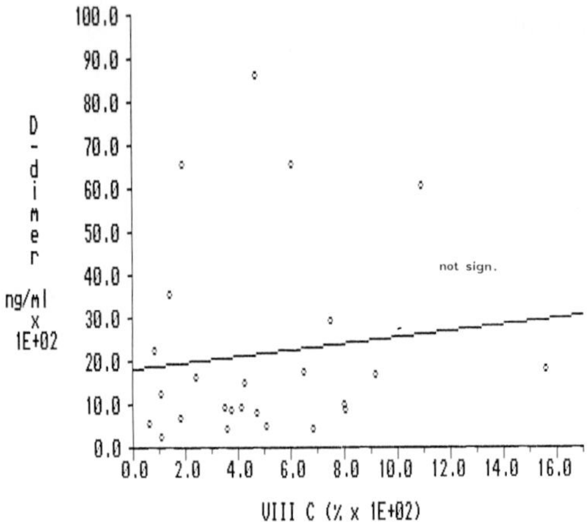

Fig. 11. Correlation of D-dimer values and factor VIII activity in healthy term neonates

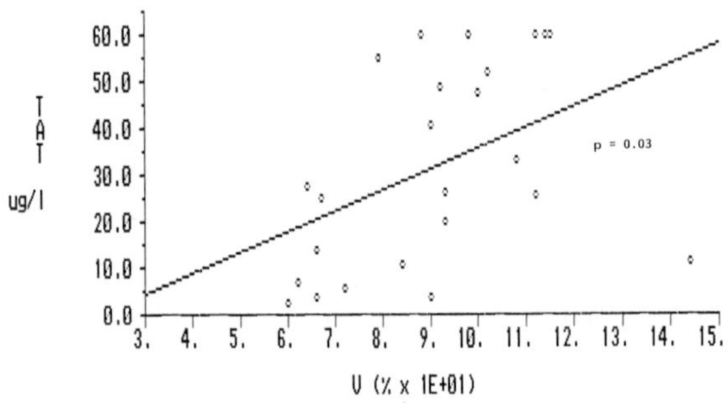

Fig. 12. Correlation of thrombin-antithrombin III complex values (*TAT*) and factor V activity in healthy term neonates

TAT values (Fig. 12). No correlations were observed between factor II activity and TAT or D-dimer.

Discussion

Our findings in healthy term neonates born after an uncomplicated pregnancy and labor are consistent with a hypercoagulable state. TAT levels are very high immediately after birth and stay high for at least 10 h after birth. A high TAT level does not necessarily mean that enough free thrombin is available to intravascularly activate procoagulant proteins. However, the possibility that in newborns intravascular activation occurs is strongly suggested by the finding of the very high D-dimer values that prove fibrin formation. It is also suggested by the very high factor VIII activity and—to a lesser extent—factor V activity that correlated with the high TAT values. Also, fibrinogen was lower immediately after birth when TAT was high and low fibrinogen was correlated with high TAT values.

This hypercoagulability obviously can be handled very well by healthy neonates; no signs of consumptive coagulopathy were observed. But, in depressed neonates and neonates with complicating disease, the hypercoagulability probably induced during birth may not be compensated and lead to DIC and consumptive coagulopathy. Our study suggests that in most sick neonates an observed hypocoagulable state may be preceded by a phase of hypercoagulability. Therefore, in neonates, management of the hypercoagulability may be more important than administration of procoagulant material.

Since antithrombin III is low in neonates, an obvious idea would be to administer antithrombin III to sick neonates. However, in an open, controlled randomized study we were not able to demonstrate a beneficial effect of a single administration of antithrombin III concentrate to preterm neonates immediately after birth. No differences between controls and the antithrombin III treated group in frequency and duration of respirator therapy, grade of IRDS, or intracranial hemorrhage were observed [11].

Summary. In neonates, signs of enhanced proteolysis have been reported. After birth, fibrinolytic activity is high and fibrinogen/fibrin degradation products are elevated. Whether this proteolysis leads predominantly to a degradation of coagulation factors or to an intravascular generation of procoagulate activity with induction of a hypercoagulabile state in the newborn has remained unclear. Clincial observations suggest the latter. We, therefore, determined thrombin-antithrombin III complex (TAT) and D-dimer immediately, 1, and 10 h after birth. Even after an uncomplicated delivery, both TAT and D-dimer were significantly elevated in neonates for several hours after birth. Our results show that during delivery the procoagulant system of the infant is activated resulting in thrombin generation.

Since AT III is low in neonates, we investigated whether administration of AT III to the neonate has a beneficial effect on morbidity and mortality from idiopathic respiratory distress syndrome (IRDS) and intraventricular hemorrhage (IVH). One single dose of AT III concentrate was administered immediately after birth in an open, controlled randomized clinical trial. No effects of AT III administration on frequency and severity of IRDS and IVH were shown.

References

1. Ekelund H, Hender U, Nilsson IM (1970) Fibrinolysis in newborns. Acta Paediatr Scand 59: 33
2. Henriksson P, Ekelund H (1975) Abnormal proteolysis in sich newborns. Acta Paediatr Scand 64: 327
3. Muntean W (1980) Die Hämostase bei Frühgeborenen und reifen Neugeborenen. Padiatr Padol 15: 109
4. Muntean W, Belohradsky BH, Klose HJ, Riegel K (1977) Faktor-VIII-Aktivität und Faktor-VIII-assoziiertes Antigen bei Neugeborenen. Klin Radiatr 189: 412
5. Sell EJ, Corrigan JJ (1973) Platelet count, fibrinogen concentration, and factor V and factor VIII level and healthy infants according to gestational age. J Pediatr 82: 1082
6. Peter M, Cate JW, Breederveld C, De Leeuw R, Emeis J, Koppe J (1984) Low antithrombin III levels in neonates with idiopathic respiratory distress syndrome: poor prognosis. Pediatr Res 3: 273

7. McDonald MM, Johnosn ML, Rumack CM, Koops BL, Guggenheim MA, Babb C, Hathaway WE (1984) Rolke of coagulopathy in newborn intracranial hemorrhage. Pedatrics 74: 26
8. Waltl H, Födisch HJ, Kurz R, Hohenauer L, Mitterstieler F, Rössler H (1973) Intracranial haemorrhage in low-birth-weight infants and prophylactic administration of coagulation-factor concentrate. Lancet II: 1284
9. Pelzer H, Schwarz A, Heimburger N (1988) Determination of human thrombin antithrombin III-complex in plasma with an enzyme-linked immunosorbent assay. Thromb Haemost 59: 101
10. Belitser VA, Pozdnjakova TM, Platonova TN, Vouvk EV (1981) Fibrin-fragment-D-complex formation. Thromb Res 21: 565
11. Muntean W, Rosegger H (1989) Antithrombin III-concentrate in preterm infants with IRDS: An open, controlled, randomized clinical trial. Thromb Haemost 62: 288a

1.8 Effect of Antithrombin III Concentrate for DIC in Obstetrics and Gynecology:

The Changes of Prostanoids in Plasma Before and After Administration

HIROSHI SUZUKI[1], MAYUMI KASAI[1], KEN SATOH[1], HAJIME IIDA[1], HIROKI SUZUKI[2], and IWAO NISHIYA[2]

Introduction

Obstetrical disseminated intravascular coagulation (DIC) is frequently acute and sometimes life threatening. However, early diagnosis and prompt treatment often save lives. We have shown in patients with gestosis that changes in vasoactive substances such as prostaglandin and prostanoid are associated with progression of the disease that induces chronic DIC [1–3]. On the other hand, DIC complicating gynecological malignant tumors are mostly seen at the terminal stage of the disease, and, therefore, active treatment for DIC has been rarely performed. However, recent advances in the anti-cancer therapy and radiotherapy for gynecological malignant tumors have prolonged the life of some patients. During chemotherapy with anti-cancer drugs, DIC sometimes develops, and active treatment for DIC is often required. In this study, we administered an antithrombin III concentrate (AT-III) to 7 patients with obstetric DIC and 10 of 15 patients treated for gynecological malignant tumors who had DIC or were expected to develop DIC. To evaluate the usefulness of this drug, the AT-III activity and various effects, especially on prostanoid, were studied.

Materials and Methods

Subjects

Obstetrical DIC

The subjects were 7 patients referred to the Iwate koji Emergency Center (Iwate Prefecture) between November 1984 and April 1986 who scored 8 or

[1]Department of Obstetrics and Gynecololgy, Iwate Prefectural Central Hospital, 1-4-1 Ueda, Morioka, 020 Japan
[2]Department of Obstetrics and Gynecology, Iwate Medical University, 19-1 Uchimaru, Morioka, 020 Japan

more according to the diagnostic criteria for obstetrical DIC established by Maki et al. [4]. The underlying disease was DIC type third-stage bleeding in 2 patients, uterine rupture in 1, abruptio placentae in 2, and eclampsia in 2 (Table 1). The test drug was BI 6013 (AT-III concentrate, 500 unit vial, Berling Research Center, Hoechst Co.). One vial of BI 6013 was dissolved in distilled water (10 ml), and 3000 units (6 vials) per day was mixed with lactic acid (500 ml) and administered by drip injection for 2 h. Patients 1–4 were treated at a dose of 3000 units only on the first disease day, and patients 5–7 were treated on the first and second disease days at a total dose of 6000 units.

Gynecological DIC

The subjects were 15 patients who were admitted to the Department of Obstetrics and Gynecology of Iwate Prefectural Hospital because of gynecological malignant tumors between 1984 and 1987 and who had received chemotherapy and radiotherapy. After these therapies, all these patients scored 5–9 according to the Diagnostic Criteria for DIC established by the Ministry of Public Welfare [5]. The underlying disease was ovarian carcinoma in 12 patients, choriocarcinoma in 1, and cervical carcinoma in 2 (Table 2). Six vials of the AT-III concentrate (3000 units) was mixed with lactic acid (500 ml) and administered by drip infusion for 2 h to 10 of the 15 patients. The remaining 5 patients used as controls were not treated with this drug. Though transfusion was performed in some patients with anemia, in principle, aprotinin or heparin was not used in combination with this concentrate; and fresh frozen plasma, platelets, or fibrinogen was not administered.

Examination Items

Before as well as 1, 3, 6, 12, 24, and 48 h after the drug administration, scoring according to the diagnostic criteria for DIC was carried out. In addition, a general blood analysis, a blood chemistry test, and an examination of electrolytes and the blood clotting system [platelet count, prothrombin time (PT), fibrinogen (Fbg), fibrinogen degradation product (FDP), α_2-plasmin inhibitor (α_2-PI), plasma protamine paracoagulation test (FMT), AT-III antigen, and prostanoid (6-keto-PGF$_1\alpha$, thromboxane B$_2$)] were done [2,3].

Evaluation and Side Effects

The efficacy of the drug was evaluated (effective or ineffective) comprehensively based on clinical symptoms, values of the coagulation test, and improvement in the prostanoid values. The safety was evaluated (presence or absence of side effects) based on clinical symptoms and changes in the values of clinical chemical examinations such as general blood analysis, blood chemistry test, and examination of electrolytes.

Table 1. Clinical profiles of 7 (obstetrics) patients' treatment with antithrombin III (*AT III*) administration, *PLT*, platelet count; *PT*, prothrombin time; *Fbg*, fibrinogen; *FDP*, fibrinogen degradation product; *APTT*, activated partial thromboplastin time; *FMT*, plasma protamine paracoagulation test; *ESR*, erythrocyte sedimentation rate

Case No	Name (Age) Diagnosis	measurement time	obstetrical DC score	clinical score	blood clotting score	PLT		PT		Fbg		FDP		APTT (sec)	α_1-PI	FMT	AT-III (%)	AT-III mg/dl	ESR		6 Keto-PGF$_{1\alpha}$ pg/ml	TXB$_2$ pg/ml	AT-III administraton (units)
						×10^4	score	(sec)	score	mg/ml	score	µg/ml	score						mm/h	score			
1	HS (30)	Before	15	7	5	6.5	1	45.0	1	55	1	40	1	75.0	87	–	70	20.7	1	1	470	960	←3000
	hemor-rhage in the	24 h	0	0	1			13.0	0	235	0	<10		35.7	122	++	109	34.2	9	1	490	390	
	IIIrd stage	48 h						14.2	0	298	0	<10		47.1	110	–	90	27.6					
2	TO (23)	Before	10	8	1	19.5	0	12.5	0	340	0	40	1	31.1	66	++	90	30.9			280	550	←3000
	uterine rupture	24 h	1	0	1	22.5	0	13.3	0	335	0	20	1	29.7	116	++	101	34.2			390	500	
		48 h																					
3	SY (25)	Before	8	3	1	15.5	0	13.0	0	262	0	40	1	36.4	95	+	78	26.5	16	0	450	280	←3000
	placental abruption	24 h	1	0	1	27.5	0	12.4	0	353	0	20	1	38.1	135	–	96	31.4	40	0	330	420	
		48 h																					
4	YS (32)	Before	13	6	3	8.3	1	20.3	1	195	0	40	1	29.6	85	+	86	29.4	22	0	220	850	←3000
	eclampsia	24 h	0	0	0	18.2	0	13.2	0	344	0	10		34.5	103	–	92	35.2	44	0	450	490	
		48 h				23.0	0	14.5	0	220	0	10		32.2	101	–	99	34.8	47	0			
5	SI (36)	Before	15	8	3	8.0	1	15.1	1	243	0			39.6	58	+	76	23.0	12	1	690	770	←3000
	hemorrhage in the IIIrd	24 h	5	4	0			14.1	0	230	0			52.4	75	+	126	37.8			780	390	←3000
	stage	48 h	1	0	1	10.9	0	11.8	0	364	0	20	1	35.6	75	+	103	31.0					
6	MK (36)	Before	11	5	2	14.0	0	24.0	1	201	0	80	1	49.5	89	+	80	27.6	19	0	570	290	←3000
	eclampsia	24 h	4	3	1	15.0	0	13.0	0	342	0	40	1	39.2	105	+	90	31.2	39	0	510	330	→3000
		48 h	2	1	1	17.8	0	12.5	0	333	0	20	1	32.2	110	–	101	32.5	32	0			
7	TS (32)	Before	15	7	3	7.9	1	15.6	1	208	0	40	1	34.9	78	+	68	25.6	18	0	360	810	←3000
	placental abruption	24 h	6	4	2	10.0	1	11.8	0	290	0	20	1	30.5	99	–	89	29.1	26	0	600	620	→3000
		48 h	1	1	0	19.3	0	12.2	0	415	0	<10		27.4	115	–	110	32.8	40	0			

Table 2a,b. Clinical profiles of (gynecology) patients **a** with and **b** without administration of antithrombin III (*AT III*). *NV DIC*, Ministry of Health and Welfare test; *PLT*, platelet count; *PT*, prothrombin time; *Fbg*, fibrinogen; *FDP*, fibrinogen degradation product; *FMT*, plasma protamine paracoagulation test

a

Case no.	Name (Age) Diagnosis	measurement time	NV DIC score	PLT ($\times 10^4$)	PT (sec)	Fbg (mg/dl)	FDP (μg/ml)	α_2-PI (%)	FMT	AT III (%)	6-Keto-PGF$_{1\alpha}$ (pg/ml)	TX-B$_2$ (pg/ml)	Administration (units)
1	A. S. (52)	Before	6	18.5	15.1	150	80	79	+	70	360	610	←3000
	ovarian cancer	24 h	4	26.0	13.2	181	40	74	–	94	420	350	
2	I. H. (60)	Before	7	12.0	16.1	308	160	104	–	83	360	590	←3000
	ovarian cancer	24 h	3	16.5	13.8	245	20	106	–	121	290	410	
3	Y. S. (72)	Before	7	12.0	16.3	271	40	118	+	86	280	890	←3000
	ovarian cancer	24 h	4	18.6	12.9	335	40	172	–	129	450	320	
4	K. Y. (48)	Before	6	15.3	40.0	180	150	75	+	77	290	790	←3000
	ovarian cancer	24 h	2	18.9	14.0	220	10	111	–	131	380	610	
5	T. A. (55)	Before	8	8.0	15.2	381	40	72	+	62	380	990	←3000
	ovarian cancer	24 h	4	14.5	11.8	390	20	110	–	138	600	380	
6	T. S. (64)	Before	6	15.3	15.0	169	40	111	+	80	370	430	←3000
	ovarian cancer	24 h	3	18.9	12.0	205	20	127	–	141	380	650	
7	M. S. (58)	Before	9	6.8	17.9	75	80	85	+	85	280	950	←3000
	ovarian cancer	24 h	4	7.3	13.0	180	10	105	–	130	210	480	
8	R. N.	Before	5	17.5	13.9	288	40	120	++	82	300	710	←3000

	[illegible] carcinoma	24 h	4	[illegible]	12.2	[illegible]	40	139	–	109	390	300	
9	K. S. (59) cervical cancer	Before	6	17.8	16.2	55	10	98	++	93	420	490	←3000
		24 h	1	25.7	12.2	489	5	145	–	161	310	580	
10	N. S. (45) cervical cancer	Before	7	9.7	15.3	260	40	101	++	70	290	810	←3000
		24 h	2	12.5	13.3	335	10	136	–	120	380	430	

b

Case no.	Name (Age) Diagnosis	measurement time	NV DIC score	PLT ($\times 10^4$)	PT (sec)	Fbg (mg/dl)	FDP (μg/ml)	α_2-PI (%)	FMT	AT III (%)	6-Keto-$PGF_{1\alpha}$ (pg/ml)	TX-B_2 (pg/ml)
1	T. K. (54) ovarian cancer	Before	7	12.0	17.5	180	40	75	+	65	250	920
		24 h	6	11.5	17.0	190	40	70	+	60	300	990
2	R. K. (43) ovarian cancer	Before	5	12.0	13.8	180	10	82	±	84.8	280	310
		24 h	4	13.6	15.1	280	10	84	±	84.4	260	350
3	K. T. (68) ovarian cancer	Before	5	12.0	15.2	350	10	80	–	78.8	360	630
		24 h	3	15.0	12.8	410	10	109	–	112.5	430	550
4	R. N. (51) ovarian cancer	Before	5	22.7	15.1	325	20	78	–	88.0	330	440
		24 h	3	23.8	14.0	335	10	102	–	81.6	350	380
5	M. K. (73) ovarian cancer	Before	6	7.8	14.3	220	20	88	±	61.4	280	950
		24 h	6	5.3	17.5	250	20	73	+	41.4	320	900

Clinical Results and Result of the Laboratory Test

In patients with severe obstetrical or gynecological DIC (Figs. 1, 2), circulatory improvement and respiratory management were performed together with treatment of the underlying disease and transfusion while the AT-III concentrate (3000–6000 units) was administered by drip infusion. Relatively good results were obtained in all the 7 patients with obstetrical DIC as shock, respiratory failure, bleeding and renal insufficiency, coagulation test values, and the prostanoid value showed apparent improvement 24 h after the drug administration. The DIC scores decreased to values below the standard. In addition, no side effects associated with the AT-III drug administration were observed in clinical chemical examinations, showing the safety of this drug. In the 5 untreated patients with gynecological DIC, delay in improvement was apparent by evaluation of clinical symptoms, coagulation test values, prostanoid values, and DIC scores.

Discussion

In obstetrical DIC, its cause is often transient, and the underlying disease is relatively readily treated. However, the pathologic condition is both acute and severe involving marked changes with time in the blood coagulation and fibrinolysis systems. Therefore, in some cases, clinical changes should be accurately evaluated, and appropriate treatment should be initiated before results of laboratory examinations are obtained. We used the diagnostic criteria by Maki et al. [4] for diagnosing obstetrical DIC and administered an AT-III drug alone at the early stage to 7 patients with a total score of 8 or more [6,7].

On the other hand, DIC in the gynecological disease may be also acute, but that due to malignant tumors is usually chronic as has been suggested by a number of reports [8,9] of only slight decreases in platelets, AT-III, plasminogen, and α_2-PI and a slight increase in FDP. Since patients with an advanced or recurrent malignant tumor are in the preliminary stage of DIC, the possible development of DIC should be taken into consideration when highly invasive treatment such as extensive pelvic operation, mass administration of antitumor drugs, and radiotherapy is performed.

We graded patients with gynecological malignant tumor, primarily ovarian tumor treated by mass administration of anticancer drugs, according to the criteria by the DIC Research Group of the Ministry of Welfare [5] and administered an AT-III to 10 patients with a score of 5 or more [10]. Since the AT-III drug was reported to increase blood AT-III activity by about 1% at a dose of 1 unit/kg body weight [11], a daily dose of 3000 units was administered by drip infusion. Theoretically, in a patient weighing 50 kg, the AT-III activity is transiently increased by 60%. However, because of a shorter half-life of AT-III in

Fig. 1a–h. Results of the laboratory tests for DIC diagnosis in obstetrics with administration of antithrombin III, $n = 7$

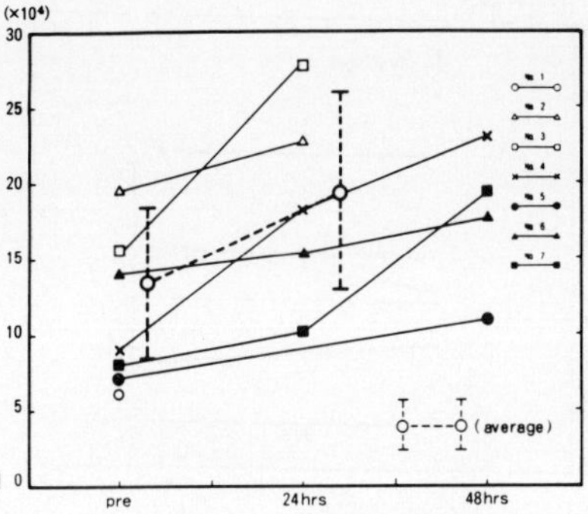

a

Changes in Platelet count

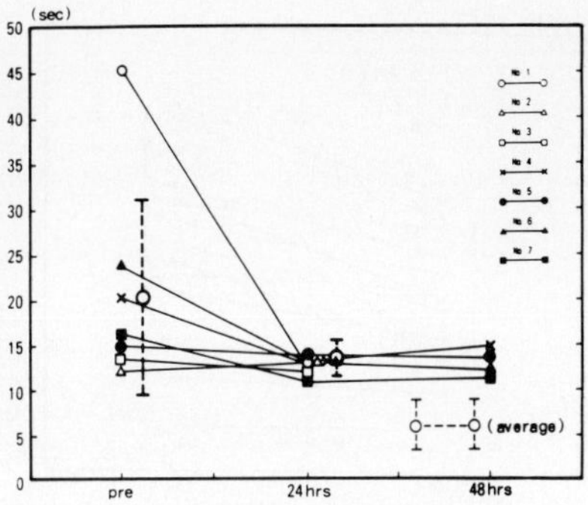

b

Changes in Protrombin

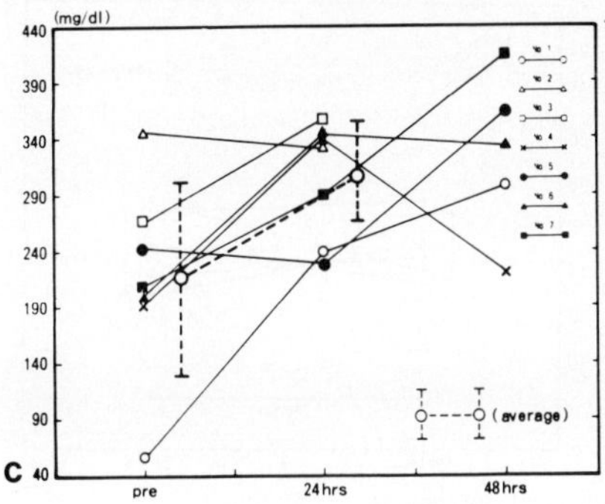

c

Changes in Fibrinogen

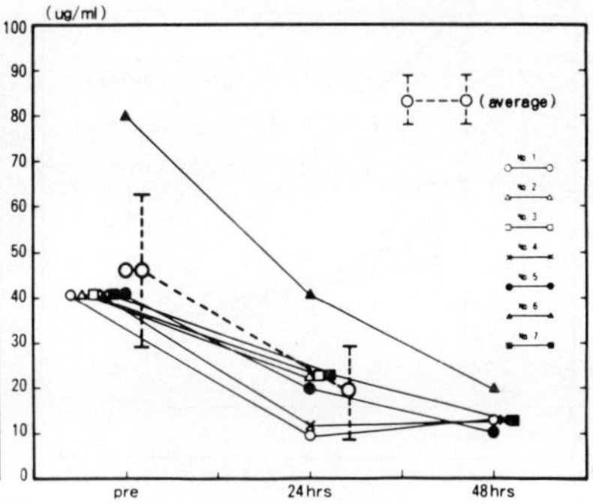

d

Changes in Fibrinoges Degradation Products

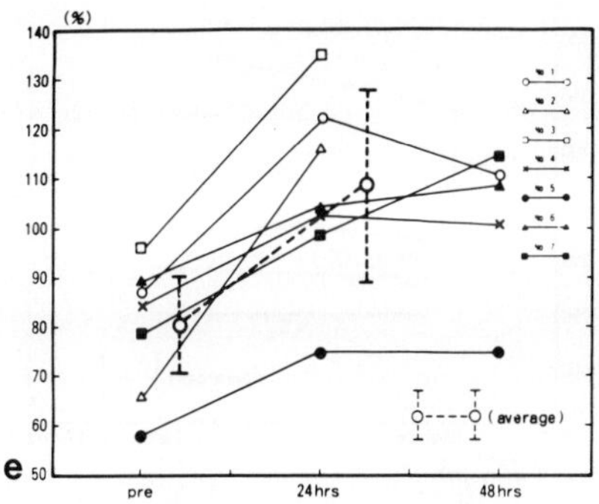

e

Changes in α_2-Plasmin inhibitor

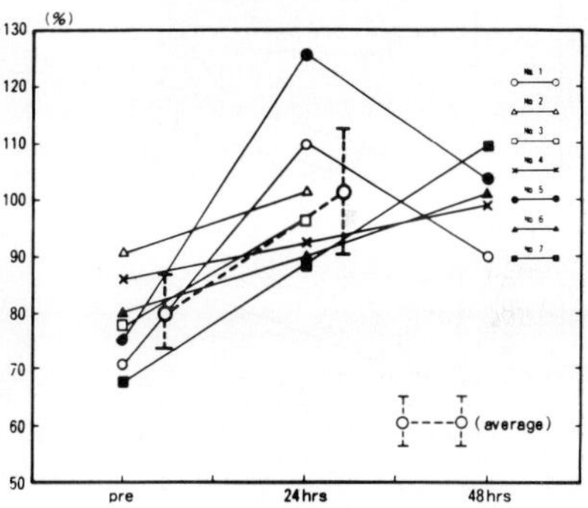

f

Changes in Antithrombin III

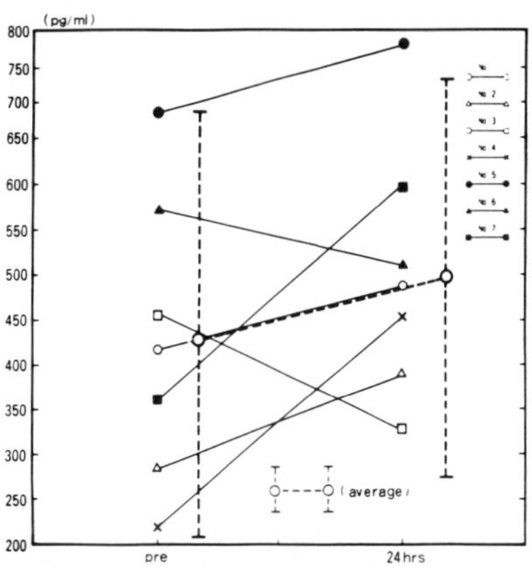

g

Changes in 6-keto-PGF$_{2\alpha}$

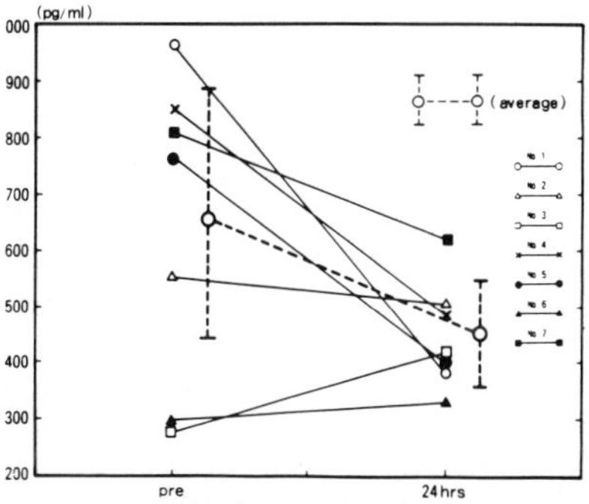

h

Changes in Thromboxane B$_2$

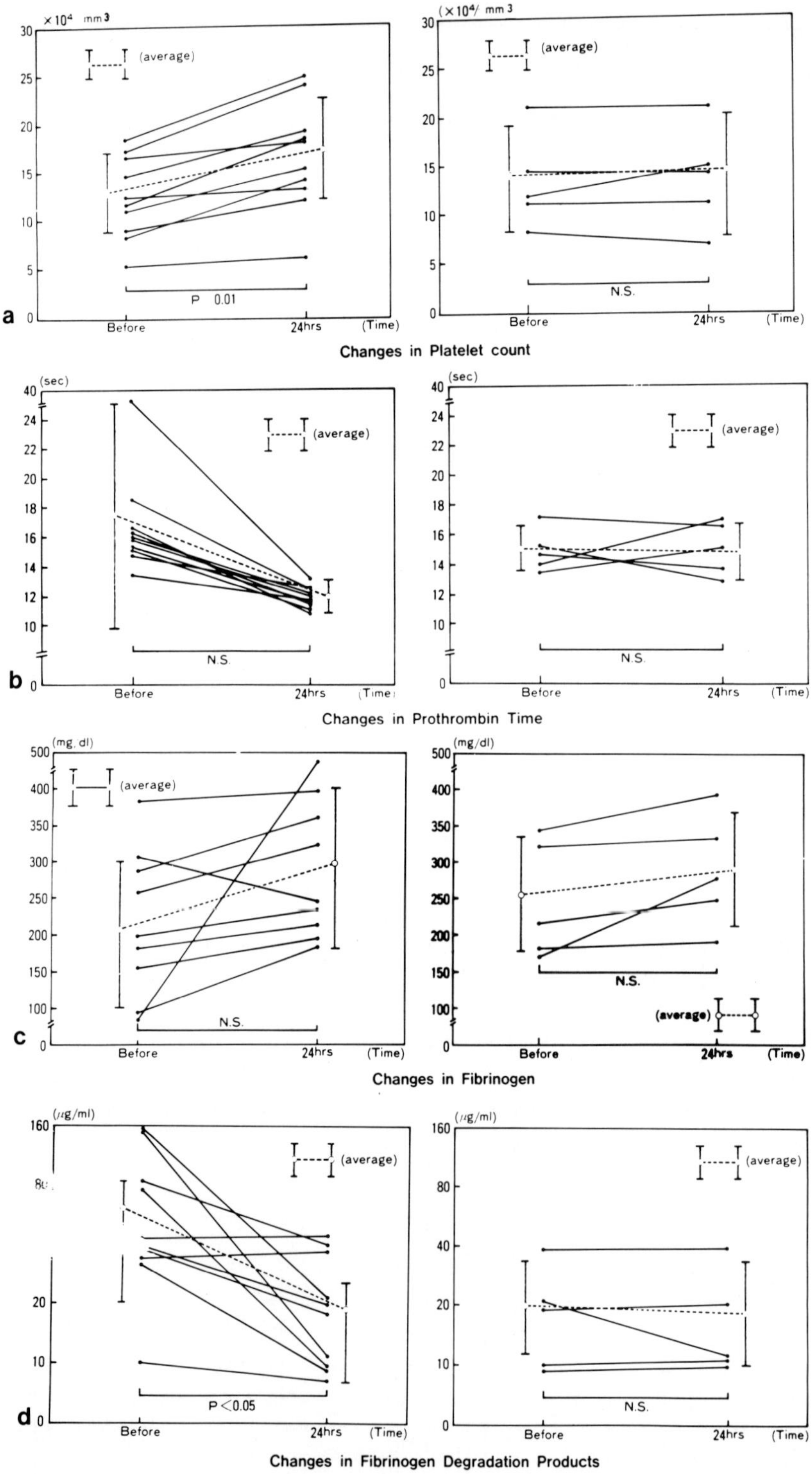

Fig. 2a–h. Results of the laboratory tests for DIC diagnosis in gynecology with (*left*, n = 10) and without (*right*, n = 5) administration of antithrombin III

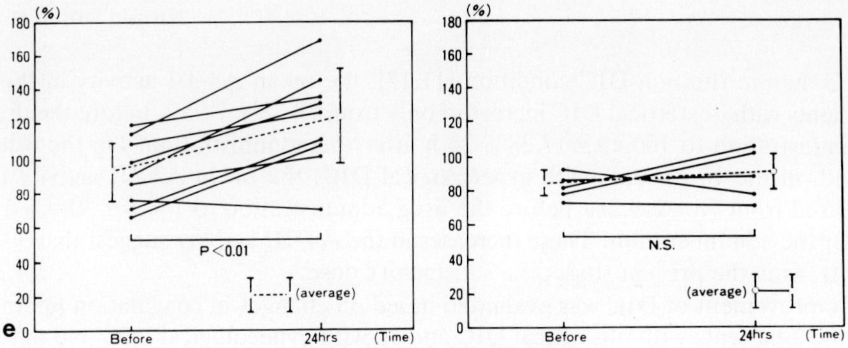

Changes in α_2-plasmin inhibitor

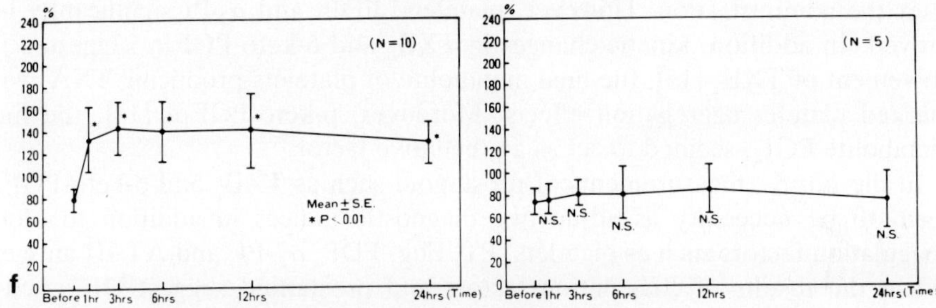

changes in Antithrombin III

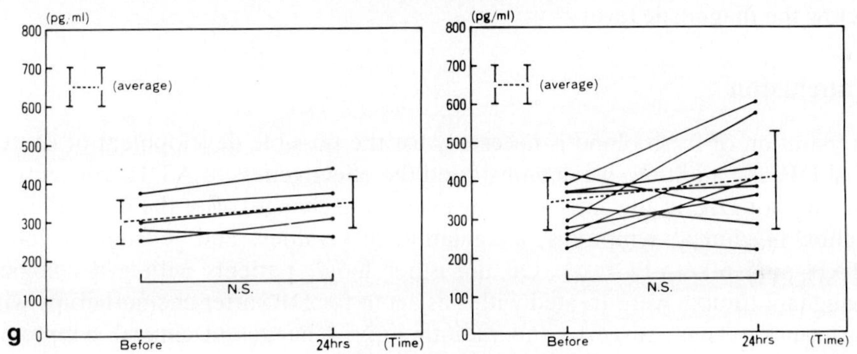

Changes in 6-Keto-Prostaglandin $F_{1\alpha}$

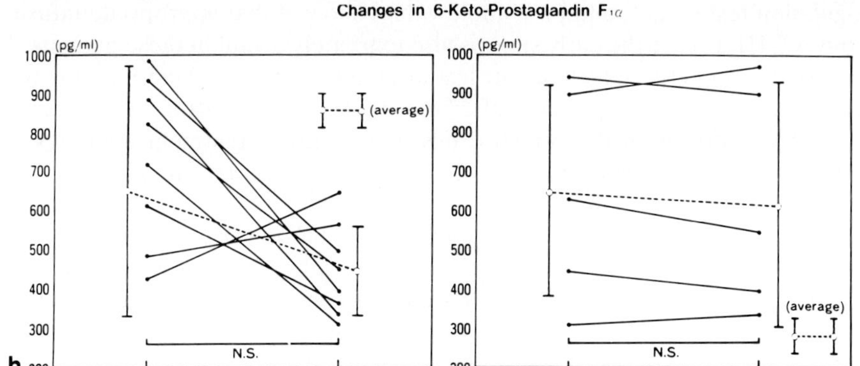

Changes in Thromboxane B_2

Fig. 2 (continued)

DIC than in the non-DIC condition [11,12], the mean AT-III activity in the 7 patients with obstetrical DIC increased only from 78.28 ± 7.95% before the drug administration to 100.43 ± 17.28% 24 h after the administration. On the other hand, in the 10 patients with gynecological DIC, the mean AT-III activity increased from 78.8 ± 9.2% before the drug administration to 134.8 ± 30.9% 1 h after the administration. These increases in the AT-III activity suggest that 3000 units, as in the present study, is a satisfactory dose.

Improvement of DIC was evaluated based on changes in coagulation findings in the 7 patients with obstetrical DIC and 10 with gynecological DIC. No difference was observed between PT or Fbg before the drug administration and that after the administration. However, platelets, FDP, and α_2-PI significantly improved. In addition, kinetic changes in TXB_2 and 6-keto-$PGF_1\alpha$ suggested involvement of TXB_2 [13], the final metabolite of platelets-producing TXA_2 with marked platelet aggregation effects. Moreover, 6-keto-$PGF_1\alpha$ [14], the final metabolite PGI_2, seemed to act as a preventive factor.

In the future, measurements of prostanoid such as TXB_2 and 6-keto-$PGF_1\alpha$ seem to be necessary as adjunctive diagnostic indices in addition to blood coagulation factors such as platelets, PT, Fbg, FDP, α_2-PI, and AT-III antigen. When the results of coagulation factors and prostanoid suggest DIC, active prophylactic anticoagulation therapy should be initiated even if the DIC score is below the diagnostic level.

Conclusion

Preparation of fresh blood is necessary for the possible development of obstetrical DIC. In addition, we demonstrated the effectiveness of AT-III concentrate infusion for DIC at the early stage by evaluating changes after the drug administration in clinical symptoms, coagulation test values, and prostanoid values (TXB_2 and 6-keto-$PGF_1\alpha$). On the other hand, patients with gynecological malignant tumors were treated with this agent for DIC after chemotherapy with anti-cancer drugs, surgery, and radiotherapy. Changes in clinical symptoms, coagulation test values, and prostanoid values showed that appropriate infusion of the AT-III drug at the early stage is also extremely useful in these patients. In patients showing DIC scores of 5 or less after chemoterapy, chemotherapy with stornger agents became possible after the infusion of this drug. These results suggest that infusion of the AT-III drugs as preventive treatment improves the prognosis of gynecological malignant tumors such as ovarian carcinoma.

Summary. The disseminated intravascular coagulation (DIC) in obstetrics was observed to have a mortal risk due to its acute and abrupt onset. However, in the case of gynecological malignancy, it sometimes has a chronic course. In the present study, the influence on the vasoactive substances in acute DIC in obstetrics and after chemotherapy in gynecological malignancy was studied after the treatment of AT-III concentrate (Behringwerke AG).

Obstetrical DIC (7 cases: 1 rupture of uterus, 2 abruptio placentae, 2 eclampsia, and 2 DIC type postpartum hemorrhage) and gynecological DIC (10 cases: 7

ovarian carcinoma, 1 chorio carcinoma, and 2 uterine carcinoma were treated with AT-III concentrate, and 3000 units per day were administered by i.v. drip infusion. Agents which are known to have influence on the coagulation and fibrinolysis systems (Aprotinim, Heparin, etc.) were not administered, in principle. Transfusion of fresh frozen plasma, fibrinogen, or platelet was also avoided. However, when hemorrhage of much volume occurred, a transfusion of a corresponding volume of fresh whole blood was allowed. Measurements of platelet count, PT, fibrinogen, serum FDP, AT-III antigen, α_2-PI activity, FMT, 6-keto-$PGF_1\alpha$, and TXB_2 were performed as coagulative tests 1, 2, 3, 6, 12, and 24 h after the administration.

Remarkable improvement in clinical findings and coagulation was observed after the administration in nearly all of the DIC patients, and a decrease in the DIC score was also found. Moreover, clinical efficacy was also observed in the changes in prostanoids.

We concluded from the study of changes of vasoactive substances that treatment with AT-III concentrate in a relatively early phase of DIC is important and effective in cases where an onset of DIC is expected not only in obstetrics, but also after chemotherapy for gynecological malignancy.

References

1. Suzuki H (1979) Studies on the clinical significance of plasma prostaglandin $F_2\alpha$ and prostaglandin $F_2\alpha$-main-urinary-metabolite. Acta Obstet Gynaecol Jpn 31: 87
2. Tsukatani E (1983) Etiology of EPH-gestosis from the viewpoint of dynamics of vasoactive prostanoid, lipid peroxides and vitamin E. Acta Obstet Gynaecol Jpn 35: 713
3. Omi K (1986) Changes in endogenous prostaglandin and affinous substances in gestosis. J Iwate Med Assoc (Morioka) 38: 67
4. Maki M, Terao T, Ikenoue K (1985) Obstetrical DIC score (in Japanese). Obstet Gynecol Ther (Tokyo) 50: 119
5. Research Group for Blood Coagulation Abnormalities (1986) In: Kobayashi N (ed) Specified diseases research report, vol 47 (in Japanese). Ministry of Public Welfare, Tokyo
6. Suzuki H, Saito K, Adachi N, Kasai M, Haga K, Tsukatani E, Ito K, Kunimoto K, Nishitani I (1987) Effects of antithrombin III concentrates on obstetrical DIC: Changes in blood prostanoid after administration (in Japanese). Obstet Gynecol (Tokyo) 54: 1219
7. Suzuki H, Kasai M, Harada K, Iida H (1987) Effect of antithrombin on obstetrical and gynaecological DIC (in Japanese). J Iwate Pref Hosp Assoc (Morioka) 27: 48
8. Nakabayashi M, Chin Z, Takeda S, Baba K, Kinoshita K, Kawana H, Sato K, Mizuno M (1984) Antifibrinolytic therapy for the ascites ovarian cancer (in Japanese). Obstet Gynecol (Tokyo) 10: 1409
9. Shinagawa N, Kagiya A, Tominra K, Takano A (1984) Gynecological malignant tumor: Diagnosis and treatment of DIC (in Japanese). Gendaiiryosha, Tokyo, pp 262–269
10. Suzuki H, Kasai M, Kubota T, Harada K, Iida H (1988) Effect on antithrombin III concentrates for DIC in gynaecological malignant tumor (in Japanese). Obstet Gynecol (Tokyo) 55: 489
11. Thalar E (1982) Antithrombin III-Konzentrate Klinische Anwendung. Hamostaseologie 3: 128

12. Takahashi K (1980) Studies on antithrombin III. II. The role for antithrombin III (AT III) in the control of disseminated intravascular coagulation (DIC). The effect of the administration of AT III concentrates in experimental DIC and in clinical DIC. Acta Haematol Jpn 43: 889
13. Samuelsson B (1976) Introduction: New trends in prostaglandin research. In: Samuelsson B, Paoletti R (eds) Advances in prostaglandin and thromboxane research, vol 1. Raven Press, New York
14. Moncada S, Gryglewski R, Bunting S, Vane JR (1976) An enzyme isolated from artteries transforms prostaglandin endperoxides to an unstable substance that inhibits platelet aggregation. Nature 263: 663

1.9 Perinatal Coagulation and Fibrinolysis

JOHN BONNAR, LEISHA DALY, and BRIAN L. SHEPPARD[1]

Introduction

In normal pregnancy extensive changes take place in the hemostatic system, involving in particular the coagulation and fibrinolytic systems. These physiological changes seem to have two major interrelated functions. First, to maintain the integrity of the expanding maternal and fetal circulations at the interface of the placenta and, secondly, to ensure the rapid and effective control of bleeding from the placental site during and after placental separation.

The overall changes in the coagulation system in normal pregnancy are in accord with a continuing low grade local activation of coagulation resulting in enhanced synthesis of fibrinogen and other clotting factors combined with a slight decrease in coagulation inhibitors. Fibrin deposition can be readily demonstrated in the utero-placental vasculature [1]. In pregnancy, the elastic lamina and smooth muscle of the expanding spiral arteries supplying the placenta are replaced by trophoblast surrounded by a matrix containing fibrin. This enables the enlargement of these vessels to accomodate an increasing blood flow to the placenta as well as reducing the pressure in the arterial blood flowing to the intervillous space of the placenta (Figs. 1, 2).

In late pregnancy, a substantial reserve of hemostatic components, especially fibrinogen and other coagulation proteins, is present in the circulating blood; in addition there is an increased blood volume. These physiological changes will provide a substantial reserve to meet the hemostatic challenge which takes place during childbirth. In the rapid process of placental separation a maternal blood flow of approximately 700mls per minute to the placental site has to be staunched by the combined effects of myometrial extravascular compression and thrombotic occlusion of the sheared maternal vessels. If one of these two mechanisms is defective serious uterine hemorrhage will occur during childbirth.

[1]Trinity College Department of Obstetrics and Gynaecology, St James's Hospital and Coombe Hospital, Dublin, Ireland

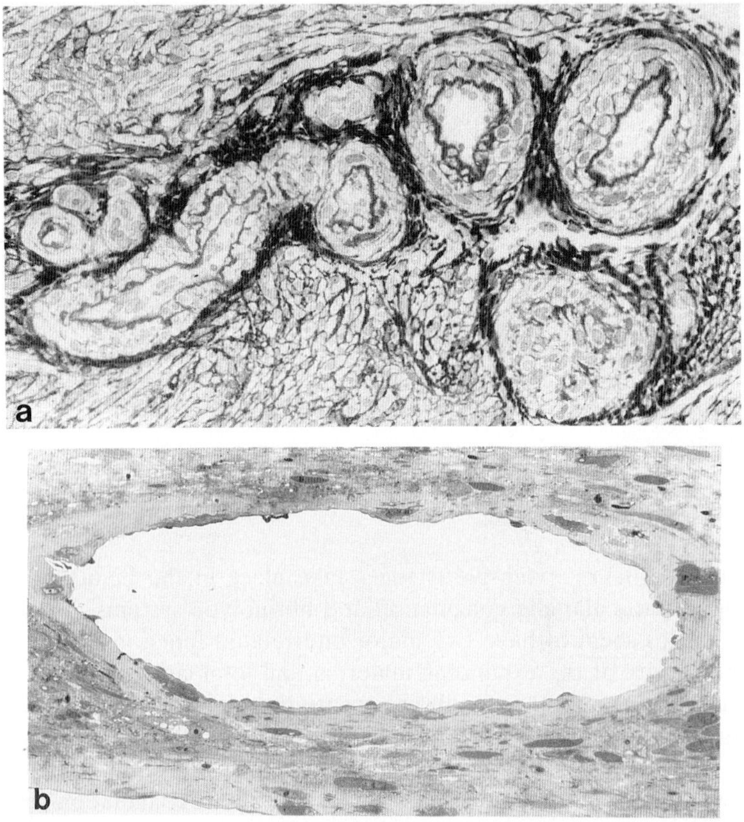

Fig. 1. The spiral artery **a** of the non-pregnant uterus, and **b** supplying the placenta at term. Large trophoblast cells form a pseudo-endothelium in parts of the vessel wall. The elastic lamina and muscle of the artery have been removed

In normal pregnancy, therefore, the coagulation and fibrinolytic systems have a central role in controlling the physiological process of fibrin deposition in the utero-placental circulation while at the same time preventing fibrin deposition in the rest of the vascular system.

The physiological changes in the hemostatic system during pregnancy establish a vulnerable state for disordered fibrin deposition both in the uteroplacental circulation and outside the uterus. Abnormal fibrin deposition is seen in pregnancies complicated by fetal growth retardation with and without pre-eclampsia. In pre-eclampsia, fibrin deposition is found in both the kidney and liver. In complications such as abruptio placentae and amniotic fluid embolism, massive intravascular coagulation can develop. The increased risk of venous thromboembolism in pregnancy is most likely due to the changes induced by pregnancy in the hemostatic system.

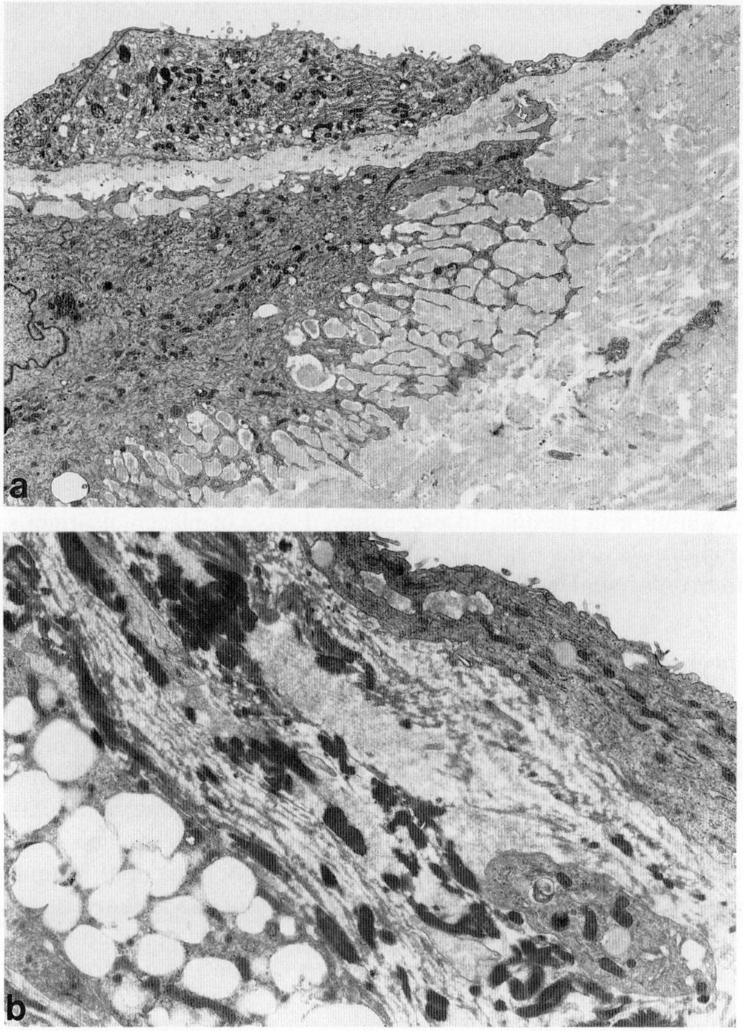

Fig. 2. **a** The spiral artery supplying the placenta: trophoblast cells are present in the wall of the vessel with deposits of fibrin at term in normal pregnancy. **b** In pregnancy complicated by pre-eclampsia and fetal growth retardation extensive fibrin deposition and lipid-laden cells are found

Coagulation and Fibrinolysis in Pregnancy

Normal pregnancy is accompanied by increases in the levels of factors VII, VIII, and X, and especially in plasma fibrinogen. The effect of pregnancy on the coagulation factors in usually evident from the first trimester and by late pregnancy, allowing for blood volume change, the amount of fibrinogen in circulation is almost double that of the non-pregnant state. Plasminogen levels increase during pregnancy and this increase in plasminogen levels during pregnancy occurs step by step with that of fibrinogen, the rise above normal levels in the third trimester being of the order of 50%–60% both with fibrinogen and plasminogen [2]. Reduced plasma fibrinolytic activity in healthy pregnant women was reported by MacFarlane and Biggs [3]. A gradual decrease of fibrinolysis during pregnancy, with the lowest values present in the third trimester, was found by Biezenski and Moore [4]. Several studies on fibrinolytic activity of plasma using clot lysis methods have confirmed fibrinolytic inhibition [1, 5–10].

Over the last five years, considerable advances have been made in our understanding of the process of fibrinolysis, but the complex relationship which exists between plasminogen activators and inhibitors during pregnancy requires further elucidation. The control of plasminogen activator may occur at the level of synthesis and release and also through its interaction with specific plasminogen activator inhibitors (PAIs). Present evidence suggests at least three distinct PAIs: PAI-1, initially called endothelial cell PA-inhibitor or fast acting PA inhibitor; PAI-2, the placental type inhibitor; and the protease nexin which also inhibits plasmin. In normal circumstances, PAI-1 seems to be the most important PA-inhibitor in plasma. In pregnancy, PAI-2 of placental origin seems to have a major role in the control of fibrinolysis during pregnancy, especially within the utero-placental circulation.

The Placental Type Plasminogen Activator Inhibitor, PAI-2

The presence of a urokinase inhibitor in the placenta was first reported by Kawano [11], who purified the inhibitor from placental homogenates. In organ culture experiments, Astedt et al. [12] showed that placental explants released inhibitors which inhibited the activation of plasminogen by urokinase, and inhibited the plasminogen activators released by kidney and fetal vessel explants. Immunohistochemically PAI-2 has been localised to the trophoblastic epithelium [13] (Fig. 3). This is in accord with our earlier observation of the absence of fibrinolytic activity from trophoblastic cells in the spiral arteries supplying the placenta in late pregnancy [4]. PAI-2 occurs in increasing amounts in maternal plasma during pregnancy and the increase is almost linear. At term, levels have been reported to be 100–300 μg/1 with a decrease to non detectable levels within about a week of delivery [14,15]. PAI-2 has a low molecular weight form estimated to be 43/48kDa [16] and a high molecular weight form estimated to be about 70kDa [17]. In maternal plasma, the high molecular weight form of PAI-2 predominates. PAI-2 is also found in amniotic fluid and umbilical cord plasma; the high molecular weight form and low molecular weight form of PAI-2 were found to be of about the same concentration in amniotic fluid but the low molecular weight form predominated in cord blood [18]. The presence of two molecular weight forms of PAI-2 may relate to the control of the placental passage and the distribution of PAI-2 between the maternal and the fetal circulation [17].

Inhibition of Fibrinolytic Activity in Pregnancy

Fibrinolytic activity decreases progressively during pregnancy, even after stimulation of plasminogen activator release by venous occlusion and remains depressed until separation of the placenta, after which it rapidly returns to non-pregnant levels [5,19,20]. In addition to the increase of PAI-2 in plasma during pregnancy, there is also an increase in the fast acting PAI-inhibitor PAI-1 [14,21]. Astedt et al. [22] showed that after removal of PAI-2 from term plasma using a PAI-2 antibody affinity column, most of the total inhibitory capacity of plasma was found to have disappeared.

Together with the increase of PAI-2 antigen during pregnancy, Kruithof et al. [14] found a marked increase of PAI-1 antigen as well as PAI-1 activity and a moderate increase of t-PA and u-PA antigen levels. The PAI-1 levels after the 20th week of pregnancy and at term were three times the non-pregnant levels. The PAI-2 levels at term showed a 25-fold increase from early pregnancy. Despite this substantial increase in PAI-1 and PAI-2 no significant change was found in plasma PA activity in diluted plasma as measured on radioactive fibrin plates. Within 1 h of delivery the level of t-PA antigen doubled and PAI-1 activity and antigen decreased and returned to control values by 3-5 days after delivery. PAI-2 decreased more slowly and remained elevated at 3-5 days after delivery. Kruithof et al [14] question the conclusions that have been drawn from the decrease of fibrinolytic activity in euglobulin precipitates.

Wright et al. [23] confirmed a marked reduction of the fibrinolytic activity of the plasma euglobulin fraction and a parallel reduction in t-PA activity in the second and third trimester with a rapid return to non-pregnant levels post-partum. This pattern was found in both resting and post-venous occlusion samples. PAI-2 antigen increased throughout pregnancy and remained at a high level up to 48 post-partum. Despite the reduction of fibrinolytic activity of the euglobulin fraction and the high level of t-PA inhibition, increased concentration of fibrin degradation products (FDP) and D-dimer was found in the third trimester. Different results on fibrinolytic activity are found depending on the methodology and whether the assay is performed on whole blood, plasma, or euglobulins. Immunological methods which can measure both free and complex antigen also give rise to problems in interpretation. The complex interrelationship of plasminogen activation and inhibition in pregnancy requires further elucidation.

The increased levels of fibrin degradation products which occur in pregnancy [24] are confirmed by the recent findings of elevated levels of x-oligomer [25]. They indicate that the fibrinolytic system remains active in the general circulation and that the inhibition of fibrinolysis is most likely confined to the utero-placental circulation both during pregnancy and for several days in the placental bed following delivery. Trophoblast, the source of PAI-2, is present in the utero-placental vessels (Fig. 2) and is known to persist for some days after delivery. This would have the advantage of perserving fibrin in the utero-placental vessels following delivery and so securing hemostasis in the highly vascular placental site.

Tissue plasminogen activator exists in two forms, the native single chain enzyme and the two chain enzyme which results from proteolytic cleavage by plasmin. The efficiency of the two forms of t-PA in the fibrinolytic process is apparently the same. PAI-1 inhibits both forms of t-PA while PAI-2 acts mainly against the two chain t-PA with only a slight effect on the single chain form.

Astedt et al. [26] have suggested that the different pattern of t-PA inhibition which occurs with PAI-2 is of physiological importance in pregnancy to protect fibrinolytic potential, by leaving the single chain t-PA essentially uninhibited in the presence of the placental inhibitor. PAI-2 will also provide an effective stop to the generation of plasmin once the necessary amount has been formed, since an excess of plasmin cleaves the single chain t-PA to the two chain enzyme which will be removed by the action of PAI-2.

Coagulation and Fibrinolysis and Pre-Eclampsia

A well-known finding in women dying with eclampsia has been widespread fibrin deposition especially affecting the kidney and the liver. In pre-eclampsia associated with fetal growth retardation we have shown an excess of fibrin deposition in the spiral arteries supplying the placenta (Fig. 2) [6,8]. This has raised the possibility that disordered fibrin deposition may be of importance in the pathogenesis of pre-eclampsia. In early studies on fibrinolysis in pre-eclampsia a diminished sensitivity to urokinase-induced fibrinolysis was found [27,28], but most investigators could find no difference between fibrinolytic activity and inhibitory activity between normal pregnancy and pre-eclampsia [29].

More recent investigations in pre-eclampsia using new methodology have been reported by Aznar et al. [30], who found that in severe pre-eclampsia that levels of the fast acting plasminogen activator inhibitor were higher than in normal pregnancy and the levels of Protein C antigen and activity were decreased. The high level of t-PA inhibitor and the reduced protein C in severe pre-eclampsia could be related to reduced fibrinolysis and persistance of microthrombi in the utero-placental circulation. In a further report, Estelles et al. [31] found that in severe pre-eclampsia the levels of PAI-1, both antigenic and functional, were increased and the levels of PAI-2, both antigenic and functional, were decreased in comparison to levels in normal pregnancy. Despite the evidence of a greater level of fibrinolytic inhibition in pre-eclampsia, most studies have shown that the levels of fibrin degradation products are increased [27,31,32]; the levels of fibrinopeptide A and B-beta peptides are also increased [33,18].

In a recent serial study we compared the findings in 28 healthy primigravidae with 15 primigravidae with pre-eclampsia during pregnancy, labor, and following delivery [34]. Plasminogen activator antigen was significantly higher in the pre-eclamptic patients and the higher levels were maintained until 3 days after delivery (Fig. 4). The levels of plasminogen activator inhibitor were lower in pre-eclampsia at 24–28 weeks gestation but not at other stages (Fig. 5). In cord blood plasminogen activator antigen and plasminogen activator inhibitor levels were higher in pre-eclampsia than in normal pregnancy (Fig. 6).

Fig. 3. Inhibition of fibrinolysis (F) at **a** the cytotrophoblast cell (T) in contrast to **b** the endothelial cell (E) in the lining of the spiral artery in pregnancy. **c** Immunological staining with PAI-2 antisera shows the inhibitor localised to the trophoblast of a decidual spiral artery

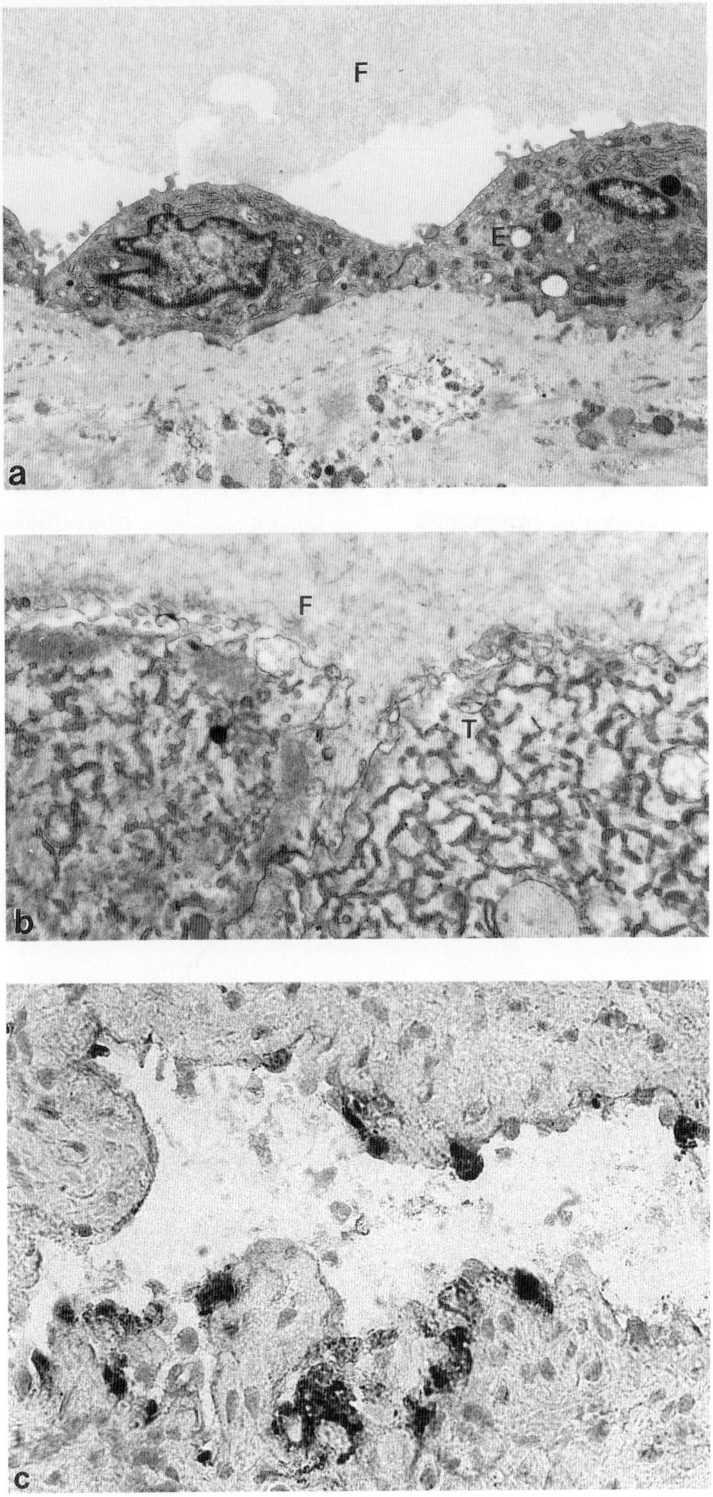
F
E
a
F
T
b
c

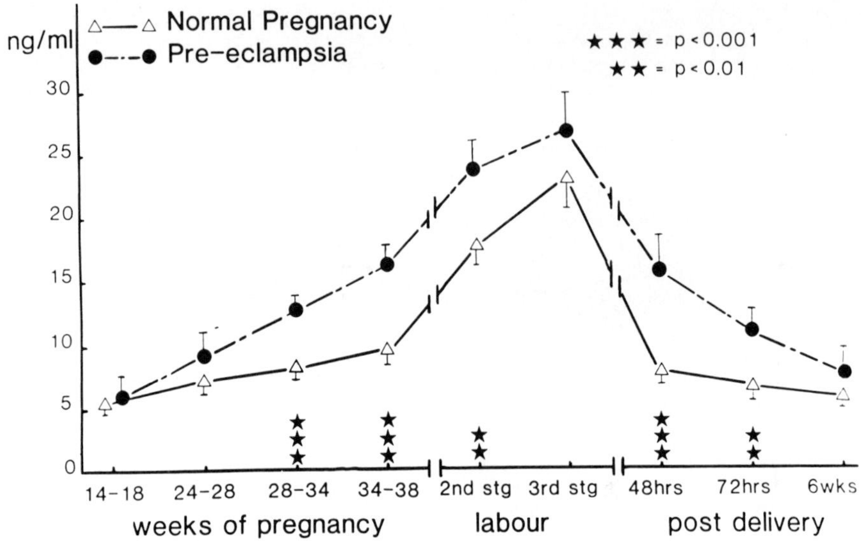

Fig. 4. Plasminogen activator level (antigen) in 28 healthy primigravidae and 15 primigravidae with pre-eclampsia

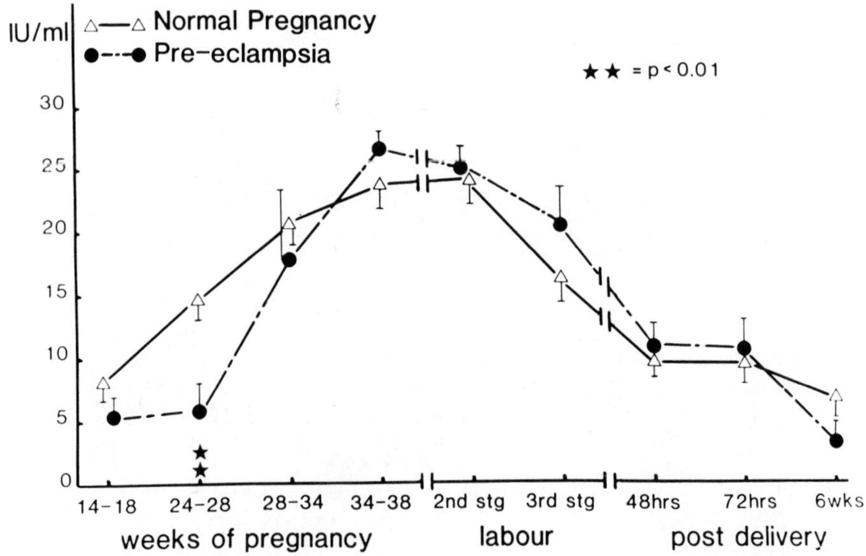

Fig. 5. Plasminogen activator inhibitor levels in 28 healthy primigravidae and 15 primigravidae with pre-eclampsia

Fig. 6a, b. Plasminogen activator antigen **a**, and plasminogen activator inhibitor **b** levels in maternal and cord blood at time of delivery in 28 healthy primigravidae and in 15 primigravidae with pre-eclampsia

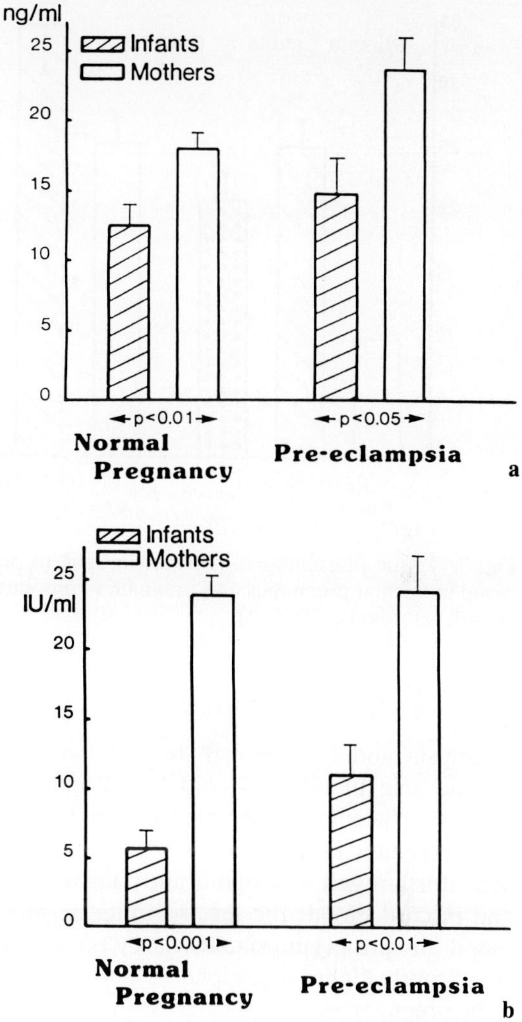

The fibrinolytic system, with its highly complex system of activators and inhibitors, is designed for local action. Studies on the circulating blood provide only a limited perception of events taking place in a specific area of the vascular system. For this reason we have endeavored to study the process in the uterus at the time of delivery.

Utero-Placental Fibrinolysis in Pre-Eclampsia and Fetal Growth Retardation

These studies have been carried out in women requiring delivery by Cesarean section. The findings in normal pregnancy and in pregnancy complicated by pre-

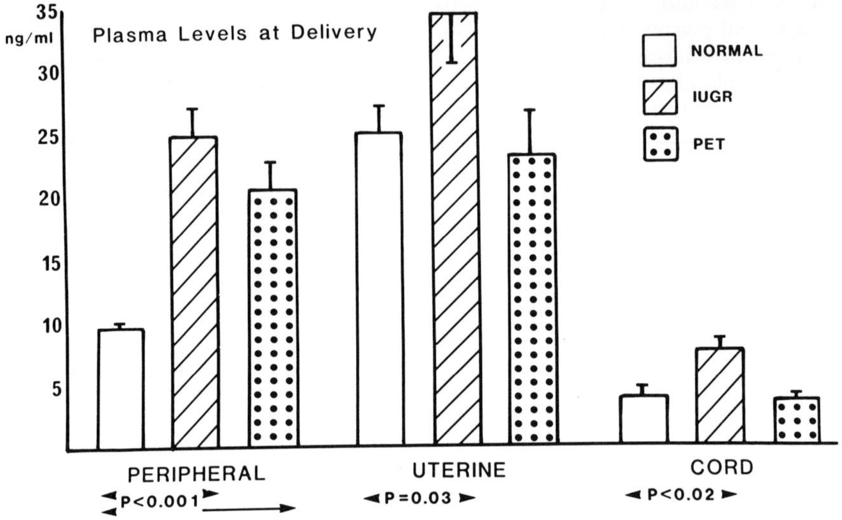

Fig. 7. Tissue plasminogen activator antigen in peripheral uterine vein blood and cord blood in normal pregnancy and pregnancy complicated by pre-eclampsia (PET) and fetal growth retardation (IUGR)

eclampsia and fetal growth retardation were compared in peripheral blood, uterine vein blood, and cord blood taken simultaneously [9]. Tissue extracts from the placenta and the placental bed of the uterus were also studied.

In pregnancies complicated by fetal growth retardation tissue plasminogen activator antigen was significantly higher in peripheral and uterine vein blood and in cord blood; the levels in uterine blood were higher than in peripheral blood. In pre-eclampsia, levels of tissue plasminogen activator antigen were significantly higher in peripheral blood (Fig. 7).

In pregnancies complicated by pre-eclampsia and fetal growth retardation plasminogen activator inhibitor (PAI-1) was higher in both peripheral and uterine vein blood, but the cord levels were similar (Fig. 8).

In pregnancies complicated by pre-eclampsia and fetal growth retardation the placental inhibitor, PAI-2 was found to be much lower in both peripheral and uterine vein blood; within each group the levels of PAI-2 in peripheral and uterine vein blood were similar (Fig. 9).

These findings would suggest that within the utero placental circulation disordered coagulation and fibrinolysis occur in pre-eclampsia and fetal growth retardation. The low levels of PAI-2 may be the result of the impaired placental function in pre-eclampsia and intrauterine fetal growth retardation or they may be due to the greater consumption of the inhibitor associated with the excess of fibrin which is present in the utero placental circulation. The higher level of t-PA antigen and PAI-I in pre-eclampsia and fetal growth retardation may be the result of enhanced fibrinolysis in the circulation which functions counteract the low grade systemic intra vascular coagulation which occurs in pre-eclampsia.

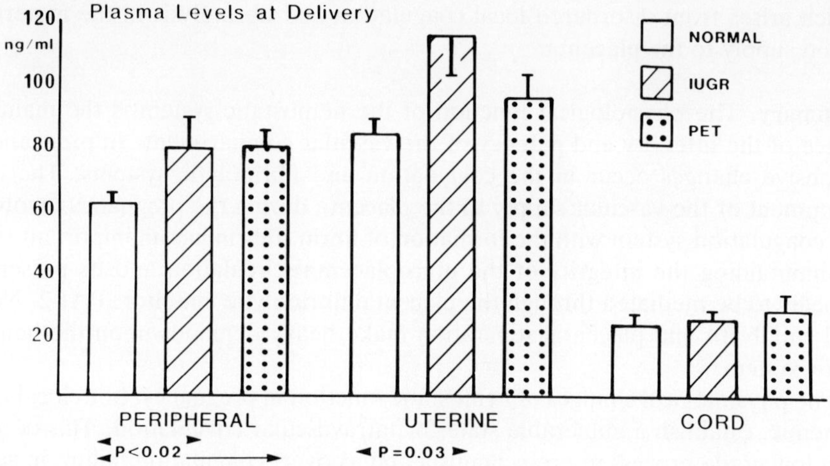

Fig. 8. Plasminogen activator inhibitor (PAI-1) in peripheral uterine vein blood and cord blood in normal pregnancy and pregnancy complicated by pre-eclampsia (PET) and fetal growth retardation (IUGR)

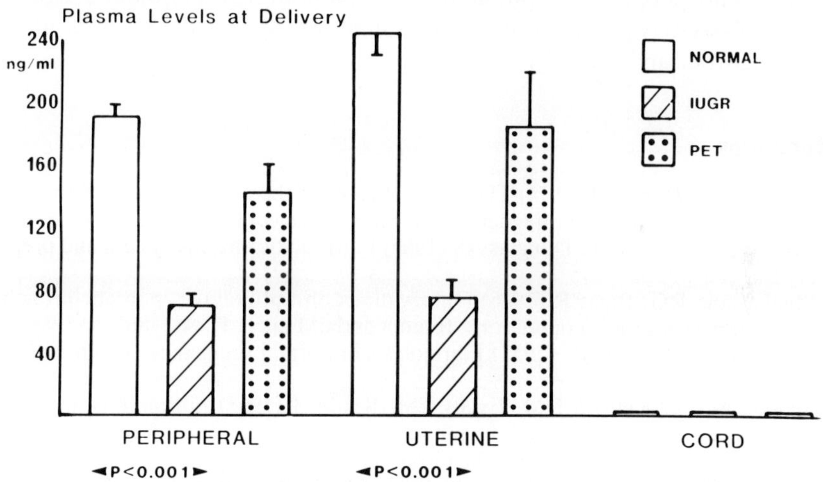

Fig. 9. Placental inhibitor (PAI-2) in peripheral and uterine vein blood in normal pregnancy and pregnancy complicated by pre-eclampsia (PET) and fetal growth retardation (IUGR)

Conclusion

Fibrin is a matrix necessary to protect the integrity of the maternal and fetal circulations at the interface of the placenta. The related disorders of bleeding and thrombosis at the placental site are responsible for a substantial proportion of fetal mortality and morbidity. Further research in this area may open up new possibilities for protecting the fetus in utero from the impaired placental function which arises from disordered local coagulation and fibrinolysis in the maternal blood supply to the placenta.

Summary. The physiological function of the hemostatic system is the maintenance of the integrity and patency of the vascular compartment. In pregnancy, extensive changes occur in the coagulation and fibrinolytic systems. The development of the vascular supply to the placenta during the pregnancy involves the coagulation system with the formation of fibrin. Fibrin has an important role in maintaining the integrity of the uteroplacental circulation and its presence appears to be mediated through the placental fibrinolytic inhibitor, PAI-2. Normal childbirth and placental separation make heavy demands upon the hemostatic system.

The physiological changes of hemostatic function in pregnancy, both local and systemic, establish a vulnerable state for intravascular coagulation. This occurs as a low grade process in pre-eclampsia and as overt coagulation failure in such complications as abruptio placentae and amniotic fluid embolism where massive intravascular coagulation can develop. Impaired placental function, and thereby impaired fetal health and growth, usually involves thrombotic occlusion of the vascular supply to the placenta.

Further knowledge of the physiology and pathology of perinatal coagulation and fibrinolysis may provide rational treatment for the vascular hazards affecting both the mother and the baby.

References

1. Sheppard B, Bonnar J (1974) The ultrastructure of the arterial supply of the human placenta in early and late pregnancy. J Obstet Gynaecol Br Cwlth 81: 497–511
2. Bonnar J, McNicol GP, Douglas AS (1969) Fibrinolytic enzyme system and pregnancy. Br Med J 3: 387–395
3. MacFarlane RG, Biggs R (1946) Observations on fibrinolysis; spontaneous activity associated with surgical operations, trauma and c. Lancet II: 862–864
4. Biezenski JJ, Moore HC (1958) Fibrinolysis in normal pregnancy. J Clin Pathol 11: 306–310
5. Shaper AG, Macintosh DM, Evans CM, Kyope J (1965) Fibrinolysis and plasminogen levels in pregnancy and the puerperium. Lancet II: 706–708
6. Sheppard BL, Bonnar J (1976) The ultrastructure of the arterial supply of the human placenta in pregnancy complicated by fetal growth retardation. Br J Obstet Gynaecol 83: 948–959
7. Sheppard BL, Bonnar J (1978) Fibrinolysis in decidual spiral arteries in late pregnancy. Thromb Haemost 39: 751–758
8. Sheppard BL, Bonnar J (1981) An ultrastructural study of utero-placental spiral arteries in hypertensive and normotensive pregnancy and fetal growth retardation. Br J Obstet Gynaecol 88: 695–705
9. Sheppard BL, Boyle C, Gleeson N, Jordan M, Daly L, Bonnar J (1990) Plasminogen activator inhibitors of the placenta and placental bed at delivery in normotensive and hypertensive pregnancy. Placental communications. Biochem Morphol Cell Aspects 199: 151–159
10. Stirling Y, Woolf, L, North WRS, Seghatchian MJ, Meade TW (1984) Haemostasis in normal pregnancy. Thromb Haemost 52: 176–182
11. Kawano T, Morimoto K, Uemura Y (1968) Urokinase inhibitor in human placenta. Nature 217: 253–254

12. Astedt B, Pandolphi M, Nilsson IM (1972) Inhibitory effect of placenta on plasminogen activation in human organ culture. Proc Soc Exp Biol Med 139: 1421–1424
13. Astedt B, Hagerstrom I, Lecander I (1986) Cellular localisation in placenta of placental type plasminogen activator inhibitor. Thromb Haemost 56: 63–65
14. Kruithof EKO, Tran-Thang C, Gudinchet A, Hauert J, Nicoloso G, Genton C, Welti H, Bachmann F (1987) Fibrinolysis in pregnancy: A study of plasminogen activator inhibitors. Blood 69: 460–466
15. Lecander I, Astedt B (1986) Isolation of a new specific plasminogen activator inhibitor from pregnancy plasma. Br J Haematol 62: 221–228
16. Astedt B, Lecander I, Brondin T, Lundblad A, Low K (1985) Purification of a specific placental plasminogen activator by monoclonal antibody and its complex formation with plasminogen activator. Thromb Haemost 53: 122–125
17. Astedt B, Lecander I, Ny T (1987) Review The placental type plasminogen activator inhibitor, PAI-2. Fibrinolysis 1: 203–208
18. Douglas JT, Shah M, Lowe GDO, Belch JJF, Forbes CD, Prentice CRM (1982) Plasma fibrinopeptide A and beta-thromboglobulin in pre-eclampsia and pregnancy hypertension. Thromb Haemost 47: 54–55
19. Astedt B (1972) On fibrinolysis in pregnancy, labour, puerperium, and during treatment with sex hormones. Acta Obstet Gynecol Scand 51: (Suppl. 8): 1–24
20. Bonnar J, McNicol GP, Douglas AS (1970) Coagulation and fibrinolytic mechanisms during and after normal childbirth. Br Med J 2: 200–203
21. Wiman B, Csemiczky, Marsk L, Robbe H (1984) The fast inhibitor of tissue plasminogen activator in plasma during pregnancy. Thromb Haemost 52: 124–126
22. Astedt B, Lecander I, Nilsson IM (1986) Depression of PA activity during pregnancy by the placenta inhibitor fibrinolysis. Proceedings of the eighth international congress on fibrinolysis, p. 185
23. Wright JG, Cooper P, Astedt B, Lecander I, Wilde JT, Preston FE, Greaves M (1988) Fibrinolysis during normal human pregnancy: complex inter-relationships between plasma levels of tissue plasminogen activator and inhibitors and the euglobulin clot lysis time. Br J Haematol 69: 253–258
24. Fletcher AP, Alkjaersig NK, Burstein R (1979) The influence of pregnancy upon blood coagulation and plasma fibrinolytic enzyme function. Am J Obstet Gynecol. 134: 743–751
25. Gaffney PJ, Creighton LJ, Callus M, Thorpe R (1988) Monoclonal antibodies to cross-linked fibrin degradation products (XL-FDP) II. Evaluation in a variety of clinical conditions. Br J Haematol 68: 91–96
26. Astedt B, Bladh B, Christensen U, Lecander I (1985) Different inhibition of one and two chain tissue plasminogen activator by a placental inhibitor studied with two tripeptide-p-nitroanilide substrates. Scand J Clin Lab Invest 45: 429–435
27. Bonnar J, McNicol GP, Douglas AS (1971) Coagulation and fibrinolytic systems in pre-eclampsia and eclampsia. Br Med J II: 12–16
28. Howie PW, Prentice CRM, McNicol GP (1971) Coagulation, fibrinolysis and platental function in pre-eclampsia, essential hypertension, and placental insufficiency. J Obstet Gynaecol Br Cwlth 78: 992–1003
29. Gow L, Campbell DM, Ogston D (1984) The fibrinolytic system in pre-eclampsia. J Clin Pathol 37: 56–58
30. Aznar J, Gilabert J, Estelles A, Espana F (1986) Finbrinolytic activity and Protein C in pre-eclampsia. Thromb Haemost 55: 314–317
31. Estelles A, Gilabert J, Aznar J, Scheef RR (1988) Plasminogen activator inhibitors type 1 and type 2 (PAI-1 and PAI-2) in normal pregnancy and in patients with severe pre-eclampsia. Fibrinolysis 2: 162
32. Giles C (1982) Intravascular coagulation in gestational hypertension and pre-eclampsia: the value of haematological screening tests. Clin Lab Haematol 4: 351–358
33. Borok Z, Weitz J, Owen J, Auerbach M, Nossel HL (1984) Fibrinogen proteolysis and platelet alpha-granule release in pre-eclampsia/eclampsia. Blood 63: 525–531
34. Daly L, Bonnar J (1989) Fibrinolytic activation and inhibition in normal pregnancy and in pre-eclampsia. To be published

1.10 The Relationship Between the Onset of Labor Mechanisms and the Blood Coagulation System

SHIGENORI SUZUKI[1], HITOMI MATSUDA[1], and WATARU SAKAMOTO[2]

Introduction

The mechanisms for the onset of labor are still unknown despite much research [1,2]. The various changes occurring during pregnancy and before delivery are sometimes considered physiological and sometimes pathological.

In the present paper we have attempted to conduct an investigation into the physiological and pathological aspects of the onset of labor in pregnant women as they may relate to disseminated intravascular coagulation (DIC). The kallikreinkinin system is directly related to the contraction of smooth muscles, dilation of blood vessels, blood coagulation, and to fibrinolytic systems.

Plasma kallikrein produces bradykinin from high molecular weight kininogen; this dilates blood vessels and causes smooth muscles to contract. Factor XII of the blood coagulation system activates the kallikrein-kinin system of the plasma; this includes the reactions depicted in Fig. 1. Accordingly, these reactions may cause uterine contractions and bring about the onset of labor.

Materials and Methods

The investigations were carried out on three systems: the kallikrein-kinin system, coagulation system, and the fibrinolytic system. We studied 51 patients with normal deliveries, seven patients with premature separation of the placenta, and five patients with missed abortion.

To determine kininogen levels in the kallikrein-kinin system we used Diniz's method (Fig. 2) and to quantify prekallikrein we applied chromesubstance S-

[1]College of Medical Technology, Hokkaido University, Kita 12-jo, Nishi 5-chome, Kita-ku, Sapporo 060, Japan
[2]Department of Biochemistry, School of Dental Medicine, Hokkaido University, Kita 14-jo, Nishi 7-chome, Kita-ku, Sapporo 060, Japan

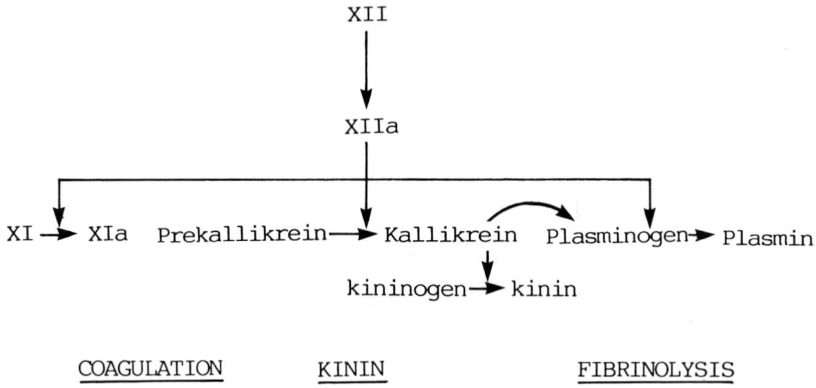

Fig. 1. Reactions by factor XII in the activation of the kallikrein-kinin system

2302. The coagulation system was observed by testing the kinetic movement of blood coagulation factors. During these investigations the levels of soluble fibrin monomer complex (SFMC) and fibrinopeptide A (FPA) were determined in order to evaluate the state of hypercoagulability.

Platelet aggregation caused by adenosine diphosphate (ADP) and its relation to the movement of fibrin/fibrinogen degradation product (FDP) was checked by aggregation-meter and the FDPL-test. For the fibrinolytic system, euglobulinolysis time was automatically monitored by the euglobulinolysis time recorder.

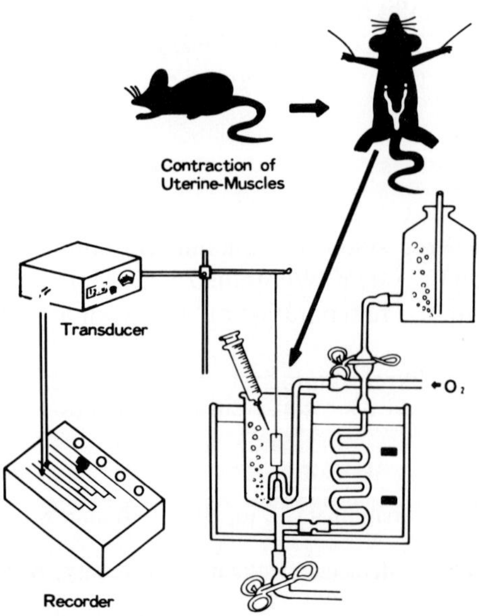

Fig. 2. Varying amounts of bradykinin were injected into rat uterine muscles and the resulting contractions were measured

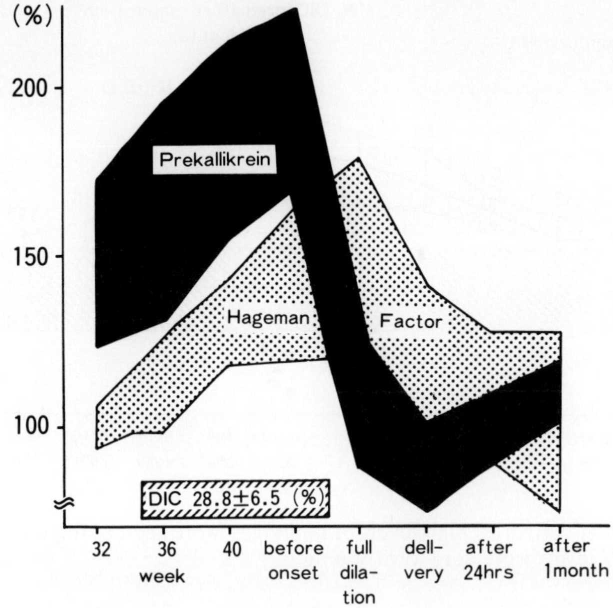

Fig. 3. Among these changes the sharp decrease in prekallikrein was the most significant observed

Results

The data for studies of the kallikrein-kinin system are shown in Figs. 3 and 4 and in Tables 1 and 2. In the latter half of pregnancy the levels of prekallikrein and kininogen increased compared to those in the non-pregnant state, but from the onset of labor until delivery, a significant decrease occurred. Prekallikrein fell from 196%–90.6%. In contrast, at the onset of labor, coagulation factor XII (Hageman factor) showed an increase of exactly the same order as the decrease in prekallikrein levels (Fig. 3). At the end of forty weeks, the values of factor XII were 131.4 ± 11.6%; these values reached 150.1 ± 30.6% at the time of full dilation of the cervix. During pregnancy the levels of kininogen increased, but they decreased after the onset of labor, especially in patients with DIC (FIg. 4).

Fluctuations in fibrinogen and other factors were also noted. At the end of pregnancy, the so-called vitamin K dependent factors, factors II, VII, IX, and X showed a 1.2 to 1.8-fold rise over the non-pregnant period (Table 3, Fig. 5). Factor V increased 1.5-fold, while factor VIII rose almost three-fold. Fibrinogen showed approximately a two-fold increase to 416 ± 51 mg/dl in the later period of pregnancy as compared to the non-pregnant state. In contrast to the pregnancy-induced increase in serum levels of these various coagulation factors, the concentration of factor XIII did not rise.

Soluble fibrin monomer complex and FPA, which directly represent enhancement of coagulation, arise from fibrinogen. Prior to the onset of labor, fibri-

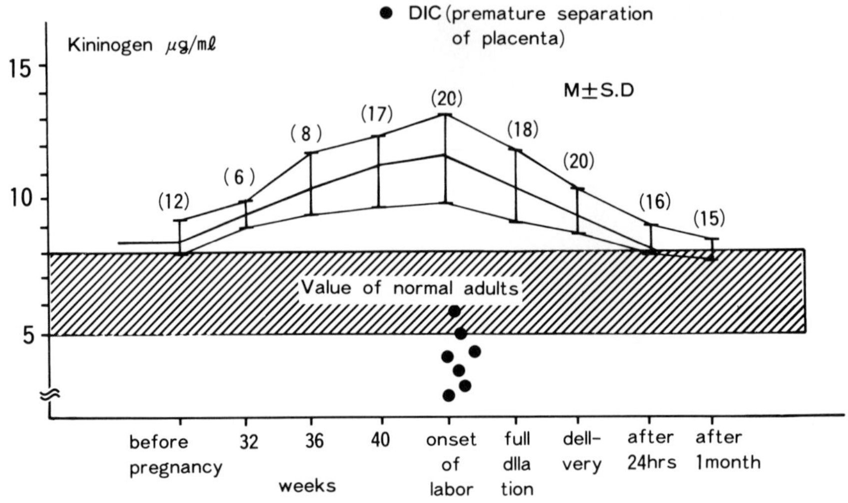

Fig. 4. In normal deliveries high levels of kininogen were seen at the onset of labor, but in cases of DIC levels were very low (<6 μg/ml)

Table 1. Changes of prekallikrein and hageman factor during pregnancy labor, and delivery

Period Factor	Cases	Hageman factor	Prekallikrein
24 W	6	100 ± 6.3	148.6 ± 25.6
32 W	8	114 ± 12.1	163.8 ± 32.4
36 W	17	131 ± 11.6	184.6 ± 28.4
Before onset	20	146 ± 18.5	196.8 ± 33.6
Full dilation	18	150 ± 30.6	100.4 ± 16.5
Delivery	20	123 ± 18.6	90.6 ± 16.8
After 24 hrs	16	110 ± 18.4	100.2 ± 15.8
After 1 month	15	100 ± 22.6	106.3 ± 16.5

Table 2. Changes of Kininogen during pregnancy, labor, and delivery

Period	Cases	Kininogen
Before pregnancy	12	8.4 ± 1.8
24 W	6	9.3 ± 0.8
32 W	8	10.1 ± 1.5
36 W	17	11.6 ± 1.8
Onset of labor	20	12.8 ± 2.0
Full dilation of cervix	18	19.3 ± 1.6
Delivery	20	8.9 ± 1.3
After 24 hrs	16	8.5 ± 0.6
After 1 month	15	7.2 ± 1.0

Table 3. Correlation of various blood coagulating factors between the late stage of pregnancy and the non-pregnant state

	Non-pregnant	Late stage of pregnancy
Fibrinogen (mg/dl)	251 ± 28	416 ± 51 ↑
Factor II (%)	91.5 ± 10.6	185 ± 24.5 ↑
Factor V (%)	89.6 ± 21.1	151 ± 28.6 ↑
Factor VII (%)	92.8 ± 8.6	176 ± 30.3 ↑
Factor VIII (%)	96.4 ± 5.4	298 ± 78.6 ↑
Factor IX (%)	97.6 ± 3.8	186 ± 39.6 ↑
Factor X (%)	95.1 ± 4.6	141 ± 23.6 ↑
Factor XI (%)	—	169 ± 113.1 ↑
Factor XII (%)	—	241 ± 101.4 ↑
Factor XIII (%)	94.6 ± 4.8	71.7 ± 5.8 ↓

Table 4. Changes of fibrinogen, SFMC fibrinopeptide A and antithrombin III before and after onset of labor $n = 48$; mean ± S.D.

	Before onset of labor	After onset of labor	
Fibrinogen (mg/dl)	368.5 ± 45.0	412.0 ± 38.5	
SFMC (%)	3.9 ± 1.1	5.0 ± 0.8	$P < 0.05$
Fibrinopeptide A (ng/ml)	12.0 ± 3.6	18.6 ± 2.5	$P < 0.05$
Antithrombin III (mg/dl)	33.0 ± 4.3	36.0 ± 7.6	

nogen serum levels increased, but this difference was not statistically significant (Table 4). However, significant increases in SFMC, from 3.9 ± 1.1% to 5.0 ± 0.8%, were seen. Increases in FPA, from 12.2 ± 3.6 ng/ml to 18.6 ± 2.5 ng/ml, were also seen while FPA in missed abortion showed remarkably low values (Table 5).

In patients at term platelet aggregation by ADP was 62.0 ± 4.6% (normal 35%–50%); this decreased to 44.0 ± 7.0% with the onset of labor. At the same time, a slight increase of FDP was seen. While FDP increased, platelet aggregation decreased, which seems to suggest an inhibiting effect by FDP on the capacity for platelet aggregation (Fig. 6, Table 6). Concerning fibrinolysis, the euglobulinolysis time was prolonged during pregnancy, being 480.3 ± 26.4 min at the end of pregnancy. However, this time decreased significantly to 356.6 ± 54.3 min at the onset of labor. Plasminogen (profibrinolysin) seemed to be activated by kallikrein at the beginning of labor (Fig. 7).

Discussion

The majority of blood coagulation factors are produced by the liver and they increase as gestation advances. Whether this is indeed a true increase or whether the increase is due to changes in the factor turnover rate is still unknown. In addition, during pregnancy, as well as in a state of hyperlipemia, the total cholesterol, serum phospholipids and serum triglycerides show high values. It is

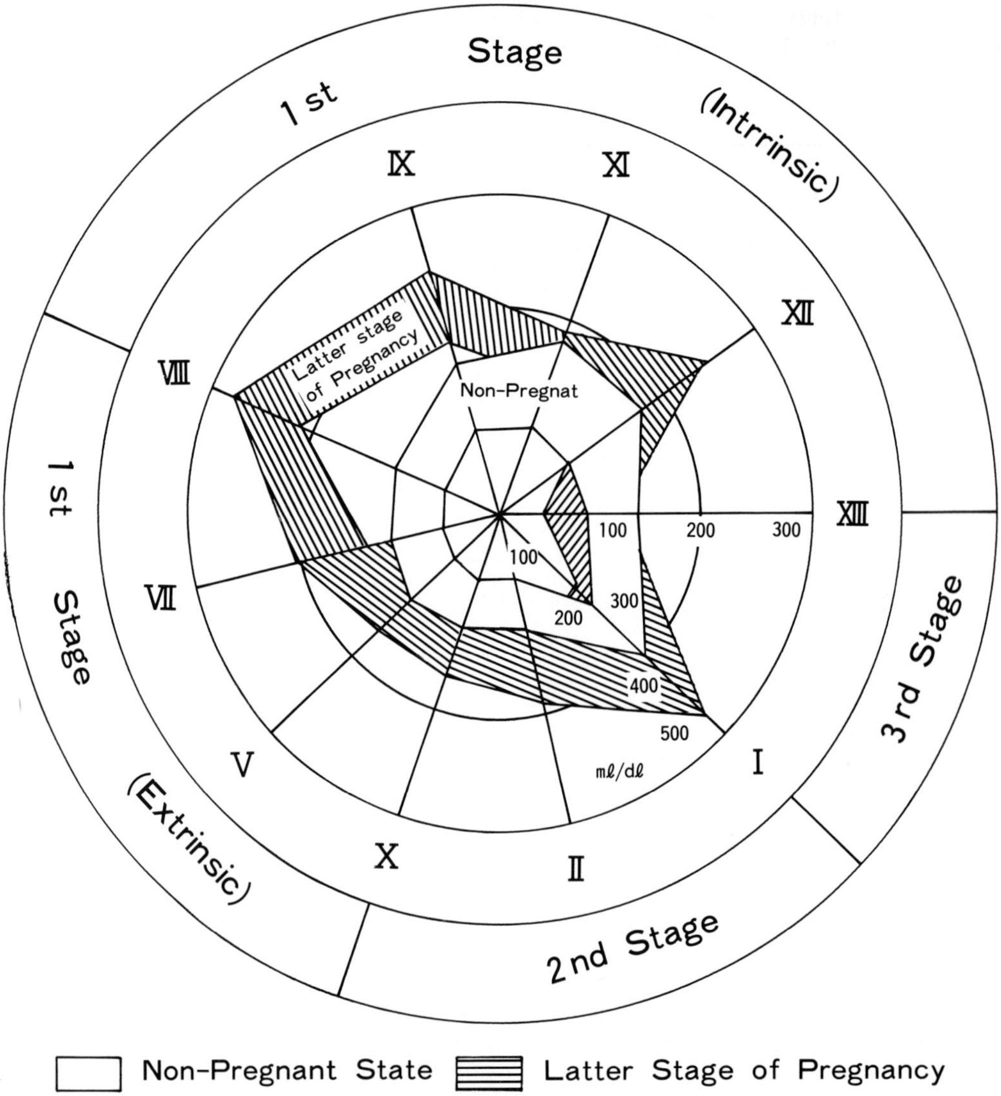

Fig. 5. In the later stage of pregnancy the level of most blood coagulation factors increases. Factor XIII is the exception and its level falls

Table 5. Changes of fibrinopeptide A in missed abortion

	Fibrinogen (mg/dl)	Fibrinopeptide A (ng/ml)
Pregnancy 15–20 wk	260.8 ± 31.6	15.1 ± 4.1
Missed abortion	320.6 ± 28.0	3.6 ± 1.4

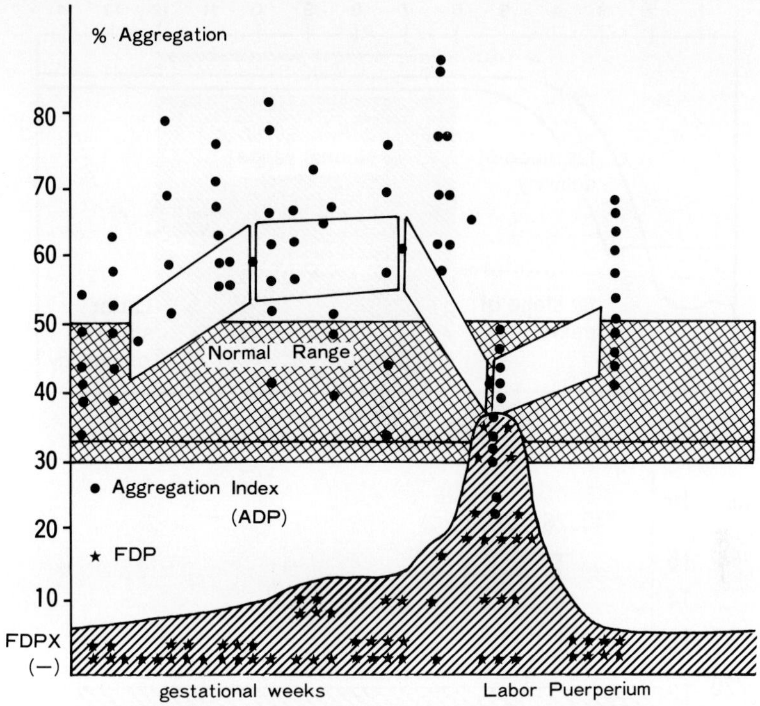

Fig. 6. The relationship between FDP and platelet-aggregation (ADP) during pregnancy and labor. During pregnancy there is an increase in the Aggregation Index but after the onset of labor this falls to its lowest point, probably due to the inhibiting effect of FDP

Table 6. Changes of platelet aggregation during pregnancy

Gestational weeks	12 16 20	24 28 32	36	40	
Values of platelet aggregation	48.6 ± 3.69	58.7 ± 53.80	60.90 ± 3.00	38.40 ± 1.21	47.60 ± 2.32
Percentage of dis-aggregation	17.6%	6.8%	2.4%	3.8%	

thought that these changes are brought about by estrogens and progesterone, which are secreted in increasing amounts by the placenta.

The definition of the term hypercoagulability is not clear. In any case, in the latter stages of pregnancy, many coagulation factors are high. However, it is noteworthy that only factor XIII does not increase; rather it decreases. The decrease in factor XIII may be the result of consumption or may be an effect of dilution (increase in plasma volume) or of another unknown mechanism; this remains to be investigated. It seems that factor XIII shows a particular change which does not depend on the alterations of the hormonal environment associated with pregnancy or with the state of hyperlipemia [3]. However, from the

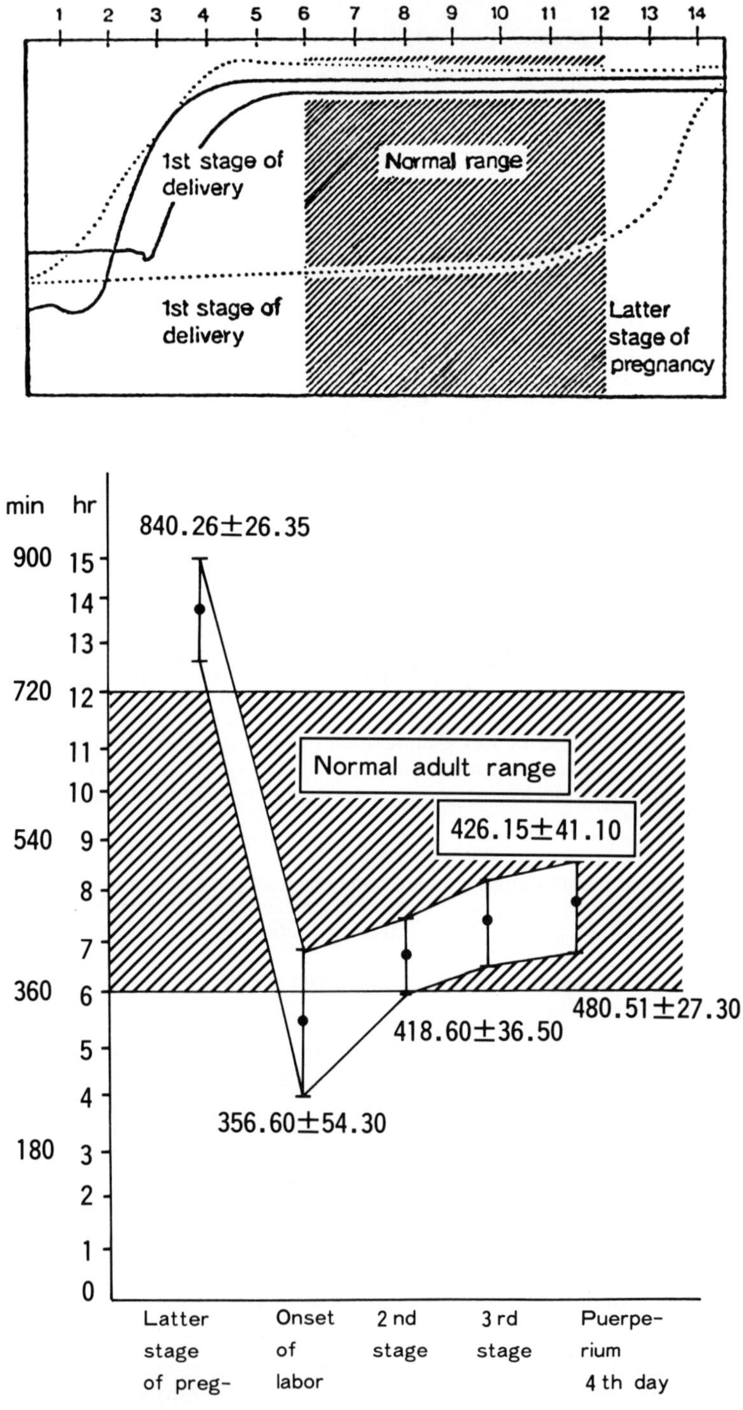

Fig. 7. During pregnancy prolongation of euglobulinlysis time was observed. However, with the onset of labor, this was significantly shortened

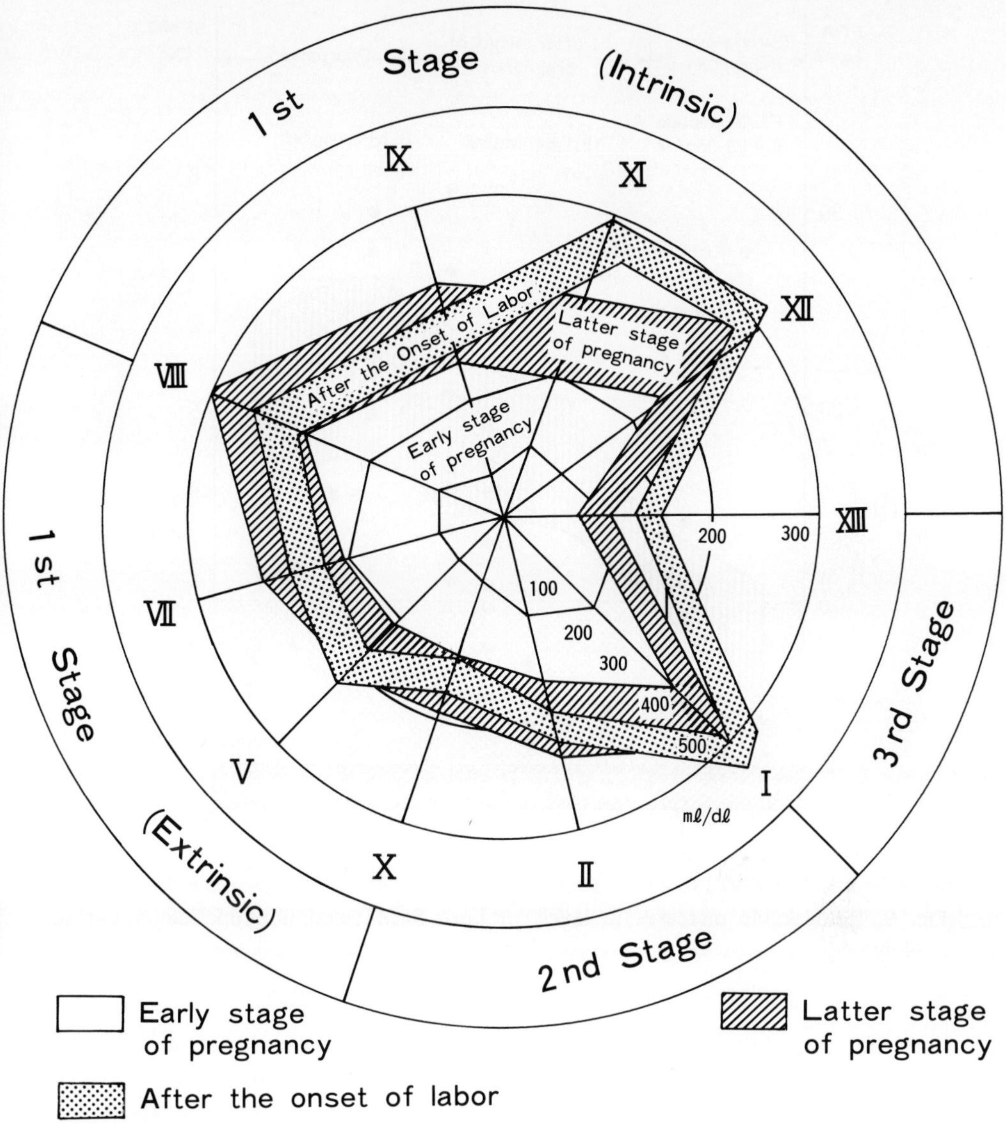

Fig. 8. Further important changes in the blood coagulation factors. Factor XIII, having decreased in the later stage of pregnancy, increases after the onset of labor due to its release from the placenta where it is formed

onset of labor until the time of delivery, factor XIII increases; therefore it might be concluded that factor XIII is formed in the placenta and is released into the bloodstream (Fig. 8). Increasing serum levels of fibrinogen as well as of SFMC could be significant in the onset of labor (Fig. 9). Even though fibrinogen levels did not show significant differences before and immediately after the onset of labor (Table 3), it is known that the accelerated erythrocyte sedimentation rate (ESR) depends mainly on an increase in fibrinogen levels. When the ESR was

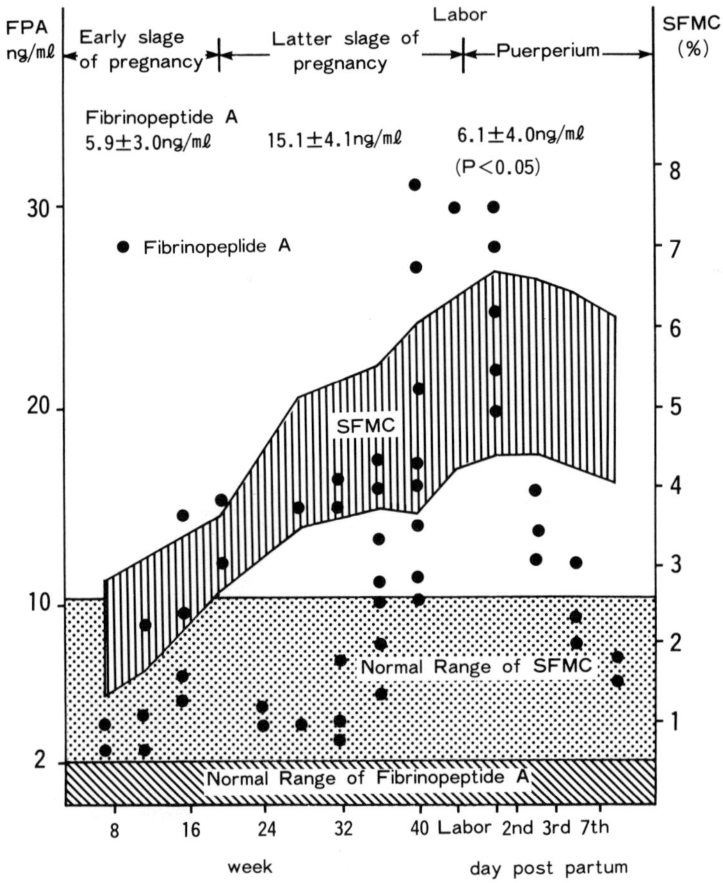

Fig. 9. Remarkable increases in levels of both SFMC and fibrinopetide A during pregnancy

determined on admission, 80% of multiparas with values over 50 mm/h delivered within 10 h, indicating that the increase of serum fibrinogen is positively associated with duration of labor and delivery (Fig. 10).

Figure 11 shows the interrelationship of the three blood clotting systems operative at the onset of labor, during labor, and during delivery. Within the coagulation system increases in fibrinogen and factor XIII were observed. Most pronounced were the changes in the Kallikrein-kinin system, which led to decreases in prekallikrein and kininogen (Fig. 11). It is thought that prekallikrein is consumed for production of bradykinin, which in turn stimulates uterine contractility. Also, the increased activity of factor XII may bring about conversion of prekallikrein to kallikrein and thereby lower serum prekallikrein levels. Plasmin is formed because of the interaction of kallikrein with plasminogen; this coincides with placental separation and FDP appears in the circulation (Fig. 11). Both bradykinin and prostaglandins act on the uterine smooth musculature and contractions may occur gradually leading to the onset of labor.

Fig. 10. Correlation between ESR and duration of normal delivery

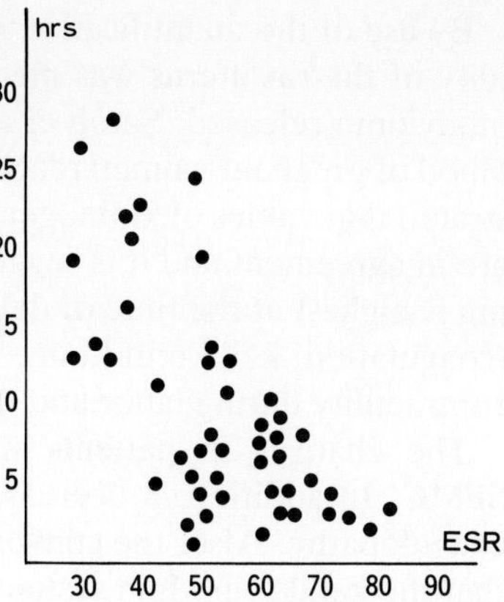

Fig. 11. Interrelationship of the three blood clotting systems operative at the onset of labor, during labor, and during delivery

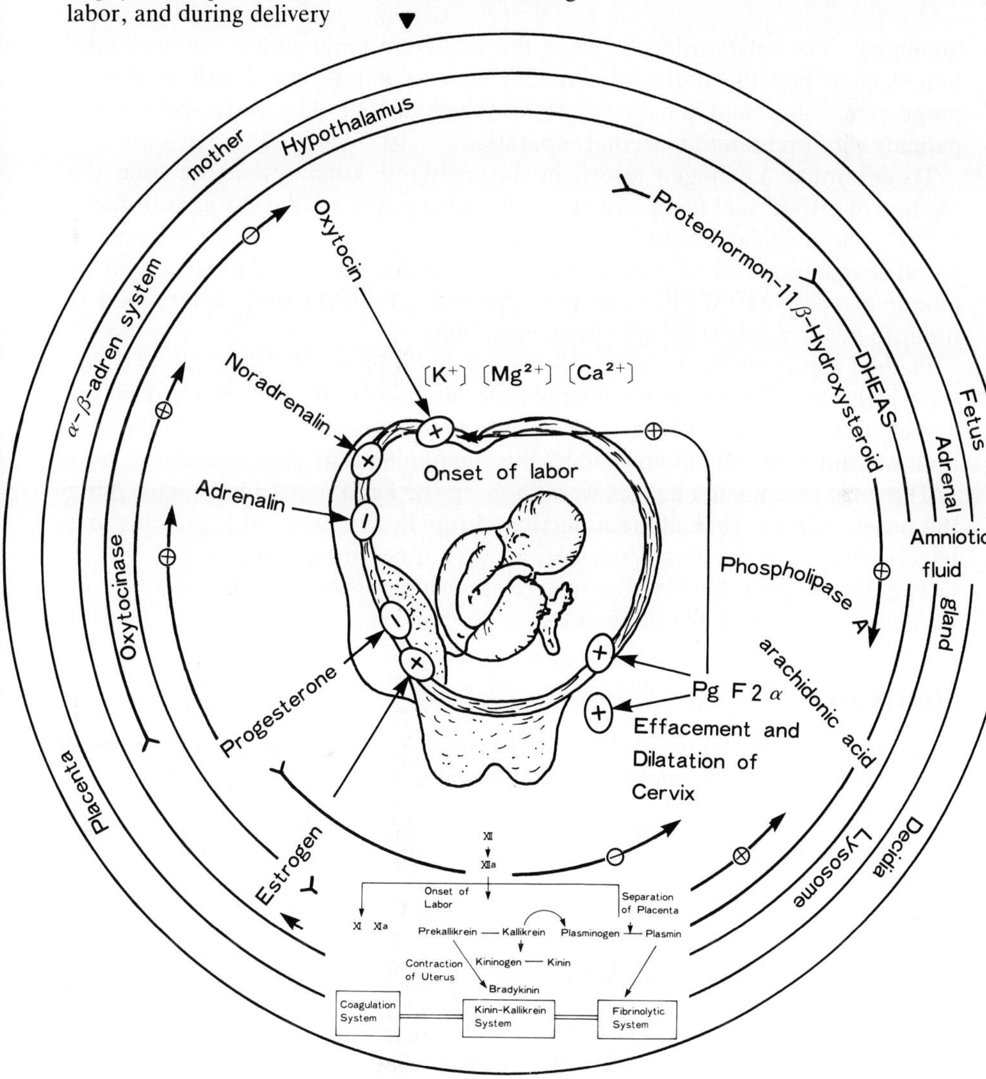

By use of the quantification method for kininogen (Diniz's method), contractility of the rat uterus was measured, allowing quantification of the amount of bradykinin released. Satoh et al. [4] reported that the amount of $PGF_2\alpha$ in the blood of pregnant women reached a peak at the time of delivery, and we demonstrated that values of kininogen are lowest at the time of delivery. These findings are in agreement and it is suggested that the sensitivity of kininogen to bradykinin is highest at the time of delivery. It seems, therefore, that the three systems (coagulation; kallikrein-kinin; fibrinolysis) are closely related and affect uterine contractility during labor and immediately post partum.

The changes in patients with DIC include rapid increases in FPA and SFMC. In addition, a decrease in the levels of the Hageman factor facilitates coagulopathy. Also, the conversion of plasminogen to plasmin strongly suggests that the kallikrein-kinin system influences DIC.

Summary. The relationship between the kallikrein-kinin system, the coagulation system, and the fibrinolytic system was evaluated on 58 patients during pregnancy, labor and puerperium. Also included in this study were seven patients with premature placental separation.

To determine kininogen levels, in the kallikrein-kinin system we used the method of DINIZ and to quantify prekallikrein we applied the chromesubstance S-2302. The coagulation system was observed by testing the kinetic movement of blood coagulation factors. Durng these investigations the levels of soluble fibrin monomer complex (SFMC) and fibrinopeptide A (FPA) were determined in order to evaluate the state of hypercoagulability.

Platelet aggregation, caused by adenosine diphosphate (ADP), relating to the movement of fibrin/fibrinogen degradation product (FDP) was checked by the aggregation-meter and FDPL-test. For the fibrinolytic system, euglobulinolysis time was automatically monitored by the euglobulinolysis time recorder.

The most prominent changes were those in the kallikrein-kinin system. After the onset of labor, prekallikrein decreased rapidly (196.8%–90.6%). This may trigger changes in the blood coagulation and fibrinolytic system.

The three systems have a close interrelationship possibly affecting uterine contractility during labor and delivery.

References

1. Keirse, MJNC (1978) Biosynthesis and metabolism of prostaglandins in the pregnant human uterus. In: Advances in prostaglandins and thromboxane research: vol 4, Raven, New York p 87
2. Huszar G, Roberts JM (1982) Biochemistry and pharmacology of the myometrium and labor: Regulation at the cellular and molecular levels. Amer J Obstet Gyencol 142: 225
3. Suzuki S (1977) Mode of influence of factor XIII on blood coagulation and fibrinolytic system in the perinatal period. Acta Obstet Gynaecol Jap., 29 (No. 12): 1762
4. Satoh K, Yasumizu T, Fukuoka H, Kinoshita K, Kaneko Y, Tsuchiya M, Sakamoto S (1979) Prostaglandin $F_2\alpha$ metabolite levels in plasma, amniotic fluid, and urine during pregnancy and labor. Amer J Obstet Gynecol 133: 886

1.11 Perinatal Problems of Thrombosis and Haemostasis

BIRGER ÅSTEDT[1]

Prevention and Treatment of Deep Vein Thrombosis in Pregnancy

Prevention and treatment of deep vein thrombosis during pregnancy presents special problems. The benefit of treatment for the original condition must be weighed against the subsequent risk of placental or fetal haemorrhage. Owing to the high risk of recurrence, prophylactic treatment is required throughout pregnancy, during delivery, and in the puerperium. At an early stage of pregnancy, the risk ot teratogenetic effects needs also to be taken into consideration.

Treatment of Deep Vein Thrombosis in Pregnancy

Diagnosis

Since thrombosis during pregnancy is a serious condition and treatment often onerous for the patient, phlebographic verification of diagnosis is essential, even where the thrombosis is clinically manifest. Usually, pelvigraphy to check the upper extent of the thrombosis may be dispensed with.

Treatment

Thrombolysis occurs when the fibrinolytic system is activated. Anticoagulant therapy with heparin inhibits the continued formation of fibrin clots and consequent extension of the thrombus. It does not, however, diminish established thrombi, which must be dealt with by the body's own fibrinolytic defences

A different principle is involved in thrombolytic treatment with streptokinase, urokinase, or the recently isolated and purified tissue and vascular plasminogen activator (t-PA). They are all plasminogen activators: they convert the pro-

[1]Department of Obstetrics and Gynecology, University Hospital, S-221 85 LUND, Sweden

enzyme, plasminogen, to the active enzyme, plasmin. Through this activation of the fibrinolytic system, which is rapid, a newly formed thrombus is soon lysed. One of the advantages of thrombolytic treatment is that venous valve function remains unimpaired [1]. Owing to the risk of hemorrhagic complications, however, thrombolytic treatment during pregnancy has won limited acceptance abroad, and is only practiced in exceptional cases here in Sweden.

Recently, however we successfully treated an acute pulmonary embolism in a pregnant woman. The patient, admitted to hospital for toxicosis, suddenly showed signs of acute pulmonary embolism which was verified by scintigram. Lung function was reduced by 75%, and since her condition was critical, to prevent permanent lung damage she was given thrombolytic treatment with streptokinase. After 2 days of treatment without hemorrhagic complications and with dramatic improvement in her clinical condition, she went into labour and a healthy child was delivered vaginally. During the actual delivery, the intravenous streptokinase infusion was temporarily suspended. The resumption of treatment resulted in massive haemorrhaging from the uterus, and treatment was switched to heparin. Subsequent lung function has been satisfactory, however, suggesting that in this respect the 2-day thrombolytic treatment was beneficial.

The value of heparin treatment in the acute phase has thus been established. The great advantage with heparin is that it does not traverse the placental membrane [2]. This is valid also for the new low molecular weight heparin preparations [3,4]. For a uniform effect, heparin is given by intravenous infusion regulated by a drip gauge. The older technique of giving heparin in intermittent intravenous boluses may be considered obsolete. After an initial dose of 100 IU/kg body weight, heparin is given intravenously by electronic infusion pump, beginning at a daily rate of 600 IU/kg body weight. Infusion should be continued for at least 5 days, the rate being adjusted daily to maintain an activated partial thromboplastin time (APTT) of about twice the control value.

Brief mention should also be made of surgical therapy, which is currently being evaluated by the vascular surgery team at the Department of Surgery, Lund University.

Once diagnosis has been established and the full extent of the thrombosis determined, an incision is made in the femoral vein just over the junction of the saphenous vein. Thrombotic material is then removed with the help of a balloon catheter-first and foremost in a proximal direction but also distally, after which an arteriovenous shunt is inserted. This is done by dividing the great saphenous vein and suturing its proximal section into the femoral artery, which effectively prevents the formation of new fibrin clots, and thus the recurrence of thrombosis. The shunt may be left in place throughout pregnancy. Eight pregnant women have so far been treated in this manner, though it is not yet possible to judge whether the surgical method is superior to heparin treatment.

Prevention of Deep Vein Thrombosis in Pregnancy

After treatment of deep vein thrombosis in pregnancy, prophylactic treatment is required throughout pregnancy, during delivery, and in the puerperium owing to the high risk of recurrence. Prophylactic treatment is also required in women with verified deep vein thrombosis during previous pregnancy. The increased risk of recurrent thrombosis has been ascribed to the depressed fibrinolytic activity during pregnancy [5,6].

Prevention of Recurrence During Pregnancy

The prophylactic options available are subcutaneous heparin therapy or the more convenient peroral treatment with coumarol. However, coumarol derivatives traverse the placental membrane to the fetus, which is thus put at risk of teratogenetic injury and haemorrhage. Teratogenetic damage, correlated to treatment with coumarol derivatives, mainly warfarin, during the first trimester, has been the subject of a number of reports. Hypoplasia of the nasal region and epiphysopathy have been mainly described, though optic atrophy, microencephaly and intrauterine growth retardation have also been reported [7–10].

Where treatment has been kept up practically throughout pregnancy, cerebral damage to the fetus is the predominant adverse effect, and it is hard to judge during which phase of pregnancy it occurred [10–17]. The prevailing consensus is, therefore, that peroral anticoagulants should not be given during the 1st trimester.

With regard to coumarol treatment during the 2nd and 3rd trimester, however, opinion is divided. According to one regimen, which has won a measure of acceptance abroad, peroral anticoagulants are given during the 2nd and 3rd trimesters up to 1 week before delivery, when a switch is made to heparin. Suspicion has been aroused that coumarol derivatives may even cause fetal damage during the 2nd and 3rd trimesters. This disorders mentioned above have also been reported where peroral anticoagulants have been given during the 2nd and 3rd trimesters only [18], and cases of intrauterine fetal mortality have also been described [19].

It is a widely held opinion that hemorrhages in the rapidly growing organism may well result in cerebral damage and microencephaly, blindness, or mental retardation [20]. Direct haemorrhagic complications were described early in the professional literature, though in some cases, perhaps, they were the result of overdosage [21–24]

Treatment of patients with heart valve prosthesis creates a special problem. Cardiologists might hesitate to change effective anticoagulant drugs. However, it should be pointed out that most embryopathies are reported in such cases [8,12,14–16] and recently as high as 25% [25]. Therefore in women with artificial heart valves also, warfarin should be replaced by heparin [25], but if so in a larger dose (see below). A new approach in anticoagulant therapy is intrauterine ultrasonic guided administration of vitamin K_1 to the child (personal communication, Dr .B. Jacobsen).

An invidious aspect of peroral anticoagulant treatment during pregnancy is that it may result in the birth of a child who seems completely healthy, but in whom cerebral damage may go undiscovered, perhaps only to be subsequently revealed by a low intelligence quotient. No follow-up studies of children born to mothers treated with coumarol derivatives during pregnancy are available.

Against this background, and with convenience of administration as its only advantage, treatment with coumarol derivatives during pregnancy is indefensible.

Since neither teratogenetic damage nor fetal hemorrhage has been reported in conjunction with heparin treatment, subcutaneous heparin treatment is the method of choice, despite the discomfort it may sometimes cause the patient due to subcutaneous infiltration. The tendency for infiltration to occur can be mitigated by using the correct injection technique, in which the skin is pierced exactly at right angle with the finest of needles.

To simplify treatment, we have taught patients to inject themselves. Low dose heparin (25 000 IU/ml for subcutaneous use) is given in 0.2 ml (5000 IU) subcutaneous injections, morning and evening, according to Kakkar [26]. The treatment of ambulant patients has been simplified by the advent of disposable syringes with standard doses of 0.2 ml heparin. After treatment of pulmonary embolism and other severe cases we have given heparin 5000 IU 3 times daily or 7500 IU twice daily. A higher dose of 10 000–12 500 IU twice daily is also required in women with artificial heart valves. After deep vein thrombosis graded compression stockings have proved helpful.

Prevention During Delivery

During delivery itself, the risk of recurrence of thrombosis is substantial and may be compared with that during surgery. Since the risk of hemorrhage is also great during delivery, prophylaxis must be appropriate, and two options are available. Either the low dose heparin may be continued throughout delivery. But where epidural anesthesia is used, many anaesthesiologists prefer prophylactic treatment with dextran rather than heparin, as the risk of hemorrhagic complications is said to be less [27]. In such cases heparin dosage is temporarily suspended about 12 h before delivery is induced. In conjunction with delivery itself, 500 ml of dextran (Rheomacrodex, Pharmacia) is given, preceded by 20 ml of the hapten Promiten, to prevent any anaphylactic reactions. A 500 ml infusion of dextran, without Promiten, is given 4 after delivery and repeated the following day, after which heparin treatment is resumed.

Prevention During the Puerperium

Since the risk of recurrence during the puerperium remains, prophylactic treatment is desirable. Although the risk of hemorrhagic complications is slight, the mother's wishes with regard to breast-feeding need to be taken into consideration, as the coumarol derivatives would be conveyed to the child via breast milk in low concentration. Should the mother opt for breast feeding, she will have to continue subcutaneous heparin treatment for about 4-8 weeks, depending upon when during pregnancy the thrombosis occurred. The concentration of warfarin in breast milk is, however, low [28]. If warfarin is to given to a nursing mother, it should be done in consultation with a pediatrician, as the child's thrombotest (TT) value will need checking in prematures and vitamin K_1 given prophylactically or as necessary. Heparin treatment may be replaced by warfarin a few days after delivery, and administration of heparin discontinued, when the TT value has reached a therapeutic level. If breast-feeding is discontinued, peroral anti-coagulants are to be preferred. The more convenient peroral treatment may be continued for 3–6 months after delivery. It should be born in mind that estrogen preparations should not be given to terminate breast-feeding, as the estrogens are known to reduce the content of fibrinolytic activators in the vessel wall, and thus impair the fibrinolytic defence system against thrombosis. Instead bromo-criptin (Pravidel, Sandoz) is recommended in a dosage of 2.5 mg twice daily for 2 weeks.

Prevention of Women with Earlier Thrombosis

A common question is whether women with a history of thrombosis should be given prophylactic treatment during pregnancy. We give such treatment in cases where earlier thrombosis has been unequivolcally verified and has occurred in conjunction with pregnancy or hormone treatment, or where there have been several thrombotic episodes. Although the juncture at which prophylactic treat-ment should be started during pregnancy must be decided individually, we generally begin around the 14th or 16th week. Prophylactic heparin treatment may also be indicated in cases of extended confinement to bed, and prophylactic dextran treatment in conjunction with surgery during pregnancy.

Additional Aspects

No coagulation analysis is necessary, other than routine tests to monitor the effect of heparin treatment (APTT), coumarol treatment (thrombotest, TT; prothrombin/proconvertin, P & P; or Stago prothrombin assay, SPA), or checks of the platelet count (see below). However, the possibility of antithrombin III deficiency should not be overlooked. In Sweden there are about 24 families with hereditary antithrombin III deficiency. Family members whose plasma anti-thrombin III content is below 50% of normal are at risk for thrombosis, and during pregnancy the concentration is reduced by a further 15%. Antithrombin III is a heparin cofactor, in the absence of which heparin is ineffective. In these rare cases in which a higher dose of heparin is required [29,30] and where anti-thrombin III must be given, consultation with one of the country's coagulation units is to be recommended, particularly as these patients are often known there already. The frequency of protein C and protein S deficiency among patients with thromboembolic complications during pregnancy is not known.

Side Effects

Although no hemorrhagic complications or thrombosis recurrence have oc-curred with this regimen to date, there have been a few cases of recurrence where, for one reason or another, prophylactic treatment has been discontinued or dispensed with. There have been some cases of urticaria during heparin treat-ment, but a switch to another heparin preparation has enabled treatment to be continued. Other known side effects of heparin treatment are osteoporosis [31,32], which requires attention though it is rare in conjunction with low dose prophylaxis, and thrombocytopenia [33–36]. The latter is an unusual side effect which appears, if at all, about 10 days after the start of treatment. We check the platelet count after the 2nd and 4th weeks of treatment, then once a month, and always before delivery. Since the development of thrombocytopenia during treatment with heparin has been shown to depend upon the primary materials used in its production, it is often sufficient to switch to another preparation.

Summary of Guidelines for Treatment and Prevention

Even in cases where a clinical diagnosis of thrombosis seems beyond doubt, it should always be verified by phlebography. However, it is usually possible to dispense with pelvigraphy to check the upper extent of the thrombosis.

Once diagnosis has been confirmed, heparin treatment is given. After an initial dose of 100 IU/kg body weight, heparin is given intravenously, preferably with an electronic infusion pump, at a daily rate of 600 IU/kg body weight for at least 5 days. The activated partial thromboplastin time (APTT) should be maintained at about twice its control value. A platelet count should be made after the 2nd and 4th weeks, then once a month, and again before delivery.

For protection against recurrence during the remainder of pregnancy, the patient should be given low dose heparin (25 000 IU/ml), 0.2 ml, i.e., 5000 IU subcutaneously, morning and evening. (N.B. Avoid coumarol preparations!) After treatment of pulmonary embolism and in other severe cases 7500-IU twice daily is recommended. The low dose heparin maybe continued throughout delivery. If epidural anesthesia is to be used heparin treatment is temporarily suspended 12 h before delivery is induced. In conjunction with delivery, 500 ml of Rheomacrodex, preceded by 20 ml of Promiten should be administered. Rheomacrodex 500 ml, without Promiten, is given 4 h after delivery and repeated the following day, after which subcutaneous heparin treatment (as outlined above) is resumed, being continued for 4-6 weeks if the patient is breast-feeding. Warfarin can be given instead, if the child's TT or SPA value is checked and vitamin K_1 is given prophylactically or as necessary. In non-nursing mothers, the simpler warfarin treatment is to be preferred, and it should be continued for 3–6 months. Note that Pravidel, rather than any of the estrogens, should be given if breast-feeding is to be discontinued.

Premature Separation of Placenta

Premature separation of placenta is a serious complication with a gloomy prognosis for fetus and child. This complication is followed by a perinatal mortality of about 35%, most of the children already dead at admission. At separation of placenta thromboplastic material might enter the maternal blood stream and thereby triggering a pathologic proteolysis with mainly activation of the coagulation mechanism as a result. If instead mainly plasminogen activators enter the

Table 1. Clinical data on the patients treated with tranexamic acid

Patient number	Acute symptom of abruptio placentae (week of pregnancy)	Therapy with tranexamic acid (weeks)	Cesarean section (week of pregnancy)	Apgar score (1 min)
1	35	3	38	8
2	26	12	38	9
3	32	1	33	9
4	32	4	36	9
5	27	10	37	8
6	29	5	34	9
Mean	30.2	5.8	36	8.7

blood stream a pathologic proteolysis with mainly activation of the fibrinolytic system might occur [37]. In a clinical series of 14 cases with premature separation of placenta the coagulation factors and components of the fibrinolytic system where analysed [38]. In most of the patients an activation of the fibrinolytic system was predominant. In six of the patients the bleeding was slight or moderate and the child immature. By treatment with the fibrinolytic inhibitor tranexamic acid (Cyklokapron) 4 g daily the bleeding ceased and the pregnancy could be prolonged with maturation of the fetus. Delivery was performed by cesarean section and all the neonates were in a good state (Table 1).

Abruptio placentae occurs in about 0.5% of the deliveries. The risk of repeated abruptio placenta increases: After one premature separation the risk is 17% and after two premature separations 25%. Such a case will be briefly described: The patient had twice before had an abruptio of the placenta resulting in death of the children. In her third pregnancy in the 26 week she came again with bleeding and signs of a premature separation of placenta. Laboratory analysis showed a normal platelet count and a normal prothrombin complex but a high concentration of fibrin degradation products indicating a pathologic proteolysis with mainly activation of the fibrinolytic system. The patient was therefore treated with the fibrinolytic inhibitor tranexamic acid, first intravenously and then per orally. By this treatment it was possible to prolong pregnancy up to the 33 week. A new bleeding now occurred, which stopped after intravenous administration of tranexamic acid. The pregnancy now had proceeded to the 34 week and cesarean section was performed. The child weighed 1.430 g and was awarded an Apgar score of 8 points and has apparently been well since birth. Signs of early abruptio were found in the placenta as well as a small fresh coagulum [39].

In the acute stage of abruptio placenta the fibrinolytic inhibitor tranexamic acid immediately should be given and cesarean section performed. In cases with partial separation of a placenta with slight bleeding and immature fetus with absence of other threatening signs, treatment with the potent fibrinolytic inhibitor tranexamic acid has proved useful to prolong pregnancy with maturation of the fetus. Thus, in cases of premature separation of the placenta, by treatment with the fibrinolytic inhibitor tranexamic acid it will be possible to reduce the perinatal mortality by this complications.

Summary. The treatment of deep vein thrombosis during pregnancy presents special problems. The benefit of treatment must be weighed against the subsequent risk of placental or fetal hemorrhage. Safe diagnosis with phlebographic verification is necessary, even where the thrombosis seems clinically manifest. Heparin has been an established treatment with the great advantage that it does not enter the fetal blood stream. In selected cases surgery or thrombolytic therapy has to be considered. Owing to the high risk of recurrence, prophylactic treatment with heparin is required throughout pregnancy. Coumarol derivatives traverse the placental membrance to the fetus and have to be avoided because of a risk for teratogenetic injury and intracranial hemorrhage in the fetus. During the puerperium, warfarin might be given because its concentration in breast milk is low. However, administration óf vitamin K_1 is recommended to prematures. Attention should be given to the side-effects of heparin i.e., thrombocytopenia and osteoporosis. The possibility of antithrombin III deficiency should not be overlooked. In such cases there is also risk of thrombosis in the newborn. In regard to premature separation of the placenta, most cases of abruptio placenta require immediate delivery by caesarian section. Analysis of the coagulation factors and components of the fibrinolytic system have shown an activation mainly of the fibrinolytic system. In cases with partial separation of placenta and immature fetus, treatment with the fibrinolytic inhibitor tranexamic acid (Cyklokapron) has proven useful to prolong pregnancy with maturation of the fetus.
Acknowledgment. Research by the clinic was supported by the Swedish Medical Research Council 04523.

References

1. Åstedt B, Robertson B, Haeger K (1974) Experience with standardized streptokinase therapy of deep venous thrombosis. Surg Gynecol Obstet 139: 387–388
2. Flessa HC, Kapstrom AB, Glueck HI, Will JJ (1965) Placental transport of heparin. Am J Obstet Gynecol 93: 570–573
3. Forestier F, Daffos F, Capella-Pavlovsky M (1984) Low molecular weight heparin (PK 10169) does not cross the placenta during the second trimester of pregnancy: study by direct fetal blood sampling under ultrasound. Thromb Res 34: 557
4. Forestier F, Daffos F, Rainaut M, Toulemonde F (1987) Low molecular weight Heparin (CY 216) does not cross the placenta during the third trimester of pregnancy. Thromb Hemost 57: 234
5. Åstedt B, Isacson S, Nilsson IM, Pandolfi M (1970) Fibrinolytic activity of veins during pregnancy. Acta Obstet Gynecol Scand 48: 171–173
6. Bonnar J, McNicol GP, Douglas AS (1970) Coagulation and fibrinolytic mechanisms during and after childbirth. Br Med J 2: 200–203
7. Bloomfield DK (1970) Fetal deaths and malformations associated with the use of coumarin derivatives in pregnancy. Am J Obstet Gynecol 107: 883–888
8. Carson M, Reid M (1976) Warfarin and fetal abnormality. Lancet 1: 1127
9. Hall GJ (1967) Warfarin and fetal abnormality. Lancet 1: 1127
10. Holtzgreve W, Carey JC, Hall BD (1976) Warfain-induced fetal abnormalities. Lancet 2: 914–915
11. DiSaia PJ (1966) Pregnancy and delivery of a patient with a Starr-Edwards mitral valve prosthesis. Obstet Gynecol 28: 469–472
12. Kerber IJ, Warr OS, Richardson C (1968) Pregnancy in a patient with a prosthetic mitral valve. JAMA 203: 157–159
13. Tejani N (1973) Anticoagulant therapy with cardiac valve prosthesis during pregnan-

cy. Obstet Gynecol 42: 785–793
14. Becker MH, Genieser NB, Finegold M, Miranda D, Spackman T (1975) Chondrodysplasia punctata. Am J Dis Child 129: 356–359
15. Fourie DT, Hay IT (1975) Warfarin as a possible teratogen. S Afr Med J 49: 2081–2083
16. Pettifor JM, Benson R (1975) Congenital malformations associated with the administration of oral anticoagulants during pregnancy. J Pediatr 86: 459–462
17. Shaul WL, Emery H, Hall GJ (1975) Chondrodysplasia punctata and maternal warfarin use during pregnancy. Am J Dis Child 129: 360–362
18. Sherman S, Hall BD (1976) Warfarin and fetal abnormality. Lancet 1: 692
19. Quenneville G, Barton B, McDevitt E, Wright IS (1959) The use of anticoagulants for thrombophlebitis during pregnancy. Am J Obstet Gynecol 77: 1135–1149
20. Warkany J (1975) A warfarin embryopathy? Am J Dis Child 129: 287–288
21. von Syndow G (1947) Hypoprothrombinemia and cerebral injury in infant after dicumarol treatment of mother. Nord Med 34: 1171–1172
22. Sach JJ, Labate JS (1949) Dicumarol in the treatment of antenatal thrombo-embolic disease: Report of a case with hemorrhagic manifestations in the fetus. Am J Obstet Gynecol 57: 965–971
23. Gordon RR, Dean T (1955) Fetal deaths from antenatal anticoagulant therapy. Br Med J 2: 719–721
24. VillaSanta U (1965) Thromboembolic disease in pregnancy. Am J Obstet Gynecol 93; 142
25. Iturbe-Alessio I, del Carmen Fonseca M, Mutchinik O, Santos MA, Zajarias A, Salazar E (1986) Risks of anticoagulant therapy in pregnant women with artificial heart valves. N Engl J Med 315: 1390–1393
26. Kakkar VV (1975) Deep vein thrombosis. Detection and prevention. Circulation 51: 8–19
27. Crawford JS (1978) Principles and practice of obstetrics anesthesia, 4th edn. Blackwell Scientific Publications, Oxford, pp 182–183
28. Orme MLE, Lewis PJ, de Swiet M, Serlin MJ, Sibeon R, Baty JD, Breckenridge AM (1977) May mothers given warfarin breast-feed their infants? Br Med J 1: 1564–1565
29. Hellgren M, Tenbgorn L, Abildgaard U (1982) Pregnancy in women with congenital antithrombin III deficiency: experience of treatment with heparin and antithrombin. Gynecol Obstet Invest 14: 127–141
30. Hellgren M, Nygårds EB, Robbe H (1982) Antithrombin III in late pregnancy. Acta Obstet Gynecol Scand 61: 187–189
31. Griffith GC, Nichols G, Asher JD, Hanagan B (1965) Heparin osteoporosis. JAMA 193: 91–94
32. Wise PH, Hall AJ (1980) Heparin-induced osteopenia in pregnancy. Br Med J 281: 110–111
33. Cines DB, Kaywin P, Bina M, Tomaski A, Schreiber AD (1980) Heparin-associated thrombocytopenia. N Engl J Med 303: 788–795
34. Chong BH, Pitney WR, Castaldi PA (1982) Heparin-induced thrombocytopenia: an association of thrombotic complications with heparin-dependent IgG antibody that induces thromboxane synthesis and platelet aggregation. Lancet 2: 1246–1248
35. Babcock RB, Wesley Dumper C, Scharfman WB (1976) Heparin-induced immune thrombocytopenia. N Engl J Med 295: 237–241
36. de Swiet M, Bulpitt CJ, Lewis PJ (1980) How obstetricians use anticoagulants in the prophylaxis of thromboembolism. J Obstet Gynecol 1: 29–32
37. Åstedt B (1988) Hemorrhagic diathesis due to pathological proteolysis. In: Renck H (ed) Bleeding and thrombotic disorders in the surgical patient. Appleton & Lange, Norwalk, pp 53–59
38. Svanberg L, Åstedt B, Nilsson IM (1980) Abruptio placenta—treatment with the fibrinolytic inhibitor tranexamic acid. Acta Obstet Gynecol Scand 59: 127–30
39. Åstedt B, Nilsson IM (1978) Recurrent abruptio placentae treated with the fibrinolytic inhibitor tranexamic acid. Br Med J 1: 756–7

1.12 Anticoagulant and Thrombolytic Therapy in the Newborn

MAUREEN ANDREW and BARBARA SCHMIDT[1]

Introduction

Pediatric thrombotic disease has its highest prevalence in the newborn period and contributes to both neonatal morbidity and mortality [1–3]. The thromboembolic complications are most frequently secondary to vascular catheters. However, spontaneous occlusion of both arterial and venous vessels in a variety of locations may also occur [2]. Currently, the anticoagulant drug, standard heparin (SH) is commonly used prophylactically to prevent catheter related thrombi [4]. Should a "clinically apparent" thromboembolic complication occur with significant limb or organ impairment, then anticoagulant and/or thrombolytic drugs are frequently used therapeutically to reestablish patency of the vessel or to prevent extension of the thrombi [5,6].

The dose schedules for the use of anticoagulant and thrombolytic drugs, in the newborn were initially modelled closely after protocols developed for and validated in the adult. The critically ill state of these infants in combination with the relative rarity of clinically apparent thrombi justified this initial approach. However, the efficacy and safety of anticoagulant and thrombolytic drugs in the newborn are likely to differ from the adult for many reasons. First, the activities of both anticoagulant and thrombolytic drugs are dependent on the endogenous concentrations of specific hemostatic components. The latter are significantly different in the newborn compared to the adult [7–9]. Second, the pharmacokinetics of many drugs including the anticoagulant drugs differ in the newborn compared to the adult [10–13]. Finally, the common locations of arterial and venous thrombi in the newborn are very different from the adult [2,14].

Current protocols for anticoagulant and thrombolytic therapy in the adult have been validated in many randomized clinical trials. This approach is hindered in the newborn by the relative rarity of symptomatic thrombosis and the

[1]Department of Pediatrics, McMaster University, Room 3N27, 1200 Main Street West, Hamilton, Ontario, L8N 3Z5, Canada

lack of data demonstrating the need for treating the more frequent asymptomatic or "clinically silent" thrombi [15–20].

In vitro studies and newborn animal models provide information which can clarify the differing responses to anticoagulant or thrombolytic drugs in the newborn. These preclinical sources of information can help refine the choice of drugs and drug dosages which can then be tested more efficiently in clinical trials. The following is a summary of data from in vitro studies and animal models on anticoagulant and thrombolytic drugs in the newborn. Suggestions as to how this information may already improve anticoagulant and thrombolytic therapy in the newborn are given.

The Procoagulant and Fibrinolytic Systems in the Newborn

The Procoagulant System

The actual components of the hemostatic system and their interactions are similar in the newborn compared to the adult. However, the absolute and relative concentrations of many coagulation and fibrinolytic proteins differ in the newborn and are dependent on the gestational and postnatal age of the infant [7–9]. As well, some coagulation proteins have modified structures (i.e., fibrinogen, von Willebrand factor, protein C); however, the clinical importance of these structural alterations is unknown at this time [21–24].

The screening tests, the activated partial thromboplastin time (APTT) and prothrombin time (PT) are frequently prolonged in the newborn reflecting the low concentrations of the four contact factors (factors XII, XI, prekallikrein [PK], and high molecular weight kininogen [HMWK]) as well as the vitamin K dependent factors (II, VII, IX, and X). The concentrations of the cofactors, factors V and VIII: C, as well as the final substrate fibrinogen, are all similar to the adult.

The generation of thrombin is a critically important step in the procoagulant side of hemostasis [25]. The differences in the concentration of the procoagulants are responsible for marked differences in the generation of thrombin in the newborn infant compared to the adult. The generation of thrombin is delayed and decreased by approximately 50% in the newborn compared to the adult [26,27]. Indeed, the thrombin generation pattern in the newborn is similar to that of an adult anticoagulated with either heparin or coumadin. The concentration of prothrombin is directly related to the amount of thrombin generated and the concentrations of other procoagulants affect the rate of thrombin generation [28].

The inhibition of thrombin itself is also important to normal hemostasis. Thrombin is inhibited by the antiproteases, antithrombin III (ATIII), heparin cofactor II (HCII) and alpha–2–macroglobulin (α_2M). At the time of birth both ATIII and HCII levels are approximately half adult values whereas α_2M is elevated above adult values. This combination results in a slower inhibition of thrombin in newborn plasma compared to adult plasma [29]. The latter is at least in part due to the low AT III level in the newnborn. The elevated level of α_2M compensates partially but not completely for the low AT III level in the newborn. The activities of both SH and LMWH are mediated by potentiating the inhibitory activity of AT III [30,31]. One would anticipate that the low level of AT III in combination with the profound differences in thrombin generation will affect the interaction of SH and LMWH in the newborn.

The Fibrinolytic System

The components of the fibrinolytic system and their interactions are similar in the newborn compared to the adult [6,32,33]. When fibrin is formed the components of the fibrinolytic system are incorporated into the fibrin clot. These include plasminogen, alpha–2–antiplasmin (α_2AP), tissue plasminogen activator (TPA), and plasminogen activator inhibitor (PAI). Plasminogen, α_2AP, and TPA all bind through lysine binding sites to fibrin, resulting in the close proximity of plasminogen to its activator TPA. TPA cleaves plasminogen to plasmin which can either degrade fibrin of fibrinogen or bind to α_2AP.

The absolute and relative concentrations of the fibrinolytic components differ in the newborn compared to the adult [6,9,33]. Most importantly, the concentration of plasminogen is approximately 50% of the adult value. The activities of all thrombolytic drugs in current use are dependent on the generation of plasmin from endogenous plasminogen in the patient. One would anticipate that the low level of plasminogen may limit the effectiveness of thrombolytic drugs in the newborn. Finally, the concentration of α_2AP, the most important inhibitor of plasmin in the adult, is 80% of the adult value. The latter may lead to alterations in the regulation of plasmin once it is generated in the newborn.

Anticoagulant Drugs in the Newborn

In Vitro Studies: Standard Heparin

Standard heparin (SH) was first prepared in the 1930s. Since that time SH has been used extensively in the initial treatment of thromboembolic complications in the adult. The efficacy of SH as an antithrombotic agent has been estabished beyond doubt in many large clinical trials. The anticoagulant and antithrombotic activities of SH are due to their catalytic enhancement of the physiologic inhibitor, antithrombin III (AT III) [34,35]. The inhibition of the thrombin mediated activation of factors V and VIII: C by AT III is the mechanism by which SH exerts its effect [36]. The latter mechanism likely applies to the newborn as well as the adult.

The antithrombotic effects of SH in the adult are monitored ultimately by clinical outcome. The anticoagulant effects of SH in certain coagulation assays (i.e., the APTT, antithrombin or factor Xa assays) correlate with the clinical outcome. Indeed, the correlation between the anticoagulant effect in vitro and the antithrombotic effect in vivo has resulted in the establishment of "therapeutic ranges" for SH therapy. In general, values below the therapeutic range indicate that the patient is not sufficiently anticoagulated and is at risk for further thromboembolic complications [37]. Values above the "therapeutic range" indicate that the patient is receiving excessive SH and may be at risk of hemorrhagic side effects [38].

The use of SH in the newborn began with the advent of neonatal intensive care units and the improved survival of premature infants. Over the last two decades SH has been primarily used to prevent catheter related thrombi and to treat clinically apparent thrombi. However, evidence has accumulated that newborn plasma responds differently to SH than adult plasma. The newborn was reported to display an increased sensitivity to SH compared to the adult in assays dependent upon the conversion of endogenous prothrombin to thrombin, i.e., the APTT, PT, and thrombin generation assays [35,26]. In contrast, resistance to SH was observed in assay systems in which excess amounts of exogenous factor Xa or thrombin were added [26,39]. The reasons for this apparent paradox were recently investigated [27]. By manipulating the ratio of AT III to (pro)thrombin in newborn plasma either sensitivity or resistance to SH could be induced using a thrombin generation assay. Under physiologic conditions normal newborn plasma is more sensitive to SH than adult plasma, due to relative excess of AT III to (pro)thrombin in the newborn (ratio of 0.6: 0.4) compared to the adult (ratio 1.0: 1.0). The sensitivity of newborn plasma to SH could be further increased by raising the AT III level in vitro. In contrast, resistance of newborn plasma to SH could be induced be reversing the ratio of AT III to (pro)thrombin (0.6: 1.0) in vitro. Thus the reported sensitivity or resistance of newborn plasma to SH is an in vitro phenomena that largely reflects the differing ratio of AT III and prothrombin in the assay systems. Which of the in vitro assays most closely reflects the in vivo antithrombotic effect of SH in the newborn is not known.

Clearly, the therapeutic ranges for SH in the adult cannot be simply extrapolated to the newborn. The APTT will tend to overestimate the amount of SH circulating in the newborn because very small amounts of SH, considered subtherapeutic in the adult, will prolong the APTT to values above the upper boundary of the therapeutic range in the adult [3,5,26]. Heparin assays based on catalysis of AT III inhibition of exogenous thrombin or factor Xa, will systematically underestimate the amount of SH present in newborn plasma due to an incomplete supplementation of the AT III level of adult values [39]. A clinical trial validating a "therapeutic range" for SH in the newborn is needed. Until such a clinical trial is performed, it seems prudent to carefully follow the clinical response to SH in combination with noninvasive monitoring, i.e., ultrasound, in an affected infant. The starting doses per kilogram of SH, (50 units per kg bolus followed by 20 units per kg) are extrapolated from the lower end of the therapeutic amounts of SH used in the adult. Laboratory monitoring in the form of an APTT or heparin assay may be helpful to ensure that the SH level is not above the adult therapeutic range as this may place the infant at risk of bleeding.

In Vitro Studies: Low Molecular Weight Heparin

Over the past decade a class of anticoagulant drugs, the low molecular weight heparins (LMWH) have been prepared from SH and offer advantages over SH.

They are at least as efficacious as SH [40–44], but cause less bleeding in animal models [40,42] and in man [43,44]. The hemorrhagic side effects of SH are due in part to the inhibition of platelet function as measured in platelet aggregation studies [45] and by prolonging the bleeding time [46]. LMWHs do not prolong the bleeding time nor do they inhibit platelet aggregation studies in vitro [45–47].

In adults, LMWHs are particularly helpful where the use of SH is problematic, i.e., in patients who require antithrombotic protection but who are particularly vulnerable to bleeding complications [43,44]. Sick immature newborns can be considered vulnerable because of the immaturity of the coagulation system, the frequency of thrombocytopenia, the inherent risk of intraventricular hemorrhage (IVH) and the need for heparin prophylaxis to maintain the patency of vascular catheters. Because the therapeutic advantages of LMWHs may also apply to the sick newborn, in vitro experiments were conducted to explore the potential benefits of LMWH's in this age group.

The anticoagulant and antithrombotic properties of LMWHs are also mediated through AT III. Although the LMWHs potentiate the inhibition of the enzyme Xa more than SH [48], the antithrombotic ability of LMWHs is clearly linked to their antithrombin activity [30,31,35]. Therefore in vitro assays were performed to determine the ability of LMWHs to catalyze the inhibition of thrombin by AT III. It was found that just as for SH, newborn plasma is more sensitive to the activity of LMWH compared to adult plasma. This sensitivity can either be amplified by increasing the AT III level to adult values or reversed by raising the concentration of prothrombin [49].

Animal Studies

The use of an appropriate animal model of newborn hemostasis is an important extension of the in vitro studies. The newborn piglet was chosen as a model of thromboembolic disorders in the newborn because of the similarities in the hemostatic system, the low level of AT III and a birth weight which facilitated a local thrombus model in vivo [50]. We have used the piglet model to explore differences in the pharmacokinetics of both SH and LMWH as well as their activities as antithrombotic agents in the newborn.

Pharmacokinetic Studies

The pharmacokinetics of SH have been extensively studied in the human adult and animal models [51–54]. Clearance of SH best fits a model based on a combination of saturable and linear nonsaturable clearance mechanism (52–54]. Cellular clearance by the endothelium and reticulo-endothelial system provide the saturable mechanisms whereas renal clearance provides the linear nonsaturable mechanism [55–58]. The clearance of SH in the newborn piglet also fits a model based on a combination of saturable and linear nonsaturable clearance [10]. This results in a clearance of SH which is dose dependent, with large amounts of SH cleared more slowly than smaller amounts. The newborn piglet has a larger volume of distribution than the adult pig resulting in a faster overall clearance of SH in the piglet. The pharmacokinetic data for SH in the newborn piglet is compatible with the more limited data available in the human newborn [11,13]. The more rapid clearance of SH in the newborn likely contributes to an increased requirement of SH per kilogram to achieve the same SH concentration in the newborn compared to the adult.

In contrast to SH, LMWHs follow a linear nonsaturable mechanism in the adult, which is mediated by the kidney [51,53,58,59]. The decreased binding of LMWH to endothelial cells likely explains the lack of a saturable clearance mechanism [55]. LMWHs consistently show a longer half-life than SH in adult humans or animal models. The clearance of LMWH in the newborn piglet also follows a linear nonsaturable mechanism, which is not dose dependent [12]. As for SH, the newborn piglet has a larger volume of distribution than the adult pig resulting in a faster overall clearance of LMWH in the piglet. As in the adult, LMWHs were cleared more slowly than SH.

Antithrombotic Studies

In order to examine the antithrombotic properties of SH and LMWH in the neonatal period, we compared the ability of these heparins to inhibit thrombus formation in the piglet with a Wessler type thrombosis model [60 and unpublished data]. SH was less effective in the newborn than in the adult in preventing a jugular vein thrombus induced by a pathologic bolus of thrombin and stasis. A possible explanation for this SH resistance in the piglet was the relative deficiency of AT III. Increasing AT III levels in vivo in piglets to adult values significantly improved the antithrombotic properties of SH in neonatal piglets. Increasing the dose of SH overcame the resistance; however, the safety of the latter approach is unproven. Using the same animal model, similar observations were made for LMWH.

The data obtained in newborn piglets do not negate the need of clinical trials in the infant. Indeed, they cast doubt on the appropriateness of our current clinical practice based on extrapolation from the adult and underscore the need for clinical trials in the newborn.

Thrombolytic Therapy

Infants who develop a serious thrombotic complication as defined by organ or limb impairment, may benefit from thrombolytic therapy. The clinical objective is to remove the clot as quickly and as safely as possible. Surgical removal of a clot in a major vessel in the infant is technically difficult and poses a considerable life threatening risk to the infant who is usually premature with multiple problems. Therefore the use of thrombolytic agents for these infants is a preferred approach if the efficacy and safety can be assured with reasonable certainty. Although thrombolytic drugs have been used extensively in the adult, there is sparse information on their effectiveness in the newborn [6].

Recently, Corrigan et al. reported that the amount of plasmin generated in newborn plasma in response to several thrombolytic drugs was slower and decreased compared to the adult [33]. We have extended these observations by testing the ability of three thrombolytic agents, urokinase (UK), streptokinase (SK), and tissue plasminogen activator (TPA) to lyse a radiolabelled fibrin clot prepared from cord or adult fibrinogen and resuspended in cord or adult plasma [61]. Lysis of a fibrin clot by one of UK, SK, or TPA in cord plasma was consistently impaired compared to the adult. If both plasminogen and the inhibitors of plasminogen were added to the newborn test system i.e., placing the newborn clot in adult plasma the newborn responded in a similar fashion to the adult to the three thrombolytic agents. However, if purified Glu-plasminogen alone was added to newborn plasma containing a newborn clot, an excessive thrombolytic response was observed in the newborn compared to the adult with all three agents. The latter observation suggested that the newborn had an impaired ability to inhibit plasmin which was unmasked when the plasminogen level was increased to adult values. Whether or not these in vitro responses will predict the clinical response of the newborn to thrombolytic agents is unknown. However, many of the published case reports document failures of thrombolytic drugs in the infant when used in comparable amounts per kg as for the adult [6]. Urokinase is the preferred drug at this time. An initial loading dose of 4,400 units per kg over 20 minutes should be followed by 4,400 units per kg per hour. Until further information is available it would seem advisable to supplement the newborn with adult plasma when a thrombolytic agent is being used. By using adult plasma both the level of plasminogen and its inhibitors will be increased which will hopefully enhance the response to thrombolytic therapy and not lead to excessive hemorrhagic side effects.

Conclusion

The physiology of the neonate's hemostatic system clearly differs from the adult and is dependent on the gestational and postnatal age of the infant. When a sick neonate develops a clinically apparent thrombotic complication which is impairing limb or organ function, anticoagulant and/or thrombolytic therapy is frequently justified in order to re-establish vessel patency as rapidly as possible. The differing concentrations of hemostatic proteins known to be critical to the effect of anticoagulant and thrombolytic drugs likely alter the efficacy and safety of these drugs when compared to the adult. The low AT III level in combination with the even lower prothrombin level alter the activity of both SH and LMWH which are dependent for their effect on the AT III concentration. Perhaps by manipulating the prothrombin to AT III ratio in the newborn, anticoagulants such as SH and LMWH can be made safer and more effective. Similarly, all thrombolytic agents are dependent upon the generation of endogenous plasmin for their thrombolytic effect. The low level of plasminogen in the newborn limits the effect of these agents in vitro. Supplementation of the newborn system with adult plasma resuls in a similar response to thrombolytic agents as for the adult.

Future clinical trials are necessary to validate and improve upon the current approach to the prevention and management of infants with thromboembolic complications.

Summary. Thromboembolic complications occur in the sick newborn infant and may require treatment with anticoagulant and/or thrombolytic drugs. Because the coagulation and fibrinolytic systems are distinctly different from the adult, the vitro and in vivo response of the newborn to these drugs can be anticipated to differ from the adult. The anticoagulant drugs, standard heparin (SH) and low molecular weight heparins (LMWH), have been studied in the newborn. Using in vitro tests, both SH and LMWH paradoxically show increased sensitivity or increased resistance compared to the adult. This is an artifact due to the differences in how these tests are conducted. In animal models, the newborn has a faster clearance of both SH and LMWH due to the increased volume of distribution in the newborn compared to the adult. Similar to the adult, LMWH has a longer half-life than SH in the newborn. Both LMWH and SH are effective antithrombotic agents in the newborn porcine model: however, their effects can be enhanced by increasing the antithrombin III (AT III) level.

The thrombolytic drugs: urokinase (UK), streptokinase (SK), and tissue plasminogen activator (TPA), have been tested in vitro using a radio-labeled fibrin clot system. The response to all three agents is decreased in the newborn due to the low plasminogen level. As well, the inhibition of plasmin is impaired in the newborn when the plasminogen level is raised to adult values by adding exogenous plasminogen.

There are important differences is the newborn's coagulation and fibrinolytic systems which affect their response to anticoagulant and thrombolytic drugs. An understanding of these differences is important to the efficacious and safe use of these drugs in the newborn.

Acknowledgments. This work was supported by a grant-in-aid from the Heart and Stroke Foundation of Ontario. Dr. Andrew is a Career Investigator of the Heart and Stroke Foundation of Ontario. Dr. Schmidt is a Scholar of the Heart and Stroke Foundation of Canada. The authors acknowledge the secretarial assistance of Mrs. Rosemary Phillis in the preparation of this manuscript, and the technical assistance of Ms. Lesley Mitchell and Mrs. LuAnn Brooker.

References

1. Schmidt B, Andrew M (1988) Neonatal thrombotic disease: prevention, diagnosis and treatment. J Pediatr 113: 407–410
2. Schmidt B, Zipursky A (1976) Thrombotic disease in newborn infants. Clin Peri 11: 461–488
3. Barnard DR, Hathaway WE (1979) Neonatal thrombosis. Am J Pediatr Hematol/Oncol 1: 235–244
4. Gilhooly JT, Lindenberg JA, Reynold JW (1986) Survey of umbilical artery catheter practices. Clin Res 34:142A

5. McDonald MM, Hathaway WE (1982) Anticoagulant therapy by continuous heparinization in newborn and older infants. J Pediatr 101: 451–457
6. Corrigan J (1988) Neonatal thrombosis and the thrombolytic system. Pathophysiology and therapy. Am J Pediatr Hematol/Oncol 10: 83–91
7. Andrew M, Paes B, Milner R, Johnston M, Mitchell L, Tollefsen DM, Powers P (1987) Development of the human coagulation system in the full term infant. Blood 70: 165–172
8. Andrew M, Paes B, Milner R, Johnston M, Mitchell L, Tollefsen DM, Castle V, Powers P (1988) Development of the coagulation system in the healthy premature infant. Blood 72: 1651–1657
9. Andrew M, Paes B, Johnston (1990) Development of the hemostatic system in the neonate and young infant. Am J Pediatr Hematol/Oncol 12: 95–104
10. Andrew M, Ofosu F, Schmidt B, Brooker L, Hirsh J, Buchanan MR (1988) Heparin clearance and ex vivo recovery in newborn piglets and adult pigs. Thromb Res 52: 517–527
11. McDonald MM, Jacobson JJ, Hay WW, Hathaway WW (1981) Heparin clearance in the newborn. Pediatr Res 15: 1015–1018
12. Andrew M, Ofosu F, Brooker L, Buchanan MR (1989) The comparison of the pharmacokinetics of a low molecular weight heparin in the newborn and adult pig. Thromb Haemostas 56: 529–539
13. Rogner G (1976) Heparin level during anticoagulant therapy in mature and premature newborn infants. Kinderarztl Prax 44: 193–200
14. O'Neill JA, Neblett WW III, Born ML (1981) Management of major thromboembolic complications of umbilical artery catheters. J Pediatr Surg 16: 972–978
15. Neal WA, Raynolds JW, Jarvis CW, Williams HJ (1972) Umbilical artery catheterization: demonstration of arterial thrombosis by aortography. Pediatr 50: 6–13
16. Goetzman B, Stadalnick RC, Bogren HG, Blankenship WJ, Ikeda RM, Thayer J (1975) Thrombotic complications of umbilical catheters: a clinical and radiographic study. Pediatr 56: 374–379
17. Olinsky A, Aitken FG, Isdale JM (1975) Thrombus formation after umbilical arterial catheterization: an angiographic study. S Afr Med J 49: 1467–1470
18. Mokrohisky ST, Levine R, Blumhagen JD, Wesenberg RL, Simmons MA (1978) Low positioning of umbilical artery catheters increases associated complications in newborn infants. N Engl J Med 299: 561–564
19. Sais OS, Rubaltalli FF, D'Elia RD (1987) Clinical and aortographic assessment of the complications of arterial catheterization. Eur J Pediatr 128: 169–179
20. Wesstrom G, Finnstrom O, Stenport G (1979) Umbilical artery catheterization in newborns. I. Thrombosis in relation to catheter type and position. Acta Pediatr Scand 68: 575–81
21. Witt I, Muller H, Kunter LJ (1969) Evidence for the existence of fetal fibrinogen. Thromb Diath Haemorrh 22: 101–109
22. Galanakis DK, Mosesson MW (1976) Evaluation of the role of in vivo proteolysis (fibrinogenolysis) in prolonging the thrombin time of human umbilical cord fibrinogen. Blood 48: 109–118
23. Greffe BS, Manco-Johnson MJ, Marlar RA (1988) Molecular differences in the forms of fetal protein C (abstr). Pediatr Res 23: 463A
24. Weinstein MJ, Blanchard R, Moake JL, Vosburgh E, Moise K (1989) Fetal and neonatal von Willebrand factor (vWF) is unusually large and similar to the vWF in patients with thrombotic thrombocytopenic purpura. Br J Haematol 72: 68–72
25. Lammle B, Griffin JH (1985) Formation of the fibrin clot: The balance of procoagulant and inhibitory factors. Clinics in Haematol 14: 281–343
26. Schmidt B, Ofosu FA, Mitchell L, Brooker L, Andrew M (1989) Anticoagulant effects of heparin in neonatal plasma. Pediatr Res 25: 405–408
27. Vieira A, Ofosu A, Andrew M (1989) Heparin sensitivity and resistance in the newborn: an explanation. Pediatr Res 25: 274A

28. Andrew M, Schmidt B, Mitchell L, Paes B, Ofosu F (1990) Thrombin generation in newborn plasma is critically dependant on the concentration of prothrombin. Thromb Haemostas 63: 27–30
29. Schmidt B, Mitchell L, Ofosu FA, Andrew M (1989) Alpha–2–macroglobulin is an important progressive inhibitor of thrombin in neonatal and infant plasma. Thromb Haemostas 62: 1074–1077
30. Holmer E, Mattson C, Nilsson S (1982) Anticoagulant and antithrombotioc effects of heparin and low molecular weight heparin fragments in rabbits. Thromb Res 25: 475–85
31. Fernandez FA, Buchanan MR, Hirsh J, Fenton JW, Ofosu FA (1987) Catalysis of thrombin inhibition provides an index for estimating the antithrombotic potential of glyucosminoglycans in rabbits. Thromb Hemostas 57: 286–293
32. Bachman F (1987) Fibrinolysis In: Verstraete M, Vermylen J, Lijen R, Arnout J (eds) Thrombosis and Hemostasis. Leuven University Press, Leuven pp 227–265
33. Corrigan JJ, Sleeth JJ, Jeter M, Lox CD (1989) Newborn's fibrinolytic mechanism: Components and plasmin generation. Am J Hematol 32: 273–278
34. Hemker HC (1987) The mode of action of heparin in plasma. In: Verstraete M, Vermylen J, Lijnen R, AnRout J (eds) Thrombosis and Hemostasis. Leuven University Press, Leuven, pp 17–36
35. Ofosu FA, Blajchman MA, Modi GJ, Smith LM, Buchanan MR, Hirsh J (1985) The importance of thrombin inhibition for the expression of the anticoagulant activities of heparin, dermatan sulphate, low molecular weight heparin and pentosan polysulphate. Br J Hematol 60: 695–704
36. Ofosu FA, Sie P, Modi GJ, Fernandez F, Buchanan MR, Blajchman MA, Boneu B, Hirsh J (1987) The inhibition of thrombin dependent feed-back reactions is critical to the expression of the anticoagulant effect of heparin. Biochem J 243: 579–588
37. Hull RD, Raskob G, Hirsh J (1986) Continuous intravenous heparin compared to intermittent subcutaneous heparin in the initial treatment of proximal vein thrombosis. New Engl J Med 315: 1109–1114
38. Levine MN, Hirsh J (1986) Hemorrhagic complications of anticoagulant therapy. Semin Thromb Hemostas 12: 39–62
39. Schmidt B, Mitchell L, Ofosu F, Andrew M (1988) Standard assays underestimate the concentration of heparin in neonatal plasma. J Lab Clin Med 112: 641–643
40. Carter CJ, Kelton JG, Hirsh J, Cerskus A, Santos AV, Gent M (1982) The relationship between the hemorrhagic and antithrombotic properties of a low molecular weight heparin in rabbits. Blood 59: 1239–45
41. Thomas DP, Merton RE, Lewis WE, Barrowcliffe TW (1981) Studies in man and experimental animals of a low molecular weight heparin fraction. Thromb Hemostas 45: 214–218
42. Andriuolo G, Mastacchi R, Barbanti M, Sarret M (1985) Comparison of the antithrombotic and hemorrhagic effects of heparin and a new low molecular weight heparin in rats. Hemostas 15: 324–330
43. Turpie AGG, Levine MW, Hirsh J, Carter C, Jay RM, Powers PJ, Andrew M, Hull RD, Gent M (1986) A randomized controlled trial of a low molecular weight heparin (Enoxaparin) to prevent deep vein thrombosis in patients undergoing elective hip surgery. New Engl J Med 315: 925–29
44. Planes A, Vochelle N, Mansat C (1987) Prevention of deep vein thrombosis after total hip replacement by enozaparin: one daily injection of 40 mg versus two daily injections of 20 mg. Thromb Hemostas (suppl 1): 415A
45. Salzman EW, Rosenberg RD, Smith MH, Lindon JN, Favreau L (1980) Effect of heparin and heparin fractions on platelet aggregation. J Clin Invest 65: 64–73
46. Heiden D, Mielke CH, Rodvien R (1977) Impairment of primary hemostasis and platelet (14C) 5–hydroxytryptamine release. Br J Hematol 36: 427–436
47. Fernandez FA, N'guiyan P, Van Ryn J, Ofosu FA, Hirsh J, Buchanan MR (1986) Hemorrhagic doses of heparin and other glygosaminoglycans induce a platelet defect. Thromb Res 43: 491–495

48. Johnson EA, Kirkwood TBL, Stirling Y, Perez-Requejo JL, Ingram GIC, Bangham DR, Brozovic M (1976) Four heparin preparations: anti Xa potentiating effects of heparin after subcutaneous injection. Thromb Hemostas 35: 586–91
49. Vieira A, Ofosu F, Andrew M (1990) Heparin sensitivity and resistance. An explanation. Thromb Haemostas (submitted)
50. Massicotte-Nolan P, Mitchell L, Andrew M (1986) A comparative study of coagulation systems in newborn animals. Pediatr Res 20: 961–965
51. Bara L, Billaud E, Gramond G, Kher A, Samama M (1985) Comparative pharmacokinetics (PK 10169) and unfractionated heparin after intravenous and subcutaneous administration. Thromb Res 39: 631–36
52. De Swart CAM, Nijmeyer B, Roelofs JMM, Sixma JJ (1982) Kinetics of intravenously administered heparin in normal humans. Blood 60: 1251–1258
53. Bratt G, Tornebohm E, Lockner D, Bergstrom K (1988) A human pharmacological study comparing conventional heparin and a low molecular weight heparin fragment. Thromb Hemostas 53: 208–11
54. Boneu B, Caranobe C, Gabaig AM, Dupouy D, Sie P (1987) Evidence for a saturable mechanism of disappearance of standard heparin in rabbits. Thromb Res 46: 835–844
55. Barzu T, Molho P, Tobelem G, Petitou M, Caen JP (1984) Binding of heparin and low molecular weight heparin fragments to human vascular endothelial cells in culture. Nou Rev Fran Hematol 26: 243–247
56. Hiebert LM, Jaques LB (1976) The observation of heparin on endothelium after injection. Thromb Res 8: 195–204
57. Barzu T, Van Rijn JLML, Petitou M, Molho P, Tobelem G, Caen J (1986) Endothelial binding sites for heparin specificity and role in heparin neutralization. Biochem J 238: 847–854
58. Palm M, Mattsson C (1987) Pharmacokinetics of heparin and low molecular weight fragment (fragmin) in rabbits with impaired renal or metabolic clearance. Thromb Hemostas 58: 932–935
59. Boneu B, Buchanan MR, Caranobe C, Gabaig AM, Dupouy D, Sie P, Hirsh J (1987) The disappearance of a low molecular weight heparin fraction (CY216) differs from standard heparin in rabbits. Thromb Res 46: 845–853
60. Schmidt B, Buchanan MR, Ofosu F, Brooker L, Hirsh J, Andrew M (1988) Antithrombotic properties of heparin in a neonatal piglet model of thrombin induced thrombosis. Thromb Hemostas 60: 289–292
61. Andrew M, Brooker L, Weitz J (1989) Fibrin clot lysis by thrombolytic agents is impaired in the newborn. XIIth International Congress on Thromb and Hemostas, Tokyo, Japan 62: 288A

1.13 Regulatory Mechanisms Controlling Prothrombin and the Development of Blood Coagulation Factors During Gestation

C. Thomas Kisker, David Bohlken, Stanley Perlman, Ann Louise Olson, Jean Robillard, and William Clarke[1]

Disorders of blood coagulation are common in newborn infants. Major hemorrhage or thrombosis was found in 40% of neonatal deaths in one survey and intraventricular hemorrhage was detected in 26% of 101 autopsies of newborn infants in another [1,2]. Thus, problems related to hemorrhage and/or thrombosis play a major role in the mortality of newborn infants, particularly premature infants. The relationship between the increased risk for hemorrhage and thrombosis and abnormalities of blood coagulation is unclear. Decreased levels of blood coagulation factor activities in the newborn are less easily defined because the range of normal in the newborn is greater than in the adult and low levels of a number of blood coagulation factor activities based upon adult standards are present even in normal full-term newborns. Furthermore, the levels of many coagulation factors (including prothrombin and factors VII, IX, and X) differ depending on the gestational age of the infant with the lowest levels found in premature infants.

Changes in the levels of prothrombin activity during gestation are similar to the changes in other coagulation factors [3]. Understanding the regulatory controls governing prothrombin development therefore should provide information helpful to understanding the overall development of hemostasis and to better evaluate the increased risks of thrombosis and hemorrhage in the newborn.

To study the normal development of prothrombin and other blood coagulation factor activities in a growing fetus, a fetal lamb model has been developed. This model allows serial blood samples to be obtained from fetuses during the third trimester of pregnancy and following delivery [4]. Studies using this fetal lamb model in our laboratory and others have demonstrated close similarities in the developmental patterns of a number of blood coagulation factor activities throughout gestation and at delivery when compared to those present in humans [4,5]. These studies have indicated that as the fetus matures it is able to produce

[1]University of Iowa Hospitals and Clinics, Department of Pediatrics, Iowa City, IA 52242, USA

all of the components of the coagulation system. Furthermore, the levels of the coagulation factor activities gradually increase with increasing gestational age. For example, the activities of the vitamin K-dependent coagulation factors, including prothrombin and factors VII, IX and X, are significantly below adult levels early in the last trimester of pregnancy (prothrombin, 30%; factor VII, 55%; factor IX, 27%; and factor X, 29%). Prothrombin, factor VII, and fibrinogen show a slight decrease in activity midway through the last trimester. Factors VIII, XI, XII, and XIII as well as prothrombin and factors VII, IX, and X then gradually increase throughout the remainder of the last trimester though many remain below adult levels even at term (factor II, 66%; factor VII, 80%; factor IX, 61%; and factor X, 65%). Additional studies by Andrew and coworkers have indicated that the process of birth itself does not contribute to the low levels of coagulation factors found in the newborns [5]. Studies in our laboratory indicated that the birth process of labor and delivery may even accelerate the production factors VIII and IX [4].

Prothrombin is synthesized as a single polypeptide chain, requires vitamin K for post-translational gamma carboxylation, and has a pattern of development similar to many other coagulation factors synthesized by the liver [4]. The regulatory mechanisms controlling the levels of prothrombin and other coagulation factors during gestation are, however, largely unexplored. To determine if the normal developmental changes in prothrombin are the result of changes in prothrombin protein concentration or changes in the specific activity of prothrombin, prothrombin antigen levels were measured using the method of Laurell in 174 samples from 25 normal fetal lambs during the last trimester of pregnancy and following spontaneous delivery. As Fig. 1 indicates, the levels of prothrombin antigen are significantly below adult levels during gestation and increase in an age-dependent pattern similar to prothrombin activity levels as presented in Fig. 2. These parallel developmental patterns do not indicate signif-

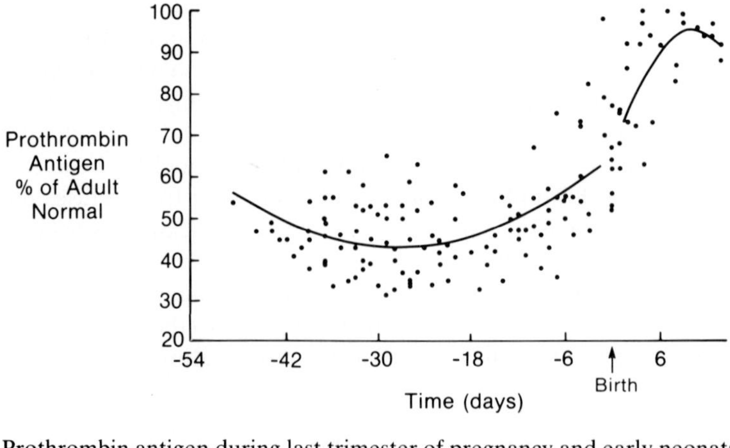

Fig. 1. Prothrombin antigen during last trimester of pregnancy and early neonatal period in 10 lamb fetuses

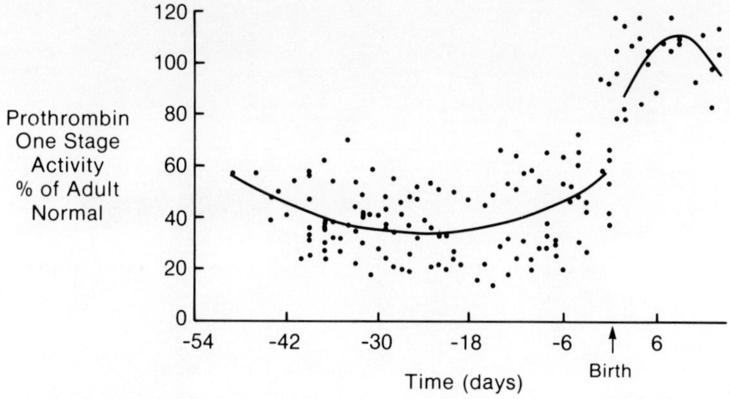

Fig. 2. Prothrombin activity during last trimester of pregnancy and early neonatal period in 10 lamb fetuses

icant changes in the specific activity of prothrombin during fetal and early neonatal development. The parallel increases in prothrombin antigen and activity could be related to increases in the quantity of prothrombin mRNA transcribed from the prothrombin gene, more rapid processing or increased stability of the mRNA transcripts, an increased rate of translation of prothrombin mRNA, an increased rate of post-translational processing of the protein, an increased transport and/or secretion of processed prothrombin, and/or an increased circulating half-life of prothrombin.

To determine the step in the biosynthetic pathway at which regulation occurs, mRNA was prepared from fetal, newborn, and adult sheep liver samples and

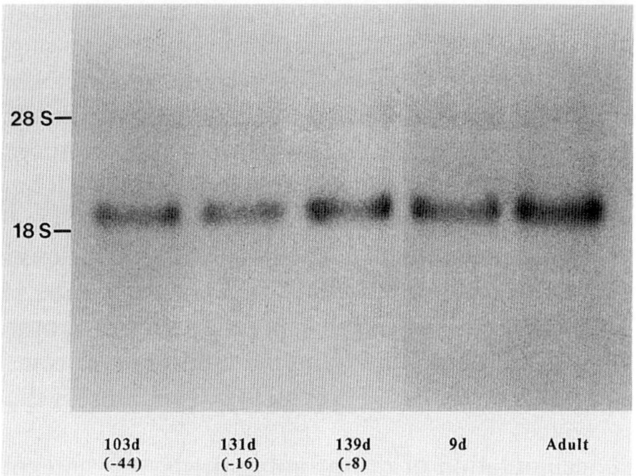

Fig. 3. Autoradiograph of Northern blot of liver RNA samples from fetal, 9-day-old newborn, and adult animals, hybridized to antisense β-actin mRNA. *d*, days; *S*, Svedberg units

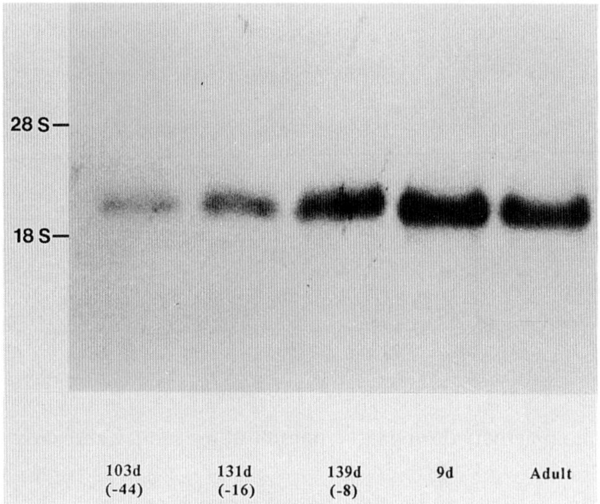

Fig. 4. Autoradiograph of Northern blot of liver RNA samples from fetal, 9-day-old, and adult animals, hybridized to antisense prothrombin mRNA. *d*, days; *S*, Svedberg units

analyzed by both slot blot and Northern blot analysis with both an antisense β-actin mRNA and an antisense prothrombin mRNA probe [6]. As shown in Fig. 3, the β-actin fraction of total mRNA remained relatively constant throughout gestation. The experiments clearly showed that there was an increased accumulation of prothrombin mRNA during gestation (Fig. 4).

It is important to note that there is no apparent difference in the molecular size of prothrombin mRNA during gestation or early neonatal development. This suggests that the differences in prothrombin antigen and activity levels during gestation are not related to the presence of a "fetal prothrombin" gene with a switch to an adult gene during late gestation and early neonatal development.

Measurements of prothrombin antigen and activity levels along with quantitation of prothrombin mRNA normalized for the amount of RNA applied to the gel or normalized to the amount of β-action mRNA present in the mRNA preparations are presented in Table 1. The quantity of prothrombin mRNA parallels the level of prothrombin antigen and activity. This parallel increase in antigen and prothrombin mRNA is also documented in Fig. 5 where the levels of prothrombin mRNA from 13 fetal and newborn lambs of various ages are superimposed on the levels of prothrombin antigen measured at the same periods of development. These findings suggest that the increases in prothrombin activity and prothrombin antigen are related to an increased rate of transcription of the prothrombin gene or to an increased processing or stability of the mRNA transcripts.

The increased accumulation of prothrombin mRNA as an explanation of the changes in prothrombin levels during gestation and early neonatal development are in contrast to the findings reported by Besmond et al. [7]. Besmond et al. studied the rates of translation of fetal and adult human prothrombin mRNAs in

Table 1. Percent of prothrombin mRNA versus prothrombin antigen activity in fetal, newborn, and adult animals

Sample	Prothrombin mRNA[a]*	Prothrombin mRNA[b]*	Prothrombin antigen*	Prothrombin activity*
Fetal (103 days)	25	26	37	28
Fetal (131 days)	41	48	47	31
Fetal (139 days)	74	94	65	55
Newborn (9 days)	100	100	97	90
Ewe	68	82	90	88

* Percentage of adult value
[a] Wormalized for amount of RNA applied to gel
[b] Wormalized for amount of β-actin mRNA present in mRNA preparation

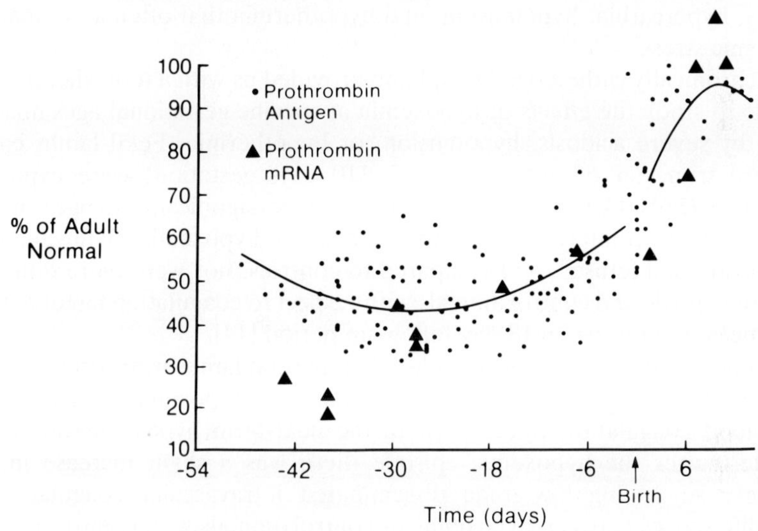

Fig. 5. Prothrombin mRNA levels (▲) superimposed on prothrombin antigen levels (•) during last trimester of pregnancy and early neonatal period. Prothrombin mRNA for individual sheep given as a percentage of adult normal

a cell-free system [7]. Their results suggested that fetal mRNA was only one-tenth as effective, thus indicating that developmental changes were related to changes in the rate of prothrombin mRNA translation rather than increased mRNA accumulation. Besmond et al.'s findings of lower molecular weight peptides synthesized by fetal as compared to adult prothrombin mRNA may indicate degradation of the fetal prothrombin mRNA during preparation. Partial degradation might also explain the decreased rate of prothrombin translation in the fetus.

The results suggesting that prothrombin synthesis is regulated at a biosynthetic step before translation will require additional measurements of the rate of transcription of the prothrombin gene as a function of gestational age and direct measures of the stability of the transcription products in fetal and adult cells.

A number of authors have reported significant changes in blood coagulation factor activities in asphyxiated infants including decreased synthesis of blood coagulation factors. For example, the studies reported by Dam et al. [8] in human infants who suffered intrauterine asphyxia showed that these infants had exceptionally low prothrombin activities. In addition, the studies by Hathaway and Henderson [9] in newborn puppies surviving prolonged periods, 18–24 h, of systemic hypoxemia demonstrated deficiencies in vitamin K-dependent factors including prothrombin and factors VII and X. Some authors have described disseminated intravascular coagulation in asphyxiated newborns [10,11], while others have found evidence of accelerated maturation of blood coagulation factors [12,13]. The variability in the results reported by different authors may reflect variations in the timing, duration, or severity of the hypoxemic episode, a variation in the maturity of the infants studied, and differences in the degree of acidosis, hypercarbia, hypotension, and hypothermia that often accompany the hypoxemic stress.

The chronically catheterized fetal lamb provided us with a tool whereby it was possible to study the effects of hypoxemia at specific gestational ages unaccompanied by severe acidosis, hypotension, or hypothermia. Fetal lambs early in the third trimester of pregnancy (107–110 days gestation) were exposed to hypoxemia (PO_2 14 mmHg/1 h). There were no significant changes in blood coagulation immediately following the exposure to hypoxemia when values from hypoxic stressed fetuses were compared to controls, nor were there differences between hypoxic and control animals with respect to coagulation factor activities when measured during an 18-day follow-up period [14].

A second study was therefore undertaken in fetal lambs near term (average 6 days prior to delivery) to determine if an episode of hypoxemia near-term might alter blood coagulation values [15]. In the near-term hypoxemic animals immediately after the hypoxemic episode there was a slight increase in fibrin monomer suggesting low-grade disseminated intravascular coagulation. No other differences between hypoxemic or control animals with regard to coagulation factor activities were seen during or 2.5 h following hypoxia. In contrast to the lack of acute changes, significant changes were apparent following delivery. Specifically, the normal post-natal increases in fibrinogen, prothrombin, and factors VII and X were significantly delayed in the hypoxic animals during the early neonatal period (Figs. 6–9). In contrast to the delayed development of fibrinogen, prothrombin, and factors VII and X; both factors VIII and IX activities were slightly but significantly increased in the hypoxemic group (Figs. 10 and 11). These findings are similar to those of Hathaway et al. [12] and Perlman and Dvilansky [16] in human infants with fetal distress and indicate that hypoxemia near-term in the absence of severe acidosis, hypotension, or hypothermia can result in a delay in the normal post-natal development of prothrombin activity as well as abnormalities in the development of other hemostatic factors. Since both factor IX and prothrombin are dependent on vitamin K and the development of factor IX activity was accelerated and prothrombin delayed, an abnormality in vitamin K metabolism is not a probable cause for these abnormalities. The precise mechanism responsible for these abnormalities is unknown at present.

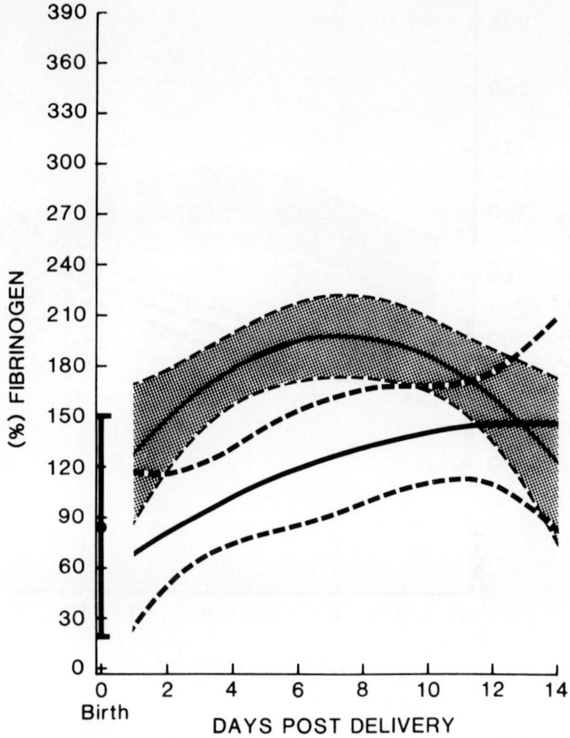

Fig. 6. Mean ± 1 SD of fibrinogen values on 14 control animals within 24 h of delivery (*bar*). *Thin dashed lines* and *shaded area* indicate regression curve and 95% confidence limits obtained on samples from the 14 control animals during 14 days after birth. *Heavy dashed lines* and *open area* indicate regression curve and 95% confidence limits obtained on samples from 6 hypoxemic animals during 14 days after birth. Groups are significantly different ($P = 0.02$)

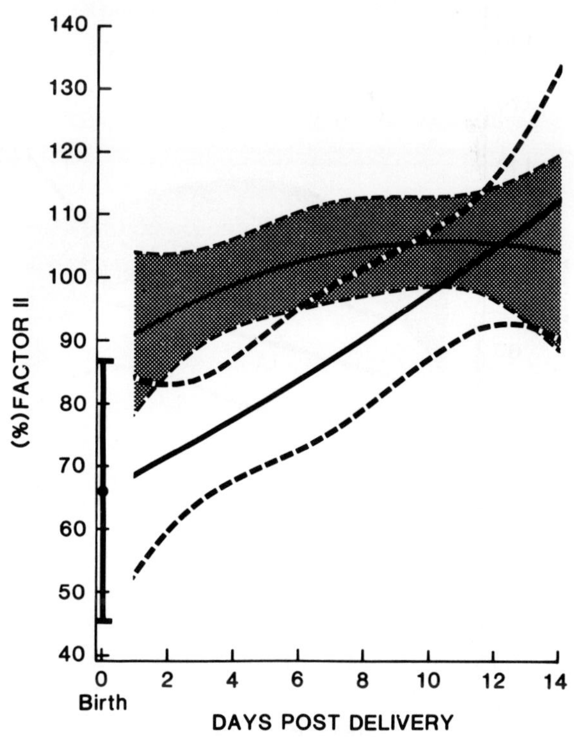

Fig. 7. Mean ± 1 SD of prothrombin values on 14 control animals within 24 h of delivery (*bar*). *Thin dashed lines* and *shaded area* indicate regression curve and 95% confidence limits obtained on samples from the 14 control animals during 14 days after birth. *Heavy dashed lines* and *open area* indicate regression curve and 95% confidence limits obtained on samples from 6 hypoxemic animals during 14 days after birth. Groups are significantly different ($P = 0.01$)

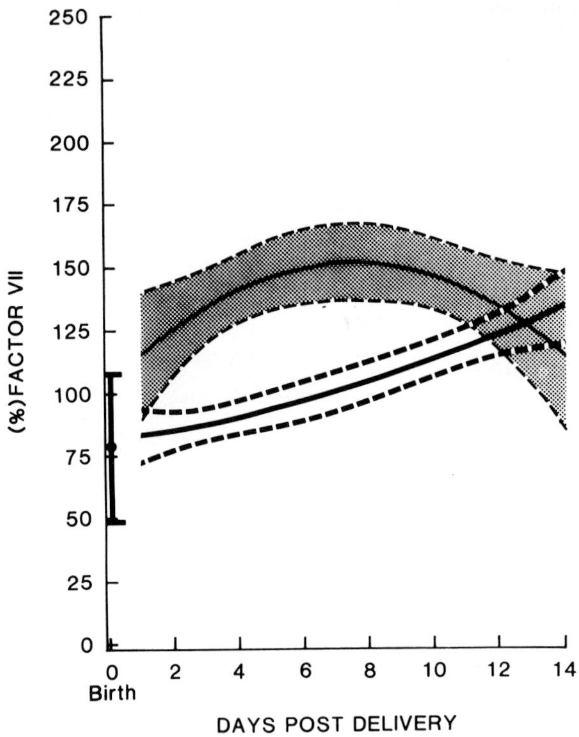

Fig. 8. Mean ± 1 SD of factor VII values on 14 control animals within 24 h of delivery (*bar*). *Thin dashed lines* and *shaded area* indicate regression curve and 95% confidence limits obtained on samples from the 14 control animals during 14 days after birth. *Heavy dashed lines* and *open area* indicate regression curve and 95% confidence limits obtained on samples from 6 hypoxemic animals during 14 days after birth. Groups are significantly different ($P = 0.01$)

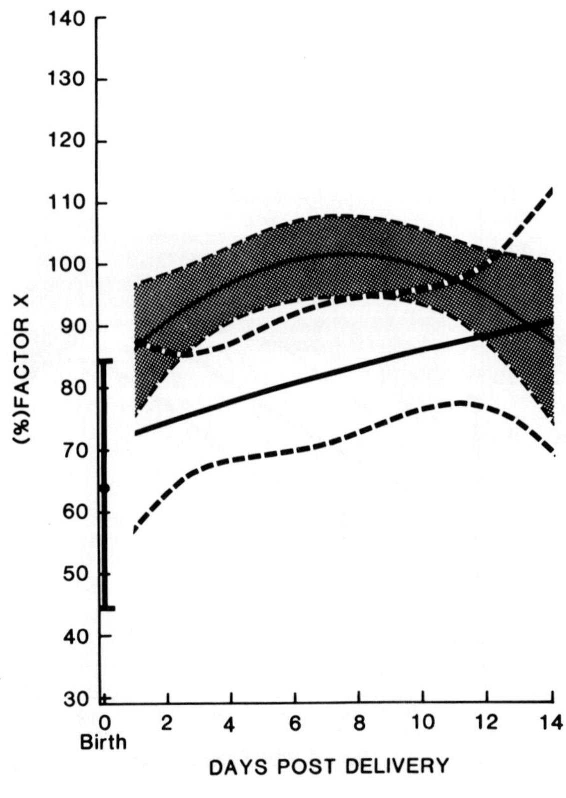

Fig. 9. Mean ± 1 SD of factor X values on 14 control animals within 24 h of delivery (*bar*). *Thin dashed lines* and *shaded area* indicate regression curve and 95% confidence limits obtained on samples from the 14 control animals during 14 days after birth. *Heavy dashed lines* and *open area* indicate regression curve and 95% confidence limits obtained on samples from 6 hypoxemic animals during 14 days after birth. Groups are significantly different ($P = 0.01$)

Fig. 10. Mean ± 1 SD of factor VIII values on 14 control animals within 24 h of delivery (*bar*). *Thin dashed lines* and *shaded area* indicate regression curve and 95% confidence limits obtained on samples from the 14 control animals during 14 days after birth. *Heavy dashed lines* and *open area* indicate regression curve and 95% confidence limits obtained on samples from 6 hypoxemic animals during 14 days after birth. Groups are significantly different ($P = 0.01$)

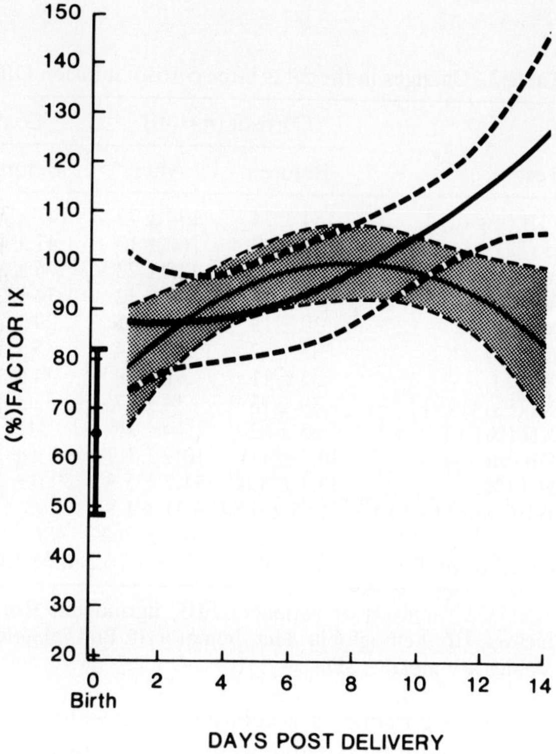

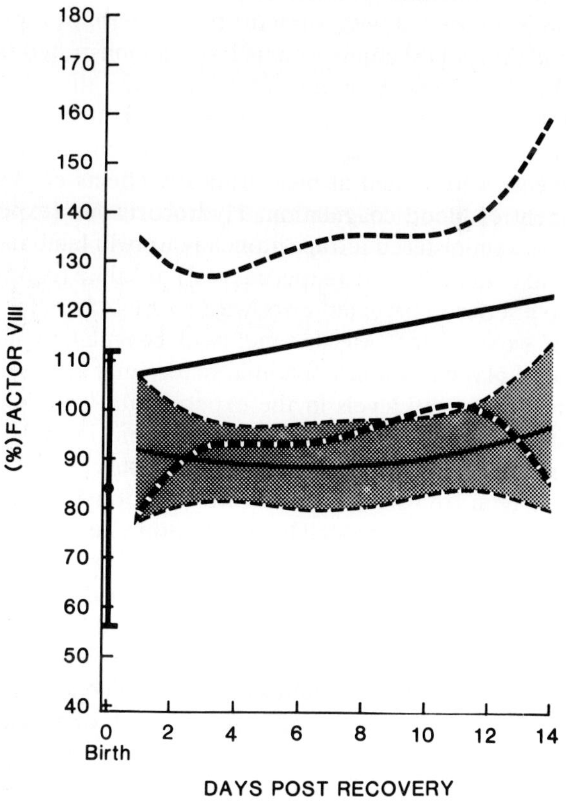

Fig. 11. Mean ± 1 SD of factor IX values on 14 control animals within 24 h of delivery (*bar*). *Thin dashed lines* and *shaded area* indicate regression curve and 95% confidence limits obtained on samples from the 14 control animals during 14 days after birth. *Heavy dashed lines* and *open area* indicate regression curve and 95% confidence limits obtained on samples from 6 hypoxemic animals during 14 days after birth. Groups are significantly different ($P = 0.01$)

Table 2. Changes in the fetus after cortisol infusion (10 sets of twins)

Test	Cortisol ($n = 10$) Before	Cortisol ($n = 10$) After	Control ($n = 10$) Before	Control ($n = 10$) After	ANOVA (P)
FIB (mg/dl)	154 ± 74	194 ± 73	147 ± 67	160 ± 62	NS
II (%)	44 ± 7	60 ± 13	47 ± 10	48 ± 11	0.001
V (%)	73 ± 15	125 ± 23	75 ± 27	91 ± 34	0.005
VII (%)	62 ± 21	88 ± 32	74 ± 21	73 ± 21	0.012
VIII (%)	30 ± 13	36 ± 25	29 ± 10	35 ± 13	NS
IX (%)	33 ± 7	47 ± 14	35 ± 12	36 ± 9	0.003
X (%)	35 ± 11	61 ± 19	44 ± 14	44 ± 16	0.001
XI (%)	39 ± 18	38 ± 17	35 ± 13	38 ± 14	NS
XII (%)	35 ± 12	44 ± 15	34 ± 9	35 ± 12	NS
Hb (gm/dl)	10.1 ± 1.4	10.9 ± 1.7	8.9 ± 1.2	10.1 ± 2.4	NS
Hct (%)	33.1 ± 4.0	34.7 ± 5.3	30.0 ± 2.2	32.5 ± 7.8	NS
WBC/mm^3 (×10^3)	2.55 ± 0.84	4.31 ± 1.8	2.96 ± 1.18	2.99 ± 1.11	0.05
Plat/mm^3 (×10^3)	488 ± 230	615 ± 360	486 ± 206	536 ± 250	NS
Cortisol (μl/dl)	0.7 ± 0.5	33.8 ± 16.2	0.65 ± 0.4	1.4 ± 0.9	0.001

ANOVA, analysis of variance; FIB, figrinogen; Roman numerals, blood coagulation factors; Hb, hemoglobin; Hct, hematocrit; Plat, platelets
Values are mean ± SD.

Were it possible to accelerate the development of blood coagulation in the fetus, it might be possible to prevent the increased risks of bleeding and thrombosis associated with immaturity and perhaps asphyxia. Studies by Liggins [17] and Avery [18] among others have demonstrated that glucocorticoids accelerate the development of the fetal lung. We therefore undertook experiments in fetal lambs of 120 days gestation, a period early in the third trimester in which the levels of coagulation factor activities are relatively stable [19]. These experiments were aimed at measuring the effects of glucocorticoids on the development of blood coagulation. Hydrocortisone (experimental) or saline (control) was administered intraperitoneally to twin lamb pairs in one set of experiments, and betamethasone (experimental) or saline (control) was given intramuscularly to a series of pregnant ewes with fetuses of similar gestational age in another set of experiments. Measurements of coagulation factor activities were done on fetal plasma samples obtained before and after glucocorticoid stimulation. The factor activity levels in the experimental and control animals were then compared. Significant increases were found in the levels of prothrombin activity and in the levels of the activities of factors V, VII, IX, and X in the plasma from the fetal lambs given direct infusions of hydrocortisone or receiving glucocorticoids indirectly through betamethasone treatment of their mothers (Tables 2 and 3).

Recent experiments measuring the levels of prothrombin messenger RNA in the livers of the glucocorticoid stimulated fetuses have suggested that the levels of messenger RNA increase in parallel with the increases in prothrombin activity [20]. Whether these increases are a reflection of increased transcription of the prothrombin gene or increased stability of prothrombin message is at present unclear.

Table 3. Changes in the fetus after *B*-methasone injections of pregnant ewes

Test	*B*-Methasone ($n = 6$)		Control ($n = 5$)		ANOVA (*P*)
	Before	After	Before	After	
FIB (mg/dl)	224 ± 218	268 ± 241	212 ± 165	221 ± 192	NS
II (%)	39 ± 5	60 ± 16	38 ± 11	36 ± 8	0.004
V (%)	79 ± 43	126 ± 32	70 ± 29	68 ± 29	0.014
VII (%)	77 ± 37	110 ± 47	72 ± 13	70 ± 16	0.001
VIII (%)	38 ± 18	38 ± 24	38 ± 15	40 ± 19	NS
IX (%)	39 ± 16	57 ± 36	39 ± 25	36 ± 19	0.052
X (%)	32 ± 11	61 ± 25	34 ± 13	34 ± 13	0.004
XI (%)	47 ± 38	46 ± 38	44 ± 21	44 ± 22	NS
XII (%)	37 ± 14	50 ± 29	39 ± 23	38 ± 19	NS
Hb (gm/dl)	10.4 ± 4	10.5 ± 0.3	10.7 ± 2.0	10.3 ± 1.2	NS
Hct (%)	33.8 ± 1.3	32.2 ± 3.3	33.8 ± 6.6	34.2 ± 6.4	NS
WBC/mm^3 ($\times 10^3$)	2.4 ± 2.9	2.7 ± 2.9	3.75 ± 3.0	3.05 ± 0.9	NS
Plat/mm^3 ($\times 10^3$)	467 ± 165	440 ± 76	353 ± 299	352 ± 56	NS

ANOVA, analysis of variance; FIB, fibrinogen; Roman numerals, blood coagulation factors; Hb, hemoglobin; Hct, hematocrit; Plat, platelets
Values are mean ± SD

Our understanding of the biosynthetic steps regulating the development of blood coagulation factors in the fetus and newborn has increased during the past few years as a result of the development of animal models and the adaptation of newer techniques in molecular biology to probe these developmental questions. Future clarification of unresolved issues regarding normal development and the factors that influence this development should help reduce the increased risks of hemorrhage and thrombosis in the fetus and newborn.

Summary. Prothrombin is known to be developmentally regulated. The fetal lamb has provided a model whereby the molecular mechanisms controlling prothrombin development can be studied. Experiments in our laboratory have indicated that the increases in prothrombin activity during gestation are reflected in increases of both prothrombin antigen levels and in liver cell prothrombin messenger RNA. We have also demonstrated increases in prothrombin activity, antigen, and messenger RNA during fetal development following the administration of glucocorticoids to the fetus. Finally near term fetal hypoxia delays the normal post natal development of prothrombin activity in the newborn lamb similar to findings in human newborns following fetal distress.

Acknowledgment. This work was supported by NIH Grant #5R01 HL39097-03 for regulatory mechanisms of prothrombin development.

References

1. Hathaway WE (1970) Coagulation problems in the newborn infant. In: Behrman R (ed) The pediatric clinics of North America, vol 17. Saunders, Philadelphia, pp 929–942
2. Valdes-Dapena MA, Arey JB (1970) The causes of neonatal mortality: An analysis of 501 autopsies on newborn infants. J Pediatr 77: 366
3. Hathaway WE, Bonnar J (1978) Physiology of coagulation in the fetus and newborn infant. In: Oliver T (series ed) Perinatal coagulation: Monographs in neonatology. Grune and Stratton, New York
4. Kisker CT, Robillard JE, Clarke WR (1981) Development of blood coagulation: A fetal lamb model. Pediatr Res 15: 1045–1050
5. Andrew M, O'Brodovich H, Mitchell L (1988) Fetal lamb coagulation system during normal birth. Am J Hematol 28: 116–118
6. Kisker CT, Perlman S, Bohlken D, Wicklund B (1988) Measurement of prothrombin mRNA during gestation and early neonatal development. J Lab Clin Med 112: 407–412
7. Besmond C, Benarous R, Kahn A (1981) Cell free synthesis of human prothrombin: immunological characterization of the translation product. Biochem Biophys Res Commun 103: 587–594
8. Dam H, Dyggve H, Larsen H, Plum P (1952) The relation of vitamin K deficiency to hemorrhagic disease of the newborn. Adv Pediatr 5: 129
9. Hathaway WE, Henderson BJ (1968) Effect of hypoxia on coagulation factors in newborn dogs. Biol Neonate 13: 26
10. Chadd MA, Elwood PC, Gray OP, Muxworthy SM (1971) Coagulation defects in hypoxic full-term newborn infants. Br Med J 4: 516
11. Chessells JM, Wigglesworth JS (1971) Coagulation studies in severe birth asphyxia. Arch Dis Child 46: 253
12. Hathaway WE, Mahasandana C, Makowski EL (1975) Cord blood coagulation studies in infants of high-risk pregnant women. Am J Obstet Gynecol 121: 51
13. Thomas DB (1975) Prenatal stress, hyaline membrane disease, and coagulation factors in low birthweight babies. Aust Paediatr J 11: 26
14. Kisker CT, Robillard JE, Clarke WR (1982) Blood coagulation changes after hypoxemia: A fetal lamb model. Pediatr Res 16: 8–12
15. Kisker CT, Robillard JE, Clarke WR (1982) Blood coagulation changes following hypoxemia in the near-term fetal lamb. Pediatr Res 16: 732–739
16. Perlman M, Dvilansky A (1975) Blood coagulation status of small-for-dates and postmature infants. Arch Dis Child 50: 424
17. Liggins GC (1969) Premature delivery of fetal lambs infused with glucocorticoids. J Endocrinol 45: 515
18. Avery ME (1975) Pharmacologic approach to the acceleration of fetal lung maturation. Br Med Bull 31: 13
19. Kisker CT, Robillard JE, Bohlken DP (1983) Glucocorticoid stimulation of blood coagulation factor activities in the fetal lamb. J Lab Clin Med 101: 569–575
20. Olson AL, Perlman S, Kisker CT (1989) Cortisol-stimulated prothrombin gene expression during gestation. (abstract) Clin Res 37: 938A

1.14 Neonatal Thrombosis:

A Critical Appraisal of the Available Evidence on Prevention, Diagnosis, and Treatment*

BARBARA SCHMIDT and MAUREEN ANDREW[1]

Introduction

Thrombotic disease in newborn infants is common and serious enough to require effective and safe prevention and treatment [1]. However, thrombotic disease in newborns is also sufficiently rare to prompt anecdotal observations rather than controlled clinical trials. While there is an abundance of case reports in the pediatric literature, there is a conspicuous paucity of well-designed studies [2]. As a result, consensus about the appropriate prophylaxis and management of neonatal thrombosis is lacking [2]. In this article, we will examine the available evidence on the efficacy and safety of heparin prophylaxis in infants with indwelling umbilical artery catheters. We will also review the management of symptomatic thrombosis, using aortic thrombosis as an example. We begin with a description of the framework which will be used to assess the strength of evidence that supports current approaches to neonatal thrombosis.

Rules of Evidence

Clinical investigators of adult cardiovascular diseases have made considerable progress through a series of randomized studies which enabled them to formulate firm recommendations on the prevention and treatment of disorders such as venous thrombosis and pulmonary embolism [3]. A working group, sponsored by the American College of Chest Physicians and the National Heart, Lung and Blood Institute, recently adopted rules of evidence on the use of antithrombotic agents in adult patients [4]. It was agreed that the strongest evidence is provided

*Reproduced in part from the *Journal of Pediatrics* 113: 407–410, 1988 with permission of The C.V. Mosby Company.

[1]Department of Pediatrics, Room 3N11G, McMaster University Medical Centre, 1200 Main Street West, Hamilton, Ontario L8N 3Z5, Canada

by randomized clinical trials with low false-positive and low false-negative errors [4]. A low false-positive error means there is only a small risk of concluding that treatment A is significantly better than treatment B when, in truth, it is not. A low false-negative error reduces the risk of concluding that treatment A is no better than treatment B when, in truth, it is. High-quality, controlled trials are sufficiently large and powerful to demonstrate a clinically important treatment benefit, if it exists. In contrast, randomized trials with high false-positive and high false-negative errors generate less convincing evidence which cannot be used to make firm treatment recommendations [4]. Nonrandomized trials with concurrent or historical controls rank lower still, since the assessment of the treatment response is inevitably biased [4]. The weakest evidence possible is provided by case reports and case series with no controls [4]. Such anecdotal evidence for the efficacy of treatment can only be convincing in diseases which, if untreated, are unequivocally fatal. Neonatal thrombosis is not one of those disorders.

Prevention of Catheter-Associated Thrombosis

The Problem

Thrombotic complications in sick newborns are frequently iatrogenic, induced by intravascular catheters [1]. Probably due to its popularity, the umbilical artery catheter dominates the literature on catheter-related thrombotic complications in the neonate. Although the incidence of severe symptomatic vessel obstruction in infants undergoing umbilical artery catheterization has not been studied prospectively, considerable amounts of data have been accumulated on the development of catheter-associated thrombi which remain clinically silent. Such thrombi have been detected at autopsy or during prospective contrast angiography in asymptomatic infants with an umbilical artery catheter in place; of 942 autopsies reported in a total of 10 pathologic studies, between 3% and 59% of the cases in each series had evidence of catheter-related thrombosis [5–14]. Two hundred and thirty-seven asymptomatic infants underwent contrast angiography in six studies altogether. Thrombosis was demonstrated in 10%–95% of cases, with a mean of 38% [15–20]. This high incidence of catheter-associated thrombosis has provided the rationale for the use of heparin prophylaxis to prevent thrombus formation and prolong catheter patency.

Efficacy of Heparin Prophylaxis

According to a recent survey, low doses of heparin are added to the infusate of umbilical artery catheters in 74% of 117 American nurseries [21]. There is strong evidence from one double-blind randomized trial that the continuous infusion of low-dose heparin prolongs the patency of umbilical artery catheters [22] (Table 1). Supportive evidence comes from three open trials in which the assessment of catheter patency was made with prior knowledge of the treatment allocation [23–25] (Table 1). None of the four studies had sufficient power to confirm or

Table 1. Demonstrated benefits and risks of heparin prophylaxis for umbilical artery catheters

Strength of evidence	Source of evidence	Efficacy		Safety
		Prolongation of catheter patency	Prevention of thrombosis	Risk of intracranial hemorrhage
High	Double-blind controlled trial with low false-positive error ($P < 0.05$)	Low-dose heparin[a] Rajani et al. [22]	—	—
Medium	Controlled trial with higher false-positive error ($P \geq 0.05$) or unblinded trial	Low-dose heparin David et al. [23] Bosque and Weaver [24] Horgan et al. [25]	High-dose heparin[b] Manco-Johnson et al. (personal communication)	—
Low	Case-control study	—	—	Lesko et al[c] [27]

[a] Low-dose heparin: < 200 U/kg/day
[b] High-dose heparin: 480–600 U/kg/day
[c] Median heparin dose: < 50 U/kg/day

refute a 50% reduction in catheter associated thrombosis [26] (Table 1). We did not attempt to perform a meta-analysis of these inconclusive trials because the diagnostic tests used to detect thrombi differed too much between studies (contrast angiography, ultrasonography, or clinical examination only). Whether low doses of heparin reduce catheter associated thrombus formation remains thus to be tested in a blinded and controlled trial with sufficient sample size to demonstrate a clinically important treatment benefit, should it exist.

Manco-Johnson et al. (personal communication) examined the effects of higher heparin doses on the incidence of catheter induced thrombosis. They conducted a trial in which infants with umbilical artery catheters were randomized to receive either 20–25 units/kg/h of heparin, or the conventional 1–2 units/ml. Seven of 25 infants in the low-dose heparin group developed thrombi which were detected by aortography and/or ultrasound, while only 1 of 20 infants in the high-dose heparin group had evidence of thrombosis ($P = 0.05$) (personal communication, June 1987). These results suggest that high doses of heparin may prevent asymptomatic catheter-induced thrombosis. However, the risk/benefit ratio of heparin in immature infants remains to be determined (Table 1).

Safety of Heparin Prophylaxis

Recently, Lesko et al. implicated heparin as a risk factor for intracranial hemorrhage in low birth weight infants [27]. Although the evidence provided against heparin in this retrospective case-control study is not very strong, the authors' hypothesis is plausible and needs to be tested in a prospective controlled clinical trial.

Management of Neonatal Aortic Thrombosis

In order to appraise the current approach to symptomatic thrombosis in the newborn infant, we reviewed all reports on aortic thrombosis published in English between 1975 and 1987 (references available on request). Aortic thrombosis is one of the more common and serious forms of neonatal thrombotic disease, which develops both spontaneously and as an iatrogenic complication of invasive monitoring. We were able to find 29 articles describing clinical and/or postmortem findings in 80 different newborns [2]. All published reports were anecdotal and therefore provide the weakest evidence possible.

Diagnosis

Figure 1 illustrates how the diagnosis of aortic thrombosis was made. Almost a quarter of all patients were not diagnosed during life. Two infants were operated on for presumed coarctation. Of the remaining infants, less than one third underwent contrast angiography, the reference test or "gold standard" for the diagnosis of large vessel obstruction. Forty percent of patients were treated solely on the basis of noninvasive imaging techniques, such as two-dimensional ultra-

Fig. 1. Diagnosis of aortic thrombosis in 80 newborn infants, reported in English between 1975 and 1987

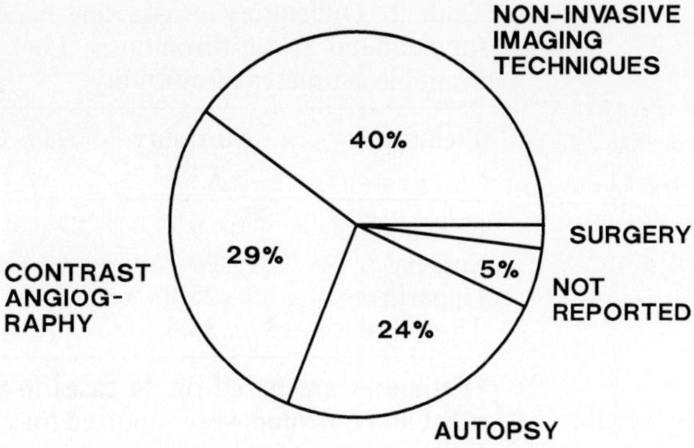

sonography (Fig. 1). However, while some of these noninvasive techniques may be very useful for the initial diagnosis as well as the follow-up of neonatal aortic thrombosis, their diagnostic efficacy remains unproven. The sensitivity and specificity of any new and promising imaging technique should be determined in a broad spectrum of consecutive infants with suspected thrombosis. In such a study all patients should receive the reference test (contrast angiography) and the noninvasive test in question, concurrently and in an unbiased fashion [28]. Even for one of the most popular techniques, ultrasonography, this has not been done, to the best of our knowledge. Vailas et al. [29] provided some data to question the sensitivity of two-dimensional ultrasonography. These authors reported that real time ultrasonography failed to visualize an aortic thrombus in 4 out of 20 cases with suspected aortic thrombosis. Three of these cases were shown to have complete aortic obstruction by contrast angiography [29].

Treatment

Fifty-nine of 80 reported infants with aortic thrombosis were diagnosed during life. Their treatment varied considerably (Fig. 2). Surgical thrombectomy or embolectomy was performed in one out of two cases. The other patients received heparin, thrombolytic agents, or no specific antithrombotic therapy at all

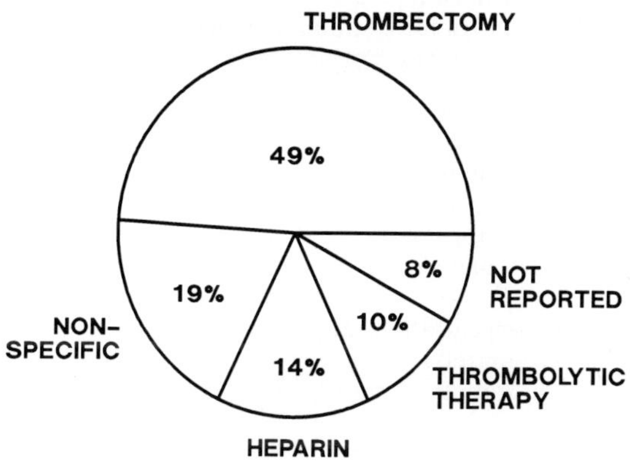

Fig. 2. Treatment of aortic thrombosis in 59 newborn infants, reported in English between 1975 and 1987

Table 2. Difficulties in assessing benefits of treatment for neonatal aortic thrombosis: Lack of confidence in available estimates of mortality[a]

Treatment	Mortality (%)	95% Confidence limits (30)
Nonspecific	9.1	0.2–41.3
Surgery	20.7	8.0–39.7
Heparin	25.0	3.2–65.1
Thrombolysis	33.3	4.3–77.7

[a]Estimates are based on 54 cases in which both treatment and outcome were reported for each individual infant.

(Fig. 2). If one compares the observed mortality rates with the different treatment approaches, one may erroneously conclude that nonspecific supportive therapy is the best therapy (Table 2). However, the 95% confidence intervals around the estimates of mortality are very large, and overlap considerably owing to the small number of cases (Table 2). More importantly, because of its anecdotal nature, the data is completely uncontrolled for confounding factors [2]. The confounding effect of "disease severity" was illustrated by Vailas et al., who categorized 20 cases of documented aortic thrombosis according to severity [29]. The only manifestation of minor thrombosis was systemic hypertension. Moderate thrombosis involved multiple signs of organ failure but preservation of a normal urine output. Major thrombosis was associated with oliguria or anuria. All infants with minor thrombosis improved without specific therapy. All infants with moderate thrombosis survived with a variety of therapies. All infants with major thrombosis died, irrespective of therapy. Table 3 summarizes patient, treatment and observer-specific confounding factors that may have biased the outcome in published case-series.

Summary. The objective of this review was to critically appraise the available evidence for the efficacy of treatment can only be convincing in diseases which,

Table 3. Difficulties in assessing benefits of treatment for neonatal aortic thrombosis: Lack of control for confounding factors

Patient	Treatment	Observer
Age of thrombus Size of thrombus	Drug dose	Reporting bias (Choice of "special" cases for publication)
Location of thrombus	Duration of drug therapy	
Severity of underlying illness	Surgical technique	
Plasma concentrations of proteins required for effective antithrombotic or thrombolytic therapy	Intensity of supportive care	

The yield of a MEDLINE literature search for articles published in English since 1975 was supplemented by additional references located in the bibliographies of listed articles. Aortic thrombosis was examined as a prototype of neonatal thrombosis. Recently adopted rules of evidence on the efficacy of antithrombotic therapy in adult patients were applied to assess the literature on the management of neonatal thrombotic disease.

For prevention of catheter-associated aortic thrombosis, there is strong evidence from controlled clinical trials that low doses of heparin prolong the patency of umbilical artery catheters. There is no good evidence that this low-dose regime also reduces catheter-associated thrombosis. Further, there is weak evidence from a case-control study that heparin, even in small doses, may be harmful to premature infants.

In diagnosis of aortic thrombosis, noninvasive imaging techniques are frequently used as definitive diagnostic tests although their reliability and validity has not been assessed adequately.

In treatment of aortic thrombosis, the risks and benefits of currently used treatment modalities are uncertain.

Acknowledgments. Dr.B. Schmidt is a Scholar of the Canadian Heart and Stroke Foundation; Dr.M. Andrew is a Career Investigator of the Canadian Heart and Stroke Foundation. This work was supported in part by Grant AN1349, the Heart and Stroke Foundation of Ontario, Canada.

References

1. Schmidt B, Zipursky A (1984) Thrombotic disease in newborn infants. Clin Perinatol 11: 461–488
2. Schmidt B, Andrew M (1988) Neonatal thrombotic disease: Prevention, diagnosis, and treatment. J Pediatr 113: 407–410
3. Hyers TM, Hull RD, Weg JG (1986) Antithrombotic therapy for venous thromboembolic disease. Summary and recommendations. Arch Intern Med 146: 467
4. Sackett DL (1986) Rules of evidence and clinical recommendations on the use of antithrombotic agents. Arch Intern Med 146: 464–465
5. Cochran WD, Davis HT, Smith CA (1968) Advantages and complications of umbilical artery catheterization in the newborn. Pediatr 42: 769–777
6. Gupta JM, Roberton NRC, Wigglesworth JS (1968) Umbilical artery catheterization in the newborn. Arch Dis Child 43: 382–387
7. Larroche JC (1970) Umbilical catheterization: its complications. Biol Neonate 16: 101–116
8. Wigger JH, Bransilver BR, Blanc WA (1970) Thrombosis due to catheterization in infants and children. J Pediatr 76: 1–11
9. Egan EA, Eitzman DV (1971) Umbilical vessel catheterization. Am J Dis Child 121: 213–218
10. Symansky MR, Fox HA (1972) Umbilical vessel catheterization: indications, management, and evaluation of the technique. J Pediatr 80: 820–826
11. Tooley WH (1972) What is the risk of an umbilical artery catheter? Pediatr 50: 1–2
12. Marsh JL, King W, Barrett C, Fonkalsrud EW (1975) Serious complications after umbilical artery catheterization for neonatal monitoring. Arch Surg 110: 1203–1208
13. Tyson JE, deSa DJ, Moore S (1976) Thromboatheromatous complications of umbilical arterial catheterization in the newborn period. Clinicopathological study. Arch Dis Child 51: 744–754

14. Joseph R, Chong A, Teh M, Wee A, Tan KL (1985) Thrombotic complication of umbilical arterial catheterization and its sequelae. Ann Acad Med Singapore 14: 576–582
15. Neal WA, Reynolds JW, Jarvis CW, Williams HJ (1972) Umbilical artery catheterization: demonstration of arterial thrombosis by aortography. Pediatr 50: 6–13
16. Goetzman BW, Stadalnik RC, Bogren HG, Blankenship WJ, Ikeda RM, Thayer J (1975) Thrombotic complications of umbilical artery catheters: a clinical and radiographic study. Pediatr 56: 374–379
17. Olinsky A, Aitken FG, Isdale JM (1975) Thrombus formation after umbilical arterial catheterization. An angiographic study. S Afr Med J 49: 1467–1470
18. Mokrohisky ST, Levine R, Blumhagen JD, Wesenberg RL, Simmons MA (1978) Low positioning of umbilical artery catheters increases associated complications in newborn infants. N Engl J Med 299: 561–564
19. Saia OS, Rubaltelli FF, D'Elia RD, Marigo A, Perale R, Audino G, Lagarjolli G, Zanardo Y, Cantarutti F (1978) Clinical and aortographic assessment of the complications of arterial catheterization. Eur J Pediatr 128: 169–179
20. Wesstrom G, Finnstrom O, Stenport G (1979) Umbilical artery catheterization in newborns. I. Thrombosis in relation to catheter type and position. Acta Paediatr Scand 68: 575–581
21. Gilhooly JT, Lindenberg JA, Reynolds JW (1986) Survey of umbilical artery catheter practices. Clin Res 34: 142A
22. Rajani K, Goetzman BW, Wennberg RP, Turner E, Abildgaard C (1979) Effect of heparinization of fluids infused through an umbilical artery catheter on catheter patency and frequency of complications. Pediatr 63: 552–556
23. David RJ, Merten DF, Anderson JC, Gross S (1981) Prevention of umbilical artery catheter clots with heparinized infusates. Dev Pharmacol Ther 2: 117–126
24. Bosque E, Weaver L (1986) Continuous versus intermittent heparin infusion of umbilical artery catheters in the newborn infant. J Pediatr 108: 141–143
25. Horgan MJ, Bartoletti A, Polansky S, Peters JC, Manning TJ, Lamont BM (1987) Effect of heparin infusates in umbilical artery catheters on frequency of thrombotic complications. J Pediatr 111: 774–778
26. Detsky AS, Sackett D (1985) When was a "negative" trial big enough? Arch Intern Med 145: 709–712
27. Lesko SM, Mitchell AA, Epstein MF, Louik C, Giacoia GP, Shapiro S (1986) Heparin use as a risk factor for intraventricular hemorrhage in low birth weight infants. N Engl J Med 314: 1156–1160
28. Hull RD, Secker-Walker RH, Hirsh J (1987) Diagnosis of deep-vein thrombosis. In: Colman RW, Hirsh J, Marder VJ, Salzman EW (eds) Hemostasis and Thrombosis. Lippincott, Philadelphia, p 1230
29. Vailas GN, Brouillette RT, Scott JP, Shkolnik A, Conway J, Wiringa K (1986) Neonatal aortic thrombosis: recent experience. J Pediatr 109: 101–108
30. Documenta Geigy: Scientific tables 6th edn (1962) Geigy Pharmaceutical, Manchester, 85–86

Part 2. Pregnancy Complicated with Coagulation Disorders

Trophoblastic Disease, Placenta, etc.

2.1 Coagulation and Fibrinolytic Activity in Trophoblastic Disease

Hiroaki Soma[1] and Hirokazu Ogawa[2]

Introduction

Trophoblastic disease can be mainly classified into hydatidiform mole, invasive mole, and choriocarcinoma. Since uterine bleeding is the most common symptom of trophoblastic disease, some patients may experience profuse bleeding after evacuation of a hydatidiform mole and bleeding from a vaginal lesion or metastatic foci of choriocarcinoma. Hydatidiform mole is one of the obstetric conditions associated with disseminated intravascular coagulation (DIC). Despite advances in the management of trophoblastic disease, hemorrhage remains a major risk in patients with trophoblastic disease. In this report, plasma concentrations of coagulation and fibrinolytic factors measured in patients with trophoblastic disease and a case report of a patient who died of DIC following chemotherapy immediately after expulsion of the mole are presented.

Materials and Methods

In 26 patients with trophoblastic disease, fibrinogen was determined according to weight methods, and fibrinogen degradation product (FDP) was assayed by latex hemagglutinin technique. Plasminogen, α_1-antitrypsin (α_1-AT), α_2-macroglobulin (α_2-MG), antithrombin-III (AT-III), and C_1-inactivator were measured using a single radial immunodiffusion technique. In 22 patients with trophoblastic disease, plasminogen activator inhibitor-2 (PAI-2) concentrations were assayed using ELISA by sandwich method with monoclonal and polyclonal antibodies.

[1] Department of Obstetrics and Gynecology Tokyo Medical College Hospital, Nishi Shinjuku 6-7-1, Shinjuku-ku, Tokyo, 160 Japan
[2] Saitama Medical School, Moroyama-cho, Iruma-gun, Saitama Prefecture, 350-04 Japan

Case Report

Case 1

The patient, a 21-year-old woman, *para* 0 had a history of complete hydatidiform mole evacuated by curettage at 29 weeks of gestation on January 16, 1972. She received chemotherapy with methotrexate (MTX) 15 mg/day for 5 days from the day after evacuation of the mole. Urinary human chorionic gonadotrophin (hCG) titer was 8 000 iu/l. The uterus was 6 cm below the umbilicus. At that time, laboratory data consisted of a hemoglobin (Hb) content of 12.6 g/dl with a hematocrit of 37%, a white cell count of 12 300/ mm^3, and a red cell count of 389×10^4/ mm^3. Chest X-ray was negative. The patient had fallen into uncontrolled hemorrhage from the nasopharyngeal region, therefore she was transferred to Tokyo Medical College Hospital under suspicion of DIC on January 27, 1972, 11 days after removal of the mole. The hematological examination data consisted of a white cell count of 3 000, Hb content of 8.4 g/dl and platelet count of 14 000. Bleeding time was 22 min and prothrombin times was 60%. Partial thromboplastin time was 63.2 s. Fibrinogen value counted 280 mg/dl (Table 1). Although blood transfusion and platelet transfusion were given repeatedly, the patient died of cyanosis and hemoptysis on January 29, 1972.

Case 2

The patient, a 40-year-old Nepalese woman, *para* 8, had continued bleeding for 5 months after 2-month history of amenorrhea. She therefore twice underwent dilation and curettage (D & C), but bloody clots were often discharged. The uterus distended over the umbilicus and ultrasonography revealed hydatidiform

Table 1. Hematological examination findings in a patient with DIC after evacuation of hydatiform mole

Date	1/24	1/25	1/26	1/28
Erythrocytes	327×10^4	284×10^4	340×10^4	283×10^4
Leucocytes	2500	2000	2400	3000
Hb (g/dl)	10.2	9.0	9.8	8.4
Platelets	0.65×10^4	0.57×10^4	0.34×10^4	0.14×10^4
Bleeding time	11′	25′	25′	22′
Clotting time	30′	8′ 30″	9′	7′
Prothrombin time				60%
PTT				63′ 2″
Fibrinogen				280 mg/dl
Plasmin				low
BUN				18.7 mg/dl
LDH				126 U/l

Blood transfusion: fresh blood transfusion, 2150 ml; platelet transfusion, 4 units
PTT, partial thromboplastin time; BUN, blood urea nitrogen; LDH, lactic dehydrogenase

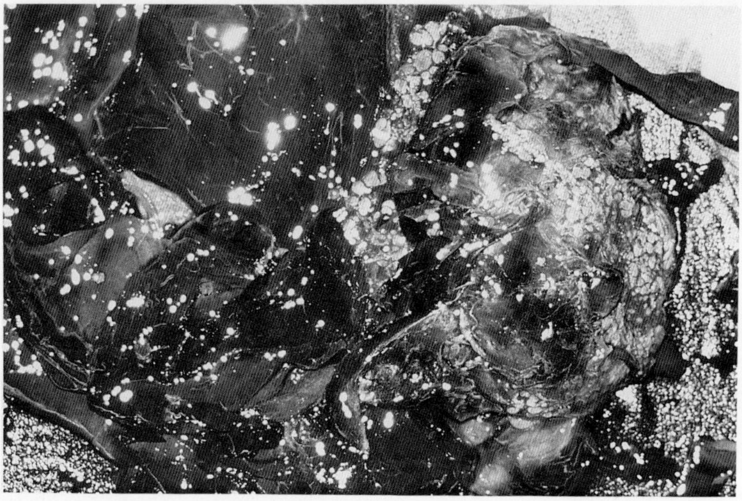

Fig. 1. Molar vesicles and large bloody clots within the uterus of a Nepalese patient

mole at 28 weeks of gestation. On January 31, 1989, total hysterectomy with bilateral salpingo-oophorectomy was carried out. The uterus being as large as overhead was filled with molar vesicles and large amounts of bloody clots (Fig. 1). Urinary hCG titer was 4 096 000 iu/l. She had received blood transfusion due to anemia.

Coagulation and Fibrinolytic Factors

In an attempt to determine whether coagulation and fibrinolytic properties of trophoblastic disease can be reflected in the occurrence of hemorrhagic disorders, coagulation and fibrinolytic factors were measured in blood samples collected from 26 patients with trophoblastic disease [1].

Fibrinogen and Plasminogen Levels

Increases in fibrinogen as well as plasminogen concentrations were found in patients with hydatidiform mole and metastatic choriocarcinoma, while decreases in fibrinogen and plasminogen values were found after removal of the moles and metastatic foci (Fig. 2).

FDP Levels

Serum FDP levels were significantly higher in both the hydatidiform mole group and the metastatic choriocarcinoma patients; after removal of tumors, FDP levels dropped (Fig. 3).

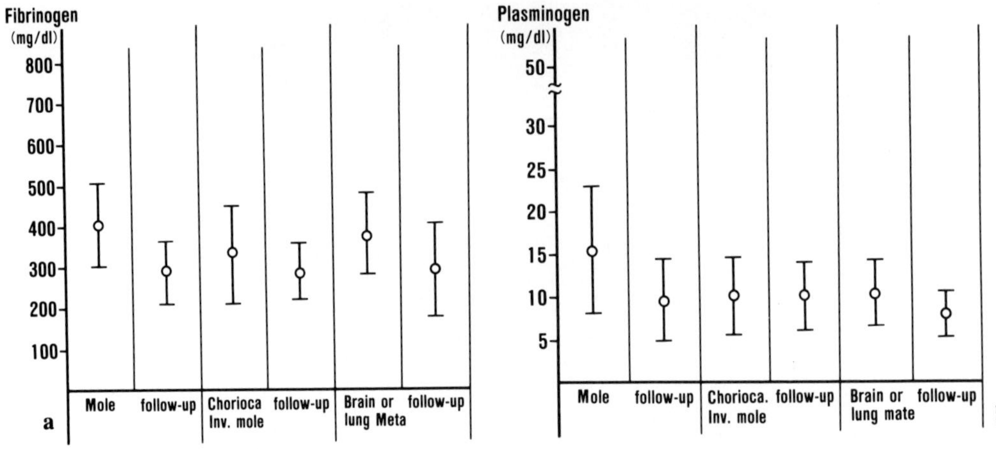

Fig. 2a. Fibrinogen and **b** plasminogen levels in trophoblastic disease patients

Fibrinolytic Inhibitor Levels

When fibrinolytic inhibitors such as α_1-AT, α_2-MG, AT-III, and C_1-inactivator were assayed in patients with trophoblastic disease, α_1-AT levels were relatively high in those with hydatidiform moles. After removal of the moles, a decline in the levels was seen. Although other fibrinolytic inhibitor levels in cases of hydatidiform mole and choriocarcinoma remain unchanged, C_1-inactivator levels appeared relatively higher in metastatic choriocarcinoma and, after treatment, the levels lowered (Fig. 4).

PAI-2 Concentrations

Plasminogen activator inhibitor-2 (PAI-2) is known to occur in placenta and in pregnancy plasma. In this report, PAI-2 levels in 13 patients with hydatidiform

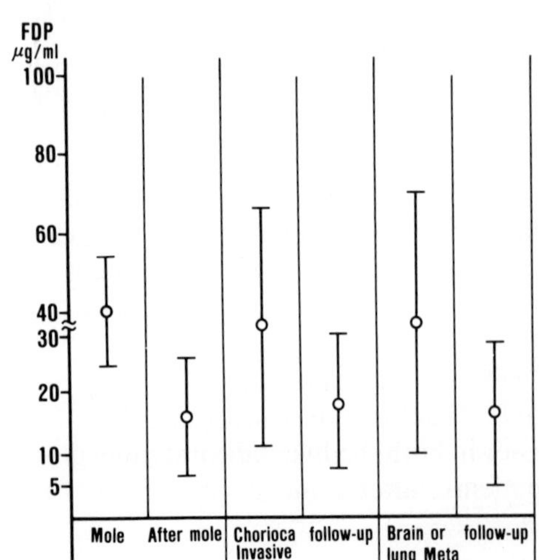

Fig. 3. Serum fibrinogen degradation product (*FDP*) levels in patients with trophoblastic disease

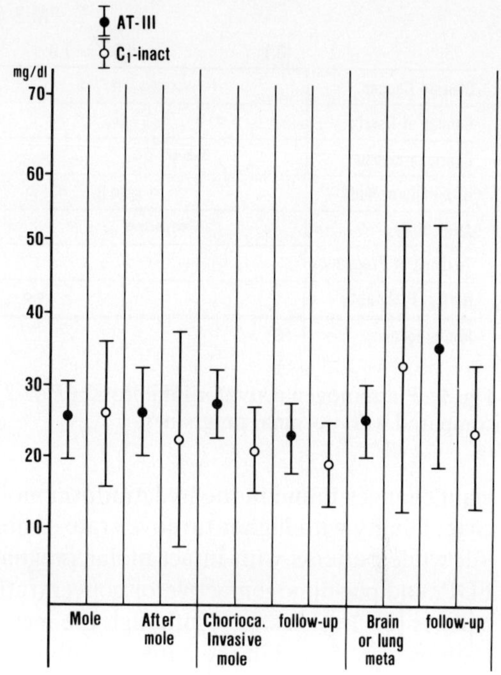

Fig. 4. Antithrombin III (*AT-III*) and C_1-inactivator levels in patients with trophoblastic disease

mole were found to be relatively lower than those in normal pregnant women, but the levels were significantly high when compared with those in choriocarcinoma and other gynecologic malignant tumors (Fig. 5). The concentrations of PAI-2 in hydatidiform mole ranged between 0.36 and 24.5 UKI μ/ml, but the levels in choriocarcinoma patients were lower than 0.5 UKI μ/ml. After evacuation of the mole, the concentrations of PAI-2 antigen decreased below the concentration of 0.5 UKI μ/ml. PAI-2 concentration in the plasma of the Nepalese patient with mole *in situ* and large bloody clots at 28 weeks of gestation was 3.65 UKI μ/ml.

Discussion and Conclusions

Hemorrhage is a frequent complication of trophoblastic disease. Excessive bleeding because of uterine atony as a complication of evacuation of hydatidiform mole is often encountered. However, until recently, DIC had been reported in few patients with hydatidiform mole [2,3]. In Nepal, the risk of hemorrhage, as seen in case 2, is often increased [4]. If such hydatidiform moles are evacuated by curettage, probably profuse bleeding would occur following evacuation. The case 1 patient would seem to indicate that the cause of uncontrolled hemorrhage due to coagulation failure such as thrombocytopenia might have been attributed to the chemotherapy given shortly after expulsion of the moles.

Few studies of coagulation and fibrinolysis in hydatidiform mole have been performed in comparison to those of normal pregnancy [5–7]. The most signif-

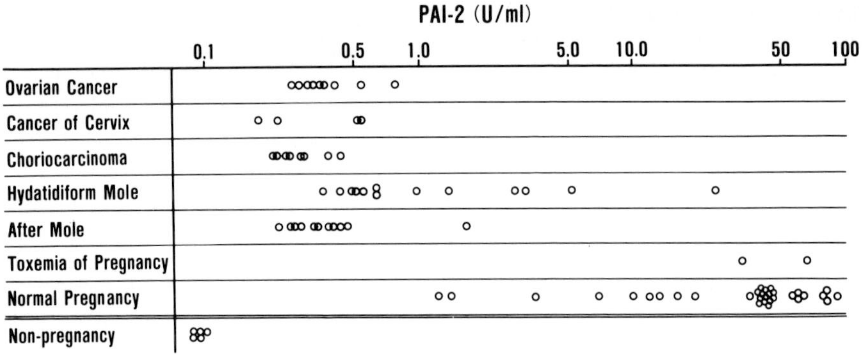

Fig. 5. Plasminogen activator inhibitor-2 (*PAI-2*) concentrations in trophoblastic disease compared with normnal pregnancy

icant changes found in the hydatidiform mole group were a latent state of hypercoagulability with higher turnover rate of fibrinogen and increased levels of FDP [6]; while patients with intact molar pregnancies had higher fibrinogen, FVIII, FDP, and plasminogen activator concentrations than controls with normal pregnancies [7]. In this study, although the increases in fibrinogen and FDP concentrations were found in the patients with hydatidiform mole and metastatic choriocarcinoma, the levels dropped shortly after removal of the tumor. However, levels of fibrinolytic inhibitors such as α_2-MG, AT-III, and C_1-inactivator (excluding α_1-AT) usually remained unchanged [1].

Increased selective inhibition of urokinase-induced fibrinolysis and variations in the fibrinolytic activity were observed in patients with trophoblastic disease. The activity of plasminogen activator is mainly balanced by two specific plasminogen activator inhibitors consisting of one which is released from endothelial cells (PAI-1) and another which is present in the placenta (PAI-2) [8]. PAI-2 was found in the trophoblast cells by means of an immunohistochemic method [9,10]. PAI-2 concentration in normal pregnancy increased gradually as pregnancy advanced. PAI-2 levels in patients with hydatidiform mole were not only significantly higher than those in other gynecologic tumors, but also significantly decreased after evacuation of the moles. Localization of PAI-2 was also immunohistochemically demonstrable in the trophoblastic layer of the hydropic villi of the mole. PAI-2 activity probably acts as a balance against activation of the fibrinolytic system in cases of hydatidiform mole.

Although it is generally considered the fibrinolytic mechanism is depressed in cancer patients, tissue Plasminogen Activator antigen and PA-inhibition were both significantly increased irrespective of the presence or absence of tumor metastasis [11]. In this study, PAI-2 levels in choriocarcinoma and other gynecologic malignant tumors were low, below 0.5 iu/ml. From these findings, it is difficult to suggest a relation between PAI-2 activity and tumor growth, but this requires further investigation.

Summary. Trophoblastic disease can be mainly classified into hydatidiform mole, invasive mole, and choriocarcinoma. These diseases are sometimes associated with hemorrhagic disorders. It is known that hydatidiform mole has a hemorrhagic tendency during evacuation of the mole and metastatic choriocarcinoma patients sometimes tend to continue bleeding disorders during chemotherapy and surgery. In this presentation, plasma concentrations of coagulation and fibrinolytic factors were measured in patients with hydatidiform mole, invasive mole, and choriocarcinoma. Additionally, a case study of a patient who died of DIC following chemotherapy immediately after the mole is presented. PAI-2 concentration in trophoblastic disease was assayed using ELISA method with a polyclonal and a monoclonal antibody against PAI-2. As a result, the PAI-2 levels of hydatidiform moles were relatively lower than those of normal pregnancies, but the levels were significantly higher when compared with those in choriocarcinoma and other gynecologic tumors. Furthermore, after evacuation of the moles the levels dropped.

References

1. Terada K (1981) Studies on hypercoagulable state and fibrinolytic activity in association with advanced gynecologic cancer. J Obstet Gynecol Neonatal Hematol 5: 179–199 (in Japanese)
2. Egley CC, Simon LR, Haddox Th (1975) Hydatidiform mole and disseminated intravascular coagulation. Am J Obstet Gynecol 121: 1122–1123
3. Talbert LM, Easterling WE Jr, Flowers CE Jr, Graham JB (1961) Coagulation defects of pregnancy including a case of a patient with hydatidiform mole. Obstet Gynecol 18: 69–76
4. Soma H, Malla D, Dali SM (1989) Clinical experience with trophoblastic diseases in Nepal. Jpn J Cancer Chemother 16: 1577–1581 (part II)
5. Goldstein, DP, Brakman P, Marshall JR (1966) The plasma fibrinolytic system in patients with trophoblastic disease and undelivered hydatidiform mole. Am J Obstet Gynecol 94: 21–28
6. López-Llera M, Espinosa ML, Ramos JN, Diaz de León M (1977) Coagulation and fibrinolysis in molar pregnancy. Am J Obstet Gynecol 127: 855–860
7. Tsakok FHM, Koh S, Ratnam SS (1976) Coagulation and fibrinolysis in intact hydatidiform molar pregnancy. Br Med J 2: 1481–1484
8. Åstedt B, Heimburger N (1988) Spezifisches Plasminogenaktivator-inhibitoren. Hamostaseologie 8: 233–239
9. Feinberg RF, Kliman HJ, Haimowitz JE, Queenan JT, Wun T-Ch, Strauss JF III (1988) Plasminogen activator inhibitor types 1 and 2 in human trophoblast. Proceedings of the 11th Rochester Trophoblast Conference with the European Placenta Group. abstract 106
10. Åstedt B, Hagerstrand I, Lecander I (1986) Cellular localisation in placenta of placental type plasminogen activator inhibitor. Thromb Haemost 56: 63–65
11. de Jong E, Knot EAR, Divet O, Iburg AC, Rijken DC, Veenhof KHN, Dooijewaard G, ten Cate JW (1987) Increased plasminogen activator inhibition levels in malignancy. Thromb Haemost 57: 140–143

2.2 Placental Protein 19 in Clinical Blood Coagulation Disorder

Masaomi Takayama[1], Keiichi Isaka[1], Yoshichika Suzuki[1], Hitoshi Funayama[1], Yasunobu Suzuki[1], Kiyoshi Akiya[1], and Hans Bohn[2]

Introduction

The human placenta is a highly functional organ able to synthesize a wide variety of biologically active proteins, including hormones, enzymes, proenzymes, activators, inhibitors, immunoregulatory factors, transport and storage proteins, receptors, and structual proteins [1]. Moreover, many proteins of unknown function have been discovered and isolated in placental extracts.

Placental tissue protein 19 (PP19) is a recently discovered protein isolated from extracts of the human term placenta by Bohn and Winckler [2]. It is a glycoprotein that contains 3.9% carbohydrate with an electrophoretic mobility between α_1-and β_1-globulin and has an isoelectric point between 4.6 and 5.4. It has a molecular weight of 36 500 (ultracentrifugation) or < 18 000 (SDS-PAGE). A term placenta contained 90 mg of PP19 [1].

We clarified the immunohistochemical localization of PP19 in the villous and extravillous trophoblastic cells of normal pregnancy and trophoblastic disease, using polyclonal anti-PP19 antibody (632 ZA) prepared by H. Bohn [3,4]. We also reported the dynamics of maternal serum PP19 concentration throughout gestation [5]. The biological function of PP19, however, remains to be clarified. In this study, we observed the circulating PP19 level in some diseases involving coagulation disorders.

Materials and Methods

Production of Monoclonal Antibody (ISTA19-1)

Two BALB/cN female mice were immunized by trophoblast obtained from a first trimester placenta. This was boosted 3 weeks later with 50 μg of purified

[1]Department of Obstetrics and Gynecology, Tokyo Medical College Hospital, 6-7-1, Nishishinjuku, Shinjuku-ku, Tokyo 160, Japan
[2]Behringwerke AG, Marburg/Lahn, Federal Republic of Germany

PP19 (225/242) injected into the mouse spleen. Three days after the boost, spleen cells were harvested and fused to myeloma cells (P3X63Ag8U.1) at a 4:1 ratio in the presence of 50% polyethylene glycol 4 000 (Merck, FRG) following the method described by Oi and Herzenberg [6]. Hybridoma culture supernatants were screened by reaction with ^{125}I-labeled PP19.

Immunostaining by Monoclonal Antibody

Formalin-fixed paraffin-embedded term placenta was immunostained by the labeled avidin-biotin technique [7] using monoclonal anti-PP19 antibody (ISTA19-1) for the first antibody, biotinylated rabbit immunoglobilin to mouse immunoglobulin (Dakopatts, Denmark) diluted 1:200, and peroxidase-conjugated avidin (Dakopatts, Denmark) diluted 1:400.

Tissue Culture

Chorionic villi obtained from therapeutic abortion at gestational week 12, were dissected and rinsed in two changes of phosphate-buffered saline (PBS) to remove blood cells, then weighed. One hundred milligrams of chorionic tissue was placed in a culture dish containing 5 ml of Minimum Essential Medium (GIBCO/BRL). The tissue was incubated in a humidified 5% CO_2 atomosphere at 37° C. After preincubation for 3 h, the medium was changed every 24 h up to 144 h and stored at −20° C until assay.

Radioimmunoassay for PP19 and Human Chorionic Gonadotropin (hCG)

Specific radioimmunoassay for PP19 was previously described [5]. Elmotec EIA-Kits [8] using monoclonal anti-hCG antibody were used for hCG assay.

Results

PP19 Localization in Placenta Demonstrated by Monoclonal Antibody

The immunohistochemical localization of PP19 in the placenta was demonstrated by monoclonal antibody (ISTA 19-1), which revealed PP19 localization identical to that revealed by polyclonal anti-PP19 antibody (632 ZA). That is, marked staining for PP19 was characteristically found in the nucleus and cytoplasm of the villous syncytiotrophoblast, in the maternal granulocyte in the intervillous space (Fig. 1), and in the extravillous cytotrophoblast-like cell in the septum and basal plate of the placenta (Fig. 2).

PP19 and hCG Concentrations in the Medium by Placental Tissue Culture

We measured the hCG and PP19 concentration in media from 3 cases of placenta tissue culture for 6 days. One of these cases (Fig. 3) showed PP19 and

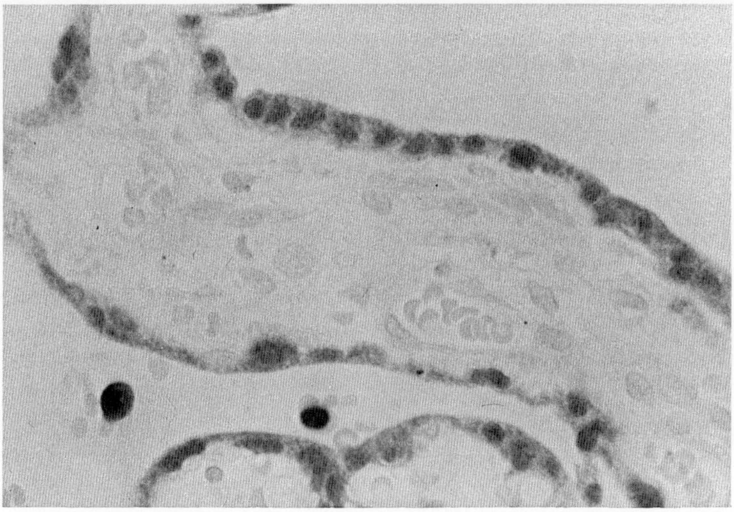

Fig. 1. The antigenic determinant detected by monoclonal antibody against placental protein (*PP19*) (ISTA19-1) was seen in the nucleus and cytoplasm of the syncytium of the chorionic villus and maternal leukocyte in the intervillous space. (Gestational week 38)

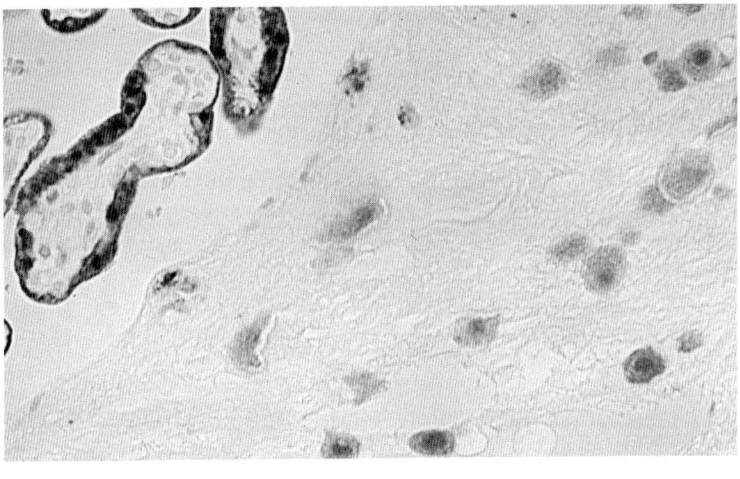

Fig. 2. Immunostaining for placental protein 19 (*PP19*) by monoclonal antibody (ISTA19-1) was seen in interstitial cytotrophoblast-like cells in the placental septum and chorionic villous syncytium. (Gestational week 38)

hCG concentrations, where hCG concentration began to rise from 10 mIU/ml/100 mg wet tissue (wt) at 72 h to 360 mIU/ml/ml/100 mg wt at 144 h, and where PP19 concentration rose from 200 ng/ml/100 mg wt at 96 h to 1400 ng/ml/100 mg wt at 144 h. Adding 0.1 m*M* cycloheximide (Sigma, USA) to the medium from day 1 to day 6, neither hCG nor PP19 increased in the medium. Two other

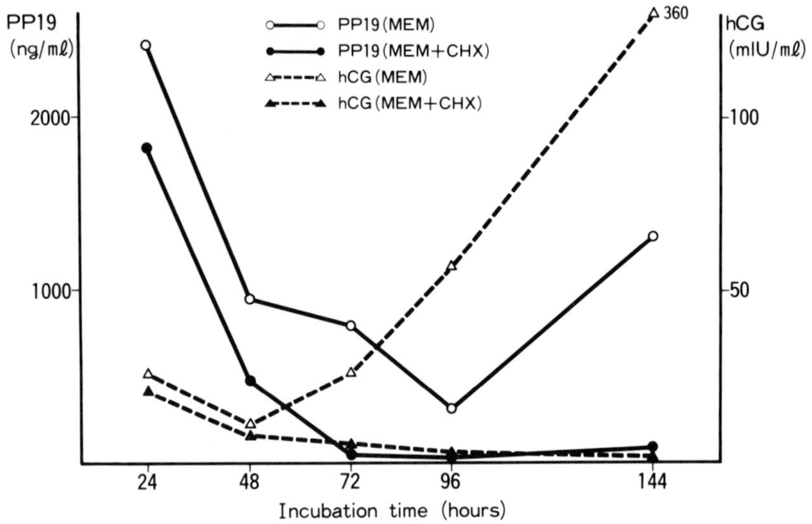

Fig. 3. Placental tissue (100 mg wet tissue) produced placental protein 19 (*PP19*) and human chorionic gonadotropin (*hCG*) in media (*MEM*) with presence and absence of 0.1 m*M* cycloheximide (*CHX*)

occasions showed similar results. These results indicate that placental explants in culture were able to synthesize and secrete both PP19 and hCG.

Serum Concentration from Men and Nonpregnant Women

Serum PP19 concentrations in nonpregnant women of reproductive age ranged from 3.4 to 6.2 ng/ml in 8 samples from the proliferative phase, and from 2.8 to 8.1 ng/ml in 7 samples from the secretory phase of the menstrual cycle. In serum samples from 12 healthy men, PP19 concentrations ranged from 2.2 to 7.8 ng/ml. No statistically significant difference was observed in levels for these groups (Fig. 4).

The PP19 Concentration in Serum, Ascites, and Fluid Tumor Content in Benign and Malignant Diseases

All serum specimens from cases with leiomyoma uteri ($n = 6$) and benign ovarian cyst ($n = 3$) showed PP19 concentrations below 10 ng/ml (Fig. 5). Two cases from pelvic endometriosis (Beecham III) showed 11 and 17 ng/ml. Two (18%) out of 11 squamous cell carcinoma of the uterine cervix in stages I and II showed 14 and 16 ng/ml. All sera from 7 cases with endometrial adenocarcinoma stage I showed below 10 ng/ml. The serum PP19 concentration in 19 ovarian adenocarcinoma cases, stages I–III, ranged from 4 to 32 ng/ml, with 11 cases (58%) showing higher than 10 ng/ml. One (20%) out of 5 metastatic choriocarcinoma cases and 3 (27%) out of 11 invasive mole cases showed concentrations above 10 ng/

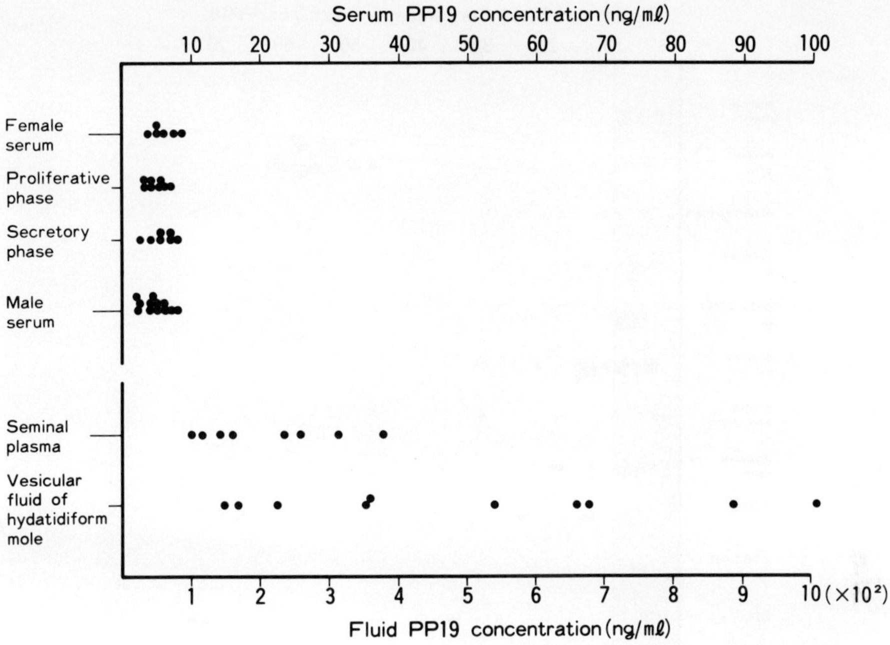

Fig. 4. Placental protein 19 (*PP19*) concentrations in sera from men and nonpregnant women, seminal plasmas, and vesicular fluids from complete hydatidiform mole

ml. The three (75%) of 4 advanced gastric adenocarcinoma cases in advanced stage showed higher concentration ranging from 12 to 23 ng/ml; however, two operable intestinal carcinoma cases showed concentrations below 10 ng/ml.

Apparently, high serum PP19 concentrations were found in 4 cases associated with disseminated intravascular coagulation (DIC) confirmed by hematological examinations such as prolonged coagulation time, prolonged activated partial thromboplastin time and prothrombin time, low platelet count, hypofibrinogenemia, and elevated circulating fibrinogen and fibrin degradation products (FDP). In three of these cases, blood samples were obtained from placental abruption or uterine rupture. Another sample was obtained from a patient with critical DIC induced by general metastasis of ovarian adenocarcinoma. Two out of 5 ascites samples and 6 out of 8 fluid contents of ovarian tumor showed PP19 concentrations ranging from 28 to 185 ng/ml, mostly seen in the ovarian carcinoma cases.

Case Associated with DIC

The patient had been treated for recurrent choriocarcinoma metastases to the lung and brain for almost one year. After the eighth course of chemotherapy by Etoposide, Methotrexate, Actinomycin D Cyclophosphamide, Vincristine, and Bleomycins, the patient had pancytopenia, liver dysfunction, and pulmonary

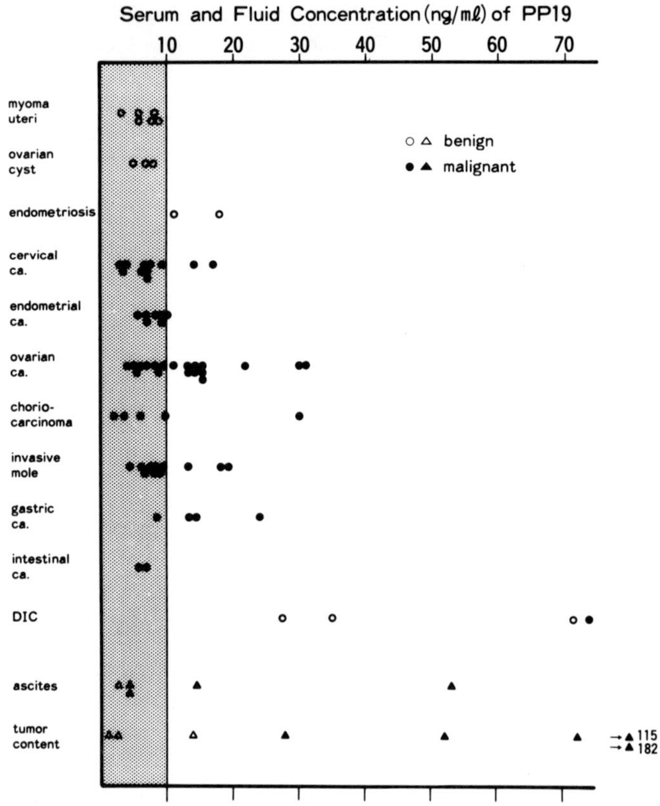

Fig. 5. Placental protein 19 (*PP19*) concentrations in sera from various diseases, ascites, and fluid contents of ovarian tumor

dysfunction by fibrosis. The urinary and serum hCG levels were relatively low, around 120 mIU/ml, and serum PP19 level was 8 ng/ml. A week later, however, the patient begun to show DIC signs; ecchymoses, decreased platelet count, increased FDP, hypofibrinogenemia, and decelerated erythrocyte sedimentation rate (ESR). The serum PP19 concentration was 36 ng/ml and urinary hCG was 800 IU/L (Fig. 6).

Discussion

We previously reported that PP19 may be a good immunohistochemical marker for detecting villous and extravillous syncytiotrophoblastic and interstital cytotrophoblast-like cells in pregnancy and trophoblastic disease due to more intense and consistent staining and a higher population of stained trophoblastic cells than hCG and pregnancy-specific β_1-glycoprotein [4]. Using monoclonal anti-PP19 antibody, we immunohistochemically demonstrated a characteristic

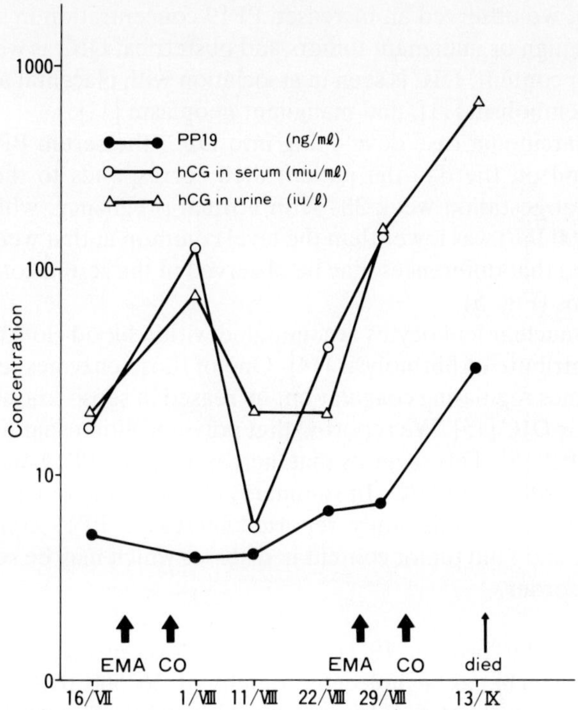

Fig. 6. The concentration of (*hCG*) in serum and urine and placental protein 19 (*PP19*) in serum in a patient with metastatic choriocarcinoma preceeding DIC

PP19 localization in the placenta (Fig. 1), which was identical to that found by using polyclonal anti-PP19 antibody [3]. That is, the PP19 localized in the nucleus and cytoplasm of villous syncytiotrophoblast and extravillous cytotrophoblast-like cell in the septum and basal plate of the placenta (Fig. 2).

Although PP19 localizes in the maternal leukocyte [3], this study clarified that placental tissue explants in culture apparently synthesized both PP19 and hCG (Fig. 3). More study is needed to determine whether the leukocyte is able to produce this protein, because a low PP19 concentration was detected from men and nonpregnant women.

It was found that the maternal serum PP19 concentration increased with gestational age, reaching a maximum of 32 ng/ml (median) at gestational week 38–39, and that the maternal serum PP19 concentration in hydatidiform mole tended to be higher than in normal pregnancy although this increase was not statistically significant [5]. However, the PP19 concentration in the vesicular fluid of complete hydatidiform mole was 10–100 times higher than the PP19 concentration in paired maternal serum. The high protein concentration in vesicular fluid also observed in hCG [9] may be due to transport at the chorionic villi, which, in the fetal membrane, may also contribute to relatively higher PP19 concentrations in amniotic fluid than in paired maternal serum [5].

In this study, we observed an increased PP19 concentration in serum in some cases having benign or malignant tumors and obstetrical DIC as well as in ascites and fluid tumor content. DIC is seen in association with placental abruption [10], amniotic fluid embolism [11], and malignant neoplasm [12].

In a choriocarcinoma case developing into DIC, the serum PP19 concentration of 36 ng/ml on the day the patient died corresponds to the serum PP19 concentration at gestation week 38–39 in normal pregnancy, while the urinary hCG level of 800 IU/l was lower than the level common at that weeks [13]. Thus, it must be noted that differences may be observed in the serum concentrations of the two proteins (Fig. 5).

Polymorphonuclear leukocytes accumulated within blood clots have proteases which may contribute of fibrinolysis [14]. One of those enzymes, elastase, which activates enzymes regulating coagulation, increased in sepsis known as an underlying disease for DIC [15]. We reported that polymorphonuclear leukocytes contained much PP19 [5]. This suggests that increased serum PP19 may be related to coagulation disorders and DIC. In summary, although the function of PP19 has not yet been clarified, this study reported increased PP19 concentrations in serum, ascites, and fluid tumor content in diseases which may be related to blood coagulation disorder.

Summary. Placental protein 19 (PP19) has a glycoprotein containing 3.9% carbohydrate, which has a molecular weight of 36 500 dalton, 1–1 electrophoretic mobility, and a 4.5–5.4 isoelectoric point [2]. This study revealed the immunohistochemical localization of PP19 in clinical coagulation disorder. Immunohistochemical staining for PP19 was done by the indirect method, and PP19 concentration was measured by RIA. PP19 was immunostained at nucleus and cytoplasm of syncytiotrophoblast and maternal leukocyte in placenta. Serum PP19 was low but detectable in nonpregnant women and in men. During pregnancy, maternal serum PP19 concentration increased from 6.2 ng/ml (median) at gestational weeks 6–7 to 34.1 ng/ml at 38–39 weeks. PP19 level in amniotic fluid ($n = 24$), ranging from 14 to 102 ng/ml, was higher than in maternal serum. Vesicular fluid of complete hydatidiform mole ($n = 12$) contained high PP19 concentration ranging from 355 to 2445 ng/ml. Increased serum PP19 concentration was observed in clinical DIC in cases associated with abruptio placentae and choriocarcinoma.

References

1. Bohn H (1985) Biochemistry of placental proteins. In: Bischof P, Klopper A (eds) Proteins of the placenta. 5th Int. Congr. on placental proteins, Annecy 1984, pp1–25 (Karger, Basel)
2. Bohn H, Winckler H (1985) Isolation and characterization of four new placental tissue proteins (PP18, PP19, PP20, PP21). Arch Gynaek 236: 235–242
3. Takayama M, Isaka K, Ogawa T, Funayama H, Yamabe S, Soma H, Bohn H (1988) Characteristic differences in immunohistochemical localization of new placental proteins (PP1, PP19, PP21) in the human placenta. Gynecol Obstet Invest 26: 274–280

4. Takayama M, Isaka K, Suzuki Y, Funayama H, Suzuki Y, Akiya K, Bohn H (1989) Comparative study of placental protein 19, human chorionic gonadotrophin and pregnancy-specific β_1-glycoprotein as immunohistochemical markers for the extravillous trophoblast in pregnancy and trophoblastic disease. Histochemistry 93: 167–173
5. Takayama M, Isaka K, Suzuki Y, Funayama H, Suzuki Y, Akiya K, Bohn H (1990) Concentration of placental protein 19 in body fluid and placental tissue. Arch Gynecol Obstet 247: 83–93
6. Oi VT, Herzenberg LA (1980) Immunoglobulin-producing hybrid cell lines. In: Mishell BB, Shiigi SM (eds) Selected methods in cellular immunology. Freeman, San Francisco, pp 351–372
7. Guesdon JL, Ternynck T, Avramias S (1979) The use of avidin-biotin interaction in immunoenzymatic techniques. J Histochem Cytochem 27: 1131–1139
8. Masuko H, Sato H, Baba M, Nobuhara M (1989) Outline of "ELMOTEC" (EIA kits) and "IMURABOT" (automatic analyzer). JJCLA 14: 208–211
9. Yuen HB (1987) Differing concentrations of human chorionic gonadotrophin and prolactin in the cyst fluid of hydatidiform mole and in amniotic fluid. Am J Obstet Gynecol 156: 400–402
10. Sutton DMC, Hauser R, Kulapong P, Bachmann F (1971) Intravascular coagulation in abruptio placentae. Am J Obstet Gynecol 109: 604–614
11. Phillips LL, Davidson EC (1972) Procoagulant properties of amniotic fluid. Am J Obstet Gynecol 113: 911–919
12. Sack GH, Levin J, Bell WR (1977) Trousseau's syndrome and other manifestations of chronic disseminated coagulopathy in patients with neoplasms: Clinical, pathophysiologic, and therapeutic features. Medicine (Baltimore) 56: 1–37
13. Mishell DR Jr, Wide L, Gemzell CA (1963) Immunologic determination of human chorionic gonadotrophin in serum. J Clin Endocrinol Metab 23: 125–131
14. Plow EF (1986) The contribution of leukocyte proteases to fibrinolysis. Blut 53: 1–9
15. Duswald K, Jochum M, Schramm W, Fritz H (1985) Released granulocyteic elastase: An indicator of pathobiochemical alterations in septicemia after abdominal surgery. Surgery 98: 892–899

2.3 Platelet Aggregation Inhibition Activity of Placental Brush Border Membrane

HIDEAKI IIOKA, I. MORIYAMA, S. AKADA, M. AKASAKI, K. NABUCHI, H. HISANAGA, K. MORIMOTO, and M. ICHIJO[1]

Introduction

Thrombus occurs frequently in the placental chorionic lumen of patients with Pre-ecclampsia (EPH) gestosis, and participation of platelets is suggested in the pathology of the diseases. In the placental tissues, there is an antiplatelet aggregating factor which plays an important role in the maintenance of microcirculation in the placenta. The brush border membrane of the placental chorioepithelium plays the part of the vasoendothelium as it is the point of direct contact with the maternal blood flow in the chorionic lumen. It has already been confirmed that a strong inhibitory action on platelet aggregation is present in the vasoendothelium, and its main active mechanism is shown to be prostacyclin (PG I_2) and ADP degrading by an ADPase-like activity which exists in edothelial membrane. Thus, it is quite possible that some inhibitory activity on platelet aggregation exists in the brush border membrane of placental chorioepithelium. We, therefore, investigated the presence of such an inhibitory activity on platelet aggregation as well as its properties using a fraction of the brush border membrane.

Method

The brush border membrane vesicles in a human placenta were isolated from the organ immediately after a normal delivery of a term pregnancy according to the method reported by Iioka et al. [1]. Proteins were measured by the methods of Lowry et al. [2].

A platelet rich plasma (PRP) was obtained by drawing citric acid-treated blood from a donor with uncomplicated pregnancy and centrifuging it at 22 °C

[1]Department of Obstetrics and Gynecology, Nara Medical University, Shijomachi 840, Kashihara City, Nara, 634 Japan

and 190 g for 7 min. Platelet aggregation was evaluated by measuring changes in the maximum aggregation rate by use of Born's nephelometry using PRP.

After incubating ^{14}C-ADP and brush border membrane vesicles at 37 °C for a fixed period, reaction was stopped by the addition of perchloric acid (0.25 M). After centrifugation, the supernatant was fractionated by thin-layer chromatography and was measured by a scintillation counter.

The brush border membrane vesicles (the final protein concentration, 20 μg/ml and 100 μg/ml) were added to the PRP (platelet rich plasma) followed by arachidonic acid (final concentration, 0.3 m*M*) and heated at 37 °C for 30 min. The reaction was stopped by the addition of trichoric acid (final concentration, 10%). After centrifugation, thiobarbituric acid (0.2 *M*) was added to the supernatant, which was heated at 100 °C for 15 min and cooled to determine absorbance at 532 nm. As a control, 10 m*M* buffer (pH 7.4) of the same volume was added instead of the brush border membrane vesicles.

Results

We studied the effect of the brush border membrane vesicles (BBMV) on platelet aggregation by varying the final concentration of BBMV. A very strong platelet aggregation inhibition activity existed in placental BBMV. In the 20–40 μg/ml protein concentration, the BBMV almost perfectly inhibited the platelet aggregation induced by ADP, arachidonic acid, and collagen; and in the 100–150 μg/ml protein concentration, the BBMV almost perfectly inhibited the platelet aggregation induced by ristocentin.

ADPase activity was studied by the methods stated above. ADP decomposition almost paralleled the time course with decomposition practically 100% after 60 s.

Changes in platelet aggregation were studied by the addition of ADP (the final concentration at the time of addition to PRP was 5 μ*M*) which had been preincubated with BBMV (the final protein concentration at the time of addition was 1 μg/ml) for 30–60 s. Platelet aggregation seen at the time of ADP addition decreased with the time course and was inhibited almost at 100% after 60 s. The time course of this ibhibition of platelet aggregation by preincubation of ADP with BBMV agreed well with that of ADP degradation by BBMV.

The effect of BBMV on malondialdehyde (MDA) production were examined by the methods described above. Production of platelet MDA was 78% of the control with BBMV at the final protein concentration of 20 μg/ml and 35% at 100 μg/ml thus proving that BBMV fraction would distinctly inhibit MDA production by platelets.

Discussion

In the present study, it was shown for the first time that an activity which would inhibit platelet aggregation was present in the brush border membrane of the placenta. The result of the study revealed that one of the anti-aggregating mechanisms of the brush border membrane was the ADP decomposition by ADPase-like activity. Also, it was found that brush border membrane possessed an activity which would inhibit arachidonic acid metabolism within the platelet.

There have already been several reports on platelet aggregation inhibiting factors in the placenta [3–7]. Although Mochizuki [7] recently succeeded in a partial purification of a platelet aggregation inhibitor (PPAI) from the microsome fraction of human placenta, this compound seems to possess different properties from the platelet aggregation inhibiting action of the brush border membrane in that it neither shows a distinct ADPase activity (an activity to decompose ADP) nor distinct inhibitory action on ristocetin-induced platelet aggregation. Meanwhile, Hutton et al. [6] showed that an inhibitor for ADP-induced platelet aggregation was present in the supernatant obtained by incubating the placental chorionic tissues. This compound, however, differed from the platelet aggregation inhibiting effect of the brush border membrane in that it would inhibit only ADP-induced platelet aggregation. It is highly possible that the presence of platelet aggregation inhibiting action in the brush border membrane, which is the direct point of contact with the maternal blood flow, plays a significant role in maintaining microcirculation in the placenta. While postacyclin action is important for inhibition of platelet aggregation in the vasoendothelium, ADPase-like activity is said to be significant as well.

On the other hand, prostacyclin productivity in the placental chorioepithelium is said to be exetremely poor in comparison to that of the vasoendothelium. Thus, it is highly possible that the platelet aggregation inhibition action in the brush border membrane, which we revealed in the present study, possesses an important meaning. It is considered to be one of the keys to elucidation of the mechanisms of maintaining microcirculation in the placenta.

Summary. To clarify the role of placental brush border in the regulation of placental microcirculation, we investigated the platelet aggregation inhibition activity of placental brush border membrane vesicles (BBMV) and obtained the following results. There existed a very strong platelet aggregation inhibition activity in placental BBMV. In the 20–40 μg/ml protein concentration, the BBMV inhibited almost perfectly the platelet aggregation induced by ADP, arachidonic acid, and collagen; and, in the 100–150 μg/ml protein concentration, the BBMV inhibited almost perfectly the platelet aggregation induced by ristocetin. There existed a very strong ADP degrading activity (ADPase activity) in the placental BBMV. The platelet aggregation activity of ADP was lost perfectly when ADP was preincubated with the placental BBMV. The placental BBMV inhibited the platelet malondialdehyde (MDA) production. In the 20 μg/ml and 100 μg/ml protein concentration of placental BBMV, 22% and 65% of platelet MDA production were inhibited, respectively.

References

1. Ioka H, Moriyama SI, Icijo M (1985) The study on placental phosphate transport mechanism (using human placental brush border membrane vesicles). Acta Obst Gynaecol Jpn 37: 2675

2. Lowry OH, Rosebrough NJ, Faro AL, Rondell RJ (1951) Protein measurement with the folin Phenol reagent. J Biol Chem 193: 265
3. Born GVR, Gross MJ (1963) The aggregation of blood platelet. J Physiol 168: 178
4. Duchesne MJD, Dao HT, Chavis C, Crastes A (1982) The human placental anti-aggregating factor is neither prostacyclin nor a prostacyclin metabolite. Prostaglandins 24: 701
5. Glassgow JG, Scade R, Pitlick FA (1978) Evidence that ADP hydrolysis by human cell is related to thrombogenic potential. Thromb Res 13: 255
6. Hutton RA, Dandona P, Chow FPR, Craft IL (1980) Inhibition of platelet aggregation by placental extracts. Thromb Res 17: 465
7. Mochizuki O (1987) Studies on platelet aggregation inhibitor isolated from the human placenta. Acta Obst Gynaecol Jpn 39: 1729

Coagulation Disorders During the Perinatal Period

2.4 Hematopoietic Malignancies During the Perinatal Period

HAJIME KOBAYASHI, SATOSHI HASHINO, KEISUKE ABE, MASANORI TANAKA, MASAHIRO IMAMURA, MASANOBU MORIOKA, KEISUKE SAKURADA, and TAMOTSU MIYAZAKI[1]

Introduction

Recently, hematopoietic malignancies have been increasing as one of the complications during pregnancy. There are some data on the effects of the hematopoietic malignancies in the mother and the fetus and of chemotherapy on the fetus and the baby [1–6]; however, it is very difficult to determine treatment of these cases due to several exceptions. We shall report here two cases of hematopoietic malignancy during pregnancy and discuss the problems encountered.

Case Reports

Case 1

In July 1987, a 24-year-old female in the 20th week of her first pregnancy underwent a routine hematological examination. At that time, she had mild anemia with a hemoglobin (Hb) value of 10.8 g/dl, but no further examination was performed. On December 24th 1987, in the 36th week of her pregnancy, she gave birth to twin male babies weighing 2620 g and 2420 g. She underwent no blood transfusion in spite of postpartum bleeding of 1280 ml. On the following day the hematological study revealed a pancytopenia with the Hb value of 9.4 g/dl, a WBC count of 2700/μl, and a platelet count of 52 000/μl. The sequence of the hematological study performed by her obstetrician showed no improvement of pancytopenia.

On March 23rd 1988, she was referred to our department. She complained of a low-grade fever and fatigue but had no bleeding tendency. A physical examination showed anemia in the conjunctiva and a slight hepatomegaly. Analysis

[1]Third Department of Internal Medicine, Hokkaido University School of Medicine, Kita-15, Nishi-7, Kitaku, Sapporo 060, Japan

revealed the following values: Hb, 6.4 g/dl; WBC, 2900/μl with marked decrease of granulocytes; and platelet count, 31 000/μl. No abnormal coagulation pattern or sign of DIC were observed. Bone marrow was hyperplastic, and 59.1% of the nucleated cells consisted of blasts. Some of them had Auer rods, and almost all of them showed positive peroxidase stain. Cytogenetic studies of these abnormal blasts demonstrated a translocation of a portion of chromosome 8–21 (t8q$^-$, 21q$^+$); therefore, this case was diagnosed acute myeloblastic leukemia (AML) which belonged to M2 of FAB classification and treated with BH-AC, daunomycin, 6-MP, and prednisolone from March 26th 1988.

By first induction therapy, complete remission (CR) was obtained. Thereafter, she received consolidation and intensification therapies. Finally, she received autologous bone marrow transplantation (BMT) in June 1989. A follow-up examination at 4 months found no clinical or hematological abnormalities and her babies were also well.

Table 1 provides a time-course of hematological examination before the admission to our department. This case was diagnosed as AML three months after the delivery, however, she appeared to have AML during the third trimester of pregnancy judging from massive bleeding and pancytopenia at the delivery. Since bleeding tendency was recognized by massive bleeding at the delivery, we have to routinely examine the platelet count as well.

Case 2

A 28-year-old female (*gravida* 3 *para* 1 *abortus* 1) in the 12th week of pregnancy underwent a routine hematological examination that showed a slight anemia with a Hb value of 10.1 g/dl on December 4th, 1988. She was started on iron pills. However, anemia and leukocytosis progressed. The Hb value was 8.7 g/dl and the WBC count was 25 600/μl on February 19th, 1989.

On March 13th, 1989, in the 26th week of pregnancy, she was referred to our department. She complained of slight fatigue but had no bleeding tendency. A

Table 1. Hematological study before admission of case 1

Date (month/day/year)	WBC (/μl)	RBC ($\times 10^4/\mu$l)	Hb (g/dl)	Hct (%)	Plt ($\times 10^4/\mu$l)
7/ 6/87	5400	315	10.8	29.5	ND
7/28/87	6500	388	12.3	34.8	ND
11/11/87	5100	342	10.4	32.1	ND
12/24/87	delivery	—	—	—	—
12/25/87	2700	298	9.4	ND	5.2
12/28/87	2800	278	8.7	27.2	9.4
1/ 2/88	2900	276	8.9	27.6	ND
2/13/88	3200	314	10.5	31.9	6.2
2/26/88	3200	311	10.7	31.6	5.1
3/ 1/88	2500	294	10.0	ND	3.7

RBC, red blood count; Hb, hemoglobin; Hct, hematocrit; Plt, platelet count physical examination showed anemia in the conjunctiva. Analysis revealed the following values: Hb, 8.5 g/dl; WBC, 35 600/μl with 4% of blasts; platelet count, 37 000/μl. Lactic dehydrogenase (LDH) (1 206 IU/l) was increased markedly. Bone marrow was hyperplastic and 5.1% of the nucleated cells consisted of blasts. Dysplasia of the three lines of hematopoietic cells was observed. A few blasts had Auer rods. Based on these findings, this case was diagnosed as myelodysplastic syndrome (MDS). According to FAB classification, this was considered to be refractory anemia with excess of blasts in transformation (RAEB in T).

During the period of pregnancy no progression of the disease was detected. The patient was observed but received only dexamethasone to prevent respiratory distress syndrome (RDS) in the fetus. An artificial delivery was induced in the 37th week of pregnancy following transfusions of erythrocyte concentrate and platelet. She had a healthy female weighing 2390 g.

Two months after the delivery, a marked leukocytosis with 50% of blasts was observed. We thought that she had AML at that time. She is receiving 6-MP as an outpatient at the present time.

Discussion

Based on the progress of medicine, patients with hematopoietic malignancies now have a better chance to have healthy pregnancies and deliveries [7]. However, it is expected that cases of pregnancy complicated by hematopoietic malignancies will increase.

Although many cases similar to case 1 have been reported in the world, our responses in Japan to such cases are completely different from those in Western countries. We usually determine the discontinuation of pregnancy on the following basis [7]:

1. When the type of leukemia has a poor prognosis
2. When a protocol of combined chemotherapy which is markedly harmful to the fetus must be chosen to prolong the mother's life
3. When infection or bleeding is anticipated
4. When there is a possibility of transfer of leukemic cells from the mother to the fetus
5. When the mother cannot be expected to live any longer

It is generally agreed that the patient is recommended to continue her pregnancy if she is more than 7 months pregnant; otherwise, to discontinue it [7–9]. We tend to give priority to treatment of leukemia over delivery of a normal newborn in our country.

By contrast, in Western countries, they have more experience with such cases; namely, they have treated a number of such cases and observed the growth of fetuses and babies [1–6]. Thus, they usually treat pregnant patients with hematopoietic malignancies except for the first trimester of pregnancy [1–6, 10]. The occurrence of malformation of the fetuses due to chemotherapy is extremely lower than we expected, based on the experimental data using animal models

[6]. According to the long-term follow-up study of the babies who were delivered by patients who had undergone chemotherapy, there are few reports of retarded children [3,5]. Since chemotherapy treatment against leukemia has markedly progressed and CR can be achieved after induction chemotherapy in more than 65% of patients with AML and in more than 79% of patients with acute lymphoblastic leukemia (ALL) who are of child-bearing age [11], it is suggested that the pregnant patients should receive chemotherapy during the second and the third trimester of pregnancy [3,6]. It is ideal that they are in CR state at their delivery; however, late in the third trimester it may not be possible to achieve remission before spontaneous labor intervenes [12]. Therefore, if the fetus is expected to survive out of the uterus, we should carry out an artificial delivery with platelet transfusion and care for infection [1,12].

Case 2 is a pregnant patient with MDS (RAEB in T). This is a rare case. MDS is a primary cytopenia with dysplastic morphology of hematopoietic cells, generally not due to bone marrow hypoplasia [13,14]. This syndrome is usually seen in the aged, ultimately leading to overt leukemia. Unfortunately, it is refractory to treatment and the main cause of death is infection and bleeding due to bone marrow failure.

RAEB in T is a high-risk group of MDS; the mean survival-time after the diagnosis is 5 months [15]. Various therapeutic modalities have given disappointing results. Since MDS is the abnormality of pluriopotent stem cells, BMT which can eradicate the malignant clone may be the most effective therapy [14,16].

This case appeared to have RAEB in T during the period of pregnancy and to have AML after the delivery. At present, there is no established treatment for this disease [14]. If we treat this patient in a similar manner to acute leukemia patients, she will have prolonged marrow suppression, thus inducing unfavorable influence on her and the fetus. Pretreatment for BMT is also dangerous to her during pregnancy although it is considered to be one of the curing treatments.

Therefore, when the disease progression is slow and mild, it is deemed wise to observe the patients without chemotherapy during the period of pregnancy and to select the therapeutic modality after the delivery. We need to increase our experience with similar cases and analyze the relationship between prognosis and the type of treatment or the timing of treatment in the future.

Summary. It is difficult to determine the proper timing of treatment for pregnant patients with malignancies, since anticancer drugs are toxic to the fetuses as well. We have recently experienced two such cases with hematopoietic malignancies. The first case is a 24-year-old patient who had anemia at 20 weeks gestation. Finally, she was diagnosed as having AML according to the hematological examinations. After the delivery, she received chemotherapy and autologous bone-marrow transplantation during the first complete remission. The second case is a 28-year-old patient who had anemia and thrombocytopenia at 12 weeks gestation. According to the hematological examinations, she was diagnosed as having RAEB-T (MDS). Since the disease was not progressive, no treatment was carried out during the pregnancy. We discuss the diagnosis and the treatment in pregnant patients with hematopoietic malignancies.

References

1. Catanzarite VA, Ferguson JE (1984) Acute leukemia and pregnancy: a review of management and outcome, 1972–1982 Obstet Gynecol Surv 39: 663–678
2. Fassas A, Kartalis G, Klearchu N, Tsatalus K, Sinacos Z, Mantalenakis S (1984) Chemotherapy for acute leukemia during pregnancy: Five case reports. Nouv Rev Fr Hematol 26: 19–24
3. Reynoso EE, Shepherd FA, Messner HA, Farquharson HA, Garvey MB, Baker MA (1987) Acute leukemia during pregnancy: The Toronto Leukemia Study Group experience with long-term follow-up of children exposed in utero to chemotherapeutic agents. J Clin Oncol 5: 1098–1106
4. Juárez S, Cuadrado Pastor JM, Feliu J, González Barón M, Ordóñez A, Montero JM (1988) Association of leukemia and pregnancy: clinical and obstetric aspects. Am J Clin Oncol 11: 159–165
5. Avilés A, Niz J (1988) Long-term follow-up of children born to mothers with acute leukemia during pregnancy. Med Pediat Oncol 16: 3–6
6. Feliu J, Juárez S, Ordóñez A, Garcia Paredes ML, González Barón M, Montero JM (1988) Acute leukemia and pregnancy. Cancer 61: 580–584
7. Kamiya T (1988) Discussion of hematological disorders complicated with pregnancy and labor. Gendai Igaku 36: 17–24 (in Japanese)
8. Tsumoto S, Ohyabu H, Sueyoshi K, Kageyama T (1981) A case of acute myelogenous leukemia occurring during the second trimester of pregnancy. Jpn J Clin Hemat 22: 1737–1742 (in Japanese)
9. Fukuda M, Fukushima Y, Miura A, Maeda H, Chida K, Fujiwara T, Higuchi S (1981) A case of acute myeloid leukemia who labored immature baby with erythroblastosis, agranulocytosis and hypoplastic bone marrow. Jpn J Clin Hemat 22: 1773–1780 (in Japanese)
10. Bartsch HH, Meyer D, Teichmann AT, Speer CP (1988) Treatment of promyelocytic leukemia during pregnancy: a case report and review of the literature. Blut 57: 51–54
11. Volkenandt M, Buchner T, Hiddemann W, Van de Loo J (1988) Acute leukemia during pregnancy. Lancet i: 1404
12. Griffiths M (1988) Acute leukemia during pregnancy. Lancet i: 586
13. Bennett JM, Catovsky D, Daniel MT, Flandrin G, Galton DAG, Gralnick HR, Sultan C (1982) Proposals for the classification of the myelodysplastic syndrome. Br J Haematol 51: 189–199
14. Yoshida Y (1988) Recent progress in treatment of hematological malignancies III. Acute leukemia (II) 2) Management of patients with myelodysplastic syndromes and atypical leukemias. J Jpn Soc Intern Med 78: 785–788 (in Japanese)
15. Mufti GJ, Stevens JR, Oscier DG, Hamblin TJ, Machin D (1985) Myelodysplastic syndromes: a scoring system with prognostic significance. Br J Haematol 59: 425–433
16. Belanger R, Gyger M, Perreanlt C, Bonny Y, St-Louis J (1988) Bone marrow transplantation for myelodysplastic syndromes. Br J Haematol 69: 29–33

References

2.5 Thrombocytopenia Associated with Type IIB von Willebrand's Disease of Pregnant Identical Twins

Masahiro Ieko[1], Megumi Yoshikawa[1], Shyouki Sakurama[1], Akira Sagawa[1], Tarou Yasukouchi[2], and Shyoichi Nakagawa

Introduction

Type II B von Willebrand's disease (vWD) is an inherited hemorrhagic disorder. The disease is characterized by the enhanced platelet aggregation at low ristocetin concentrations in the patient's platelet-rich plasma (PRP). This characteristic suggests that type II B vWD may induce a marked decrease in the platelet count under some conditions. We found pregnant identical twin mothers with marked thrombocytopenia. The twins also had type II B vW disease as well as systemic lupus erythematosus (SLE). We will report about these two cases with a recommendation for an appropriate therapy for thrombocytopenia associated with pregnancy in patients with type II B vWD disease.

Methods

VIII: C was measured using a one-stage method. VIII R: Ag was quantitated by rocket immunoelectrophoresis. Ristocetin co-factor activity (RCof) was measured using von Willebrand Reagent (Behringwerke AG, Marburg, FRG). Multimeric assays were performed by thin layer 1.2% agarose gel electrophoresis in the presence of 0.1% sodium dodecylbenzenesulfonate using the discontinuous buffer system. Von Willebrand factor (vWF) multimers were visualized directly on the gel using an immunoperoxidase technique.

[1]Second Department of Internal Medicine, Hokkaido University School of Medicine, Sapporo, 060 Japan
[2]Department of Internal Medicine, Higashi Nippon Gakuen University School of Dentistry, Toubetsu, Hokkaido, 061–02 Japan

Case Histories and Results

Case 1

The proband (Fig. 1, II-2) has been under treatment with prednisolone for SLE since she was 20 years old. She became pregnant with her first child at the age of 23 years. In the third trimester of pregnancy, her platelet count began to fall below the normal range. Anti-DNA antibody and CH_{50} remained unchanged. Bone marrow aspiration revealed the normal count of megakaryocytes. Furthermore, antiplatelet antibody and lupus anticoagulant were not present. Her platelet count became as low as 65 000/μl in the 39th week of pregnancy. Large-dose γ-globulin and prednisolone were administered, keeping in mind the possibility of an immune thrombocytopenic reaction. However, these treatments failed, and her platelet count decreased further to 47 000/μl. Labor was immediately induced and she bore a healthy boy. Interestingly, her platelet count increased sharply and spontaneously to 352 000/μl on the third postpartum day.

Eight months after her delivery, we examined the platelet aggregation studies. It showed 0.6 mg/ml ristocetin induced the aggregation of the patient's platelet. No spontaneous platelet aggregation was observed in the patient's PRP.

Factor VIII activity and Factor VIII related antigen were within the normal range throughout the clinical course. RCof decreased markedly as delivery drew near. However, its activity returned to the normal range immediately after delivery (Table 1).

VWF in her plasma lacked the large-sized multimers during the third trimester of pregnancy and immediately after parturition. However, these multimers gradually returned to the normal components thereafter (Fig. 2).

Case 2

The proband's sister (Fig. 1, II-3) has also been under treatment for SLE. She became pregnant with her first child about 1 year after the proband's delivery and followed almost the same course as that of the proband. In the 39th week of pregnancy, her platelet count decreased to 60 000/μl with genital hemorrhage.

Table 1. Changes in von willebrand factor and platelet count (patient II-2)

Date		Platelet count ($\times 10^4/\mu$l)	BT (min)	VIII:C (%)	VIIIR:Ag (%)	R Cof (%)
May/17/84		37.4	4.0	180	83	112
Jun/16/86	gw 15th	27.9	6.5	120	98	26
Nov/27/86	delivery	4.7	—	107	83	17
Jul/27/87		33.2	4.5	115	87	83
Normal		12.0–40.0	3.0–5.0	70–140	60–140	60–140

BT, bleeding time (Duke's methods); gw, gestational week; R Cof, ristocetin co-factor activity

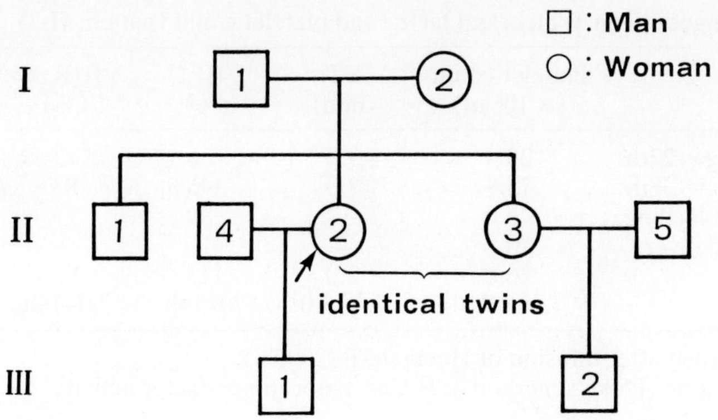

	age	ⅧR : Ag	R Cof	vWF multimer
I −1	56 y	107	160	normal
I −2	51 y	87	45	large components(−)
II −1	25 y	87	71	normal
III −1	1 y	98	146	normal
III −2	2 m	133	150	normal
		(%)	(%)	

Fig. 1. Pedigree of family with type II B von Willebrand's disease (vWD). Decreased ristocetin co-factor activity (*RCof*) and deficient large-sized von Willebrand factor (*vWF*) multimers were noted in the mother (*I-2*) of the patients (*II-2* and *II-3*) as well

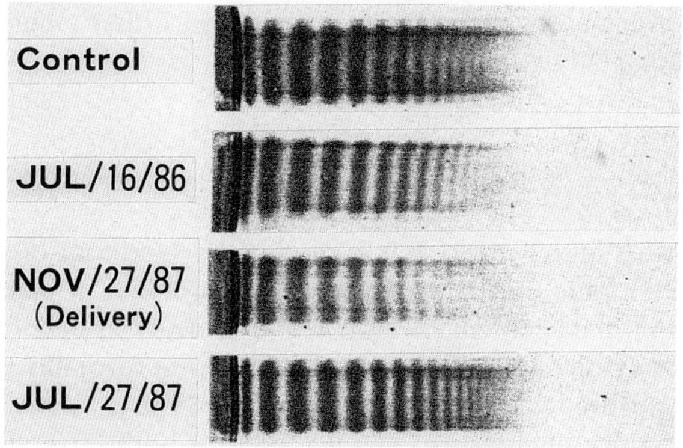

Fig. 2. Changes in von Willebrand factor multimers (patient II-2). Large-sized von Willebrand factor multimers showed a deficiency in the third trimester of her pregnancy and immediataly after parturition, but returned to the normal range thereafter

Table 2. Changes in von Willebrand factor and platelet count (patient II-3)

Date		Platelet count ($\times 10^4/\mu l$)	BT (min)	VIII:C (%)	VIIIR:Ag (%)	R Cof (%)
May/30/88	gw 22th	28.4	5.0	86	77	44
Sep/19/88	gw 38th	13.9	7.0	146	83	47
Oct/4/88	bleeding	6.0	—	89	77	35
Oct/5/88	delivery*	10.8	—	—	—	150
Oct/10/88		26.8	2.0	123	92	84
Normal		12.0–40.0	3.0–5.0	70–140	60–140	60–140

*Values recorded after infusion of Haemate-P (2000 u).
BT, bleeding time (Duke's methods); R Cof, ristocetin co-factor activity; gw, gestational week

A pasteurized factor VIII concentrate, Haemate P, was infused at a dose of 2000 units. On the following day, the platelet count increased to 102000/μl. However, she underwent cesarean section because of threatened fetal distress and delivered a healthy boy. The platelet count was 108000/μl immediately after parturition but thereafter showed sharp improvement.

Platelet aggregation in her PRP was induced at 0.4 mg/ml ristocetin and spontaneous platelet aggregation was observed in the 34th week of her pregnancy.

Factor VIII activity and factor VIII related antigen in the sister's plasma were within the normal range throughout the period under study. RCof decreased in the third trimester of pregnancy. However, 1 day after the infusion of the factor VIII concentrate, RCof showed a 150% increase (Table 2).

The patient's plasma lacked the large multimers in the third trimester of her pregnancy. However, these multimeric components were restored after treatment. There was no difference in large-sized vWF multimers between the patient's postpartum plasma and normal plasma (Fig. 3).

Further investigations were carried out to clarify coagulation functions of family members. A decrease in RCof activity and a deficiency in large multimers of plasma vWF were observed in the twins' mother. Other members showed no evidence of abnormality in their plasma (Fig. 1).

Comments

The identical twins had Type II B vWD with the symptom of marked thrombocytopenia developing during pregnancy. The problem in this study was that long-term routine management of SLE led to a delay in elucidating the exact cause of thrombocytopenia. All pregnant women with thrombocytopenia should be tested for the presence of Type II B vWD.

It has not been documented yet how to treat for both thrombocytopenia and the resultant bleeding tendency that is caused by Type II B vWD. For the second case we administered a Factor VIII concentrate. As a result, this concentrate normalized RCof and vWF multimeric conponents. Therefore, this concentrate

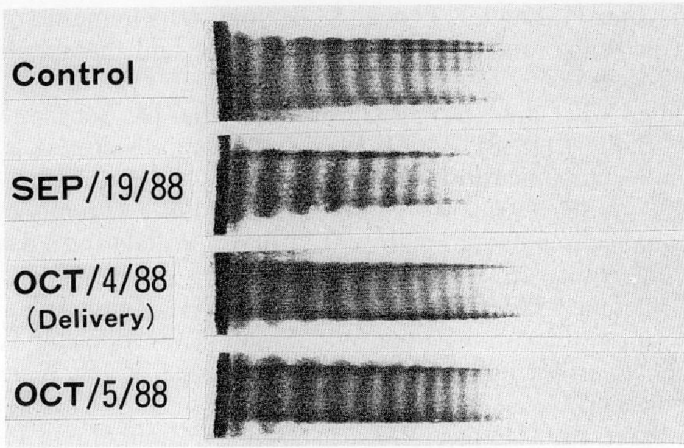

Fig. 3. Changes in von Willebrand factor multimers (patient II-3). Large-sized von Willebrand factor multimers showed a deficiency in the third trimester of pregnancy, but were restored by a factor VIII concentration administered immediately before parturition

prevented the further decrease of platelet count and treated succesfully the hemorrhagic tendency occurring during pregnancy. We consider this concentrate useful for improving both thrombocytopenia as well as the bleeding tendency caused by Type II B vWD.

Summary. Marked thrombocytopenia was detected during the pregnancy of one of identical twins suffering from systemic lupus erythematosus (SLE). Her platelet count decreased in the third trimester of pregnancy and returned to normal immediately after delivery. Laboratory examinations revealed the decreased of ristocetin co-factor activity and the lack of large multimers of von Willebrand factor (vWF) in plasma samples of the third trimeser. These abnormalities improved after delivery. Investigation of family members revealed that the identical twins inherited type II B vWD from their mother.

The other twin became pregnant about 1 year later and followed almost the same course observed in the proband. The bleeding tendency surfaced a few days before delivery. Subsequently, a Factor VIII concentrate (Haemate P) was administered for the purpose of competing with her variant vWD. After treatment, a further decrease in the platelet count was prevented and the hemorrhagic tendency was improved.

While the exact mechanism of thrombocytopenia during pregnancy still remains unclarified, it seems evident that the Factor VIII concentrate would be effective in treating thrombocytopenia associated with Type II B vWD.

References

1. Giles AR, Hoogendoorn H, Benford K (1987) Type II B von Willebrand's disease presenting as thrombocytopenia during pregnancy. Br J Haematol 67: 349–353
2. Gralnick HR, Williams SB, McKeown LP, Rick M (1985) Von Willebrand's disease with spontaneous platelet aggregation induced by abnormal plasma von Willebrand factor. J Clin Invest 76: 1522–1529

3. Kyrle PA, Niessner H, Dent J, Panzer S, Brenner B, Zimmerman TS, Lechner K (1988) II B von Willebrand's disease: pathogenetic and therapeutic studies. Br J Haematol 69: 55–59
4. López-Fernández MF, López-Berges C, Martín-Bernal JA, Sánchez R, Villarón LG, Díez-Jarilla J, Batlle J (1988) Type II B von Willebrand's disease associated with a complex thrombocytopenic thrombocytopathy. Am J Hematol 27: 291–298
5. Rick ME, Williams SB, Sacher RA, McKeown LP (1987) Thrombocytopenia associated with pregnancy in a patient with type II B von Willebrand's disease. Blood 69: 786–789
6. Ruggeri ZM, Mannucci PM, Lombardi R, Federici AB, Zimmerman TS (1982) Multimeric composition of factor VIII/von Willebrand factor following administration of DDAVP: Implication for pathophysiology and therapy of von Willebrand's disease subtypes. Blood 59: 1272–1278
7. Ruggeri ZM, Pareti FI, Mannuçci PM, Ciavarella N, Zimmerman TS (1980) Heightened interaction platelets and factor VIII/von Willebrand factor in a new subtype of von Willebrand's disease. N Engl J Med 302: 1047–1051
8. Saba HI, Saba HR, Dent J, Ruggeri ZM, Zimmerman TS (1985) Type II B Tampa: a variant of von Willebrand disease with chronic thrombocytopenia, circulating platelet aggregates, and spontaneous platelet aggregation. Blood 66: 282–286
9. Takahashi H, Tatewaki W, Nagayama R, Hanano M, Tamura M, Yamaguchi T, Takizawa S, Wada K, Shibata A (1987) Heated-treated factor VIII/von Willebrand factor concentrate in platelet-type von Willebrand's disease. Haemostasis 17: 353–360
10. Takahashi H, Tsukada T, Tatewaki W, Hanano M, Sanada M, Shibata A (1987) Von Willebrand factor fragment in type II B von Willebrand's disease: Demonstration of two different forms of fragments. Haemostasis 17: 182–188

2.6 Management of Pregnancy Complicated with Idiopathic Thrombocytopenic Purpura: A Review of 16 Cases

TAKEHIKO MATSUYAMA, KATSUHIKO IWASAKI, and AKIKAZU FUJII[1]

Introduction

Idiopathic thrombocytopenic purpura (ITP) is an autoimmune disorder related to the destruction, mostly in the spleen, of platelets coated with antibody which belongs, usually, to the IgG class. Normalization of platelet value after both acute and chronic ITP may occur spontaneously, but recovery by surgical or pharmaceutical treatment is preferred for several reasons. Primary goals are to decrease the production of antibodies or to modify the production of phagocytosing macrophages quantitatively or qualitatively. The etiology of primary ITP is unknown, but it follows secondarily to various other diseases, especially viral infections. Since ITP is common in young women in their reproductive years, it does occasionally complicate pregnancy. On one hand, fertility is not affected by the disease [10], but on the other, the percentage of spontaneous abortions is reported to be relatively high, between 7% and 30% [1,5,10]. The course of ITP does not seem to be influenced by pregnancy [2,9,10], while perinatal mortality can be up to 20% [1,2,6–8]. According to several reports [1,2,6–8], obstetrical management of ITP during pregnancy should be attempted in order to increase maternal platelet count throughout the pregnancy thus bringing it to term and preventing complications during labor. Karpatkin et al. [6] demonstrated that steroids are effective in increasing maternal and fetal platelet value. Recently, Imbach et al. [3,4] introduced treatment with high-dose intravenous immunoglobulin.

Two problems are addressed in this paper. One concerns the minimum platelet value needed for good results and the required management during pregnancy. The other concerns treatment for prevention of complications during delivery.

[1]Department of Obstetrics and Gynecology, Takai University School of Medicine, Bouseidai, Isehara, Kanagawa, 259-11 Japan

Table. 1. Pregnancies complicated by idiopathic thrombocytopenic purpura

Case	Age (years)	Pregnancy history	PLT and treatment (trimester) 1st	2nd	3rd	Treatment for delivery	PLT before delivery
1	26	1 − 0 − 0 = 1	2.6 PSL10 mg/d	20.0 PSL 10 mg/d	26.4 PSL 10 mg/d	PSL 10 mg/dl	26.0
2*	33	2 − 0 − 2 = 2	27.1 PSL 20 mg/d	27.8 PSL 20 mg/d	28.1 PSL 20 mg/d	PSL 20 mg/dl	28.1
3	27	0 − 0 − 0 = 0	1.0 PSL 10 mg/d	5.0 PSL 10 mg/d ACTH-Z 0.2 ml	0.7 PSL 30 mg/d ATCH-Z 0.3 ml	PSL 60 mg/d ACTH-Z 1.0 ml Fresh blood 2000 ml Platelets 11IU	10.8
4	22	0 − 0 − 0 = 0	? (−)	? (−)	4.8 (−)	PSL 30 mg/d	11.8
5*	26	1 − 0 − 1 = 1	6.8 (−)	8.8 (−)	8.4 (−)	PSL 20 mg/d	9.7
6	36	3 − 0 − 8 = 3	8.4 (−)	6.4 (−)	7.9 (−)	γ-gl. 15 g × 6	10.1
7	39	3 − 0 − 1 = 3	19.3 (−)	19.6 (−)	20.2 (−)	(−)	20.2
8	27	0 − 0 − 1 = 0	? (−)	? (−)	2.4 (−)	PSL 10 mg/d	2.9
9	25	0 − 0 − 0 = 0	12.1 (−)	? (−)	14.0 (−)	(−)	14.0
10	25	0 − 0 − 0 = 0	? (−)	? (−)	0.2 (−)	PSL 60 mg/d γgl. 25 g × 2	0.6
11*	29	0 − 1 − 0 = 0	10.9 PSL 10 mg/dl	5.2 PSL 20 mg/dl	5.1 PSL 20 mg/d	γ-gl. 20 g × 5	9.3
12	33	1 − 0 − 1 = 1	14.9 (−)	17.9 (−)	18.5 (−)	(−)	18.5
13	21	0 − 0 − 0 = 0	8.0 (−)	5.4 (−)	6.3 (−)	PSL 20 mg/d	5.9
14	22	0 − 0 − 0 = 0	1.3 (−)	2.0 (−)	3.3 PSL 30 mg/d	PSL 20 mg/d γ-gl. 12.5 g × 3	10.1
15	35	2 − 0 − 0 = 2	4.8 (−)	4.8 (−)	8.1 (−)	γ-gl. 50 g × 1	16.2
16	28	0 − 0 − 0 = 0	5.7 (−)	4.8 (−)	6.1 (−)	γgl. 50 g × 1	7.6

*Same patient as case above
PLT, platelet count (× 10 000); AP-S, Apgar score; PSL, prednisolone; (−), no treat-

Patients and Results

Of the approximately 7 000 deliveries in our hospital during the past 10 years, 16 were complicated with ITP (Table 1). Two patients had not been diagnosed

PLT after delivery	Delivery style	Duration of pregnancy	Time required	Blood loss (ml)	Infant			Other
					Sex	AP-S	Weight	
22.1	Vaginal	38W5d	4h51min	190	F	9	2 716	+ SLE
27.8	Vaginal	36W5d	2h50min	230	M	9	2 812	+ SLE
2.5	Vaginal	38W0d	11h13min	412	M	9	3 135	
4.0	Vaginal	38W6d	9h37min	292	F	9	2 580	Referral
12.9	Vaginal	38W6d	7h21min	260	F	9	2 141	
13.7	Cesarean	34W6d	—	422	F	4	1 910	
15.8	Cesarean	39W1d	—	170	F	9	2 394	
2.9	Cesarean	33W1d	—	408	F	0	1 545	Fetal distress Referral
16.5	Vaginal	38W4d	10h30min	150	F	7	2 396	
2.0	Vaginal	29W2d	3h52min	380	F	0	716	Fetal death Referral
10.3	Vaginal	37W4d	6h22min	156	F	8	2 696	
28.5	vaginal	36W6d	3h37min	312	M	9	3 440	
11.0	Cesarean	40W1d	—	168	M	7	2 944	Referral
13.8	Vaginal	37W2d	9h22min	466	M	9	2 986	Referral
13.7	Vaginal	37W1d	2h56min	454	M	8	3 515	Infant's PLT 3.5
9.4	Vaginal	38W3d	13h00min	424	F	9	3 010	

ment; W, week; d, day; SLE, systemic lupus erythematosus; ACTH-Z, adrenocortico tropic hormone; γ-gl., γ-globulin

as having ITP before coming to our hospital (cases 8, 10). To analyze our data on these 16 cases, we classified them into two groups according to pregnancies: an untreated group and a treated group (by prednisolone [PSL]). We further classified them into three groups according to treatment during delivery: (1) an untreated group, (2) a PSL-treated group, and (3) a γ-globulin-treated group.

Table 2. Management during pregnancy (untreated cases)

Case	Age (years)	Pregnancy history	Platelet count (trimester) 1st	2nd	3rd	Other
4	22	0 − 0 − 0 = 0	?	?	48 000	Referral
5	26	1 − 0 − 1 = 1	68 000	88 000	84 000	
6	36	3 − 0 − 8 = 3	84 000	64 000	79 000	
7	39	3 − 0 − 1 = 3	193 000	196 000	202 000	
8	27	0 − 0 − 1 = 0	?	?	24 000	Referral
9	25	0 − 0 − 0 = 0	121 000	?	140 000	
10	25	0 − 0 − 0 = 0	?	?	2 000	Referral
12	33	1 − 0 − 1 = 1	149 000	179 000	185 000	
13	21	0 − 0 − 0 = 0	80 000	54 000	63 000	Referral
15	35	2 − 0 − 0 = 2	48 000	48 000	81 000	
16	28	0 − 0 − 0 = 0	57 000	48 000	61 000	

Table 3. Management during pregnancy (treated cases)

Case	Age (years)	Pregnancy history	Platelet count (trimester) and treatment 1st	2nd	3rd	Other
1	26	1 − 0 − 2 = 1	26 000 PSL 10 mg	200 000 PSL 10 mg	264 000 PSL 10 mg	+ SLE
2	33	2 − 0 − 2 = 2	271 000 PSL 20 mg	278 000 PSL 20 mg	281 000 PSL 20 mg	+ SLE
3	27	0 − 0 − 0 = 0	10 000 PSL 10 mg	50 000 PSL 10 mg ACTH-Z 0.2 ml	7 000 PSL 30 mg ACTH-Z 0.3 ml	
11	29	0 − 1 − 0 = 0	109 000 PSL 10 mg	52 000 PSL 20 mg	51 000 PSL 20 mg	
14	22	0 − 0 − 0 = 0	13 000 (−)	20 000 (−)	33 000 PSL 30 mg	Referral

All dosages shown are daily.
PSL, prednisolone; ACTH-Z, adrenocorticotropic hormone; SLE, systemic lupus erythematosus

During Pregnancy

Table 2 lists the 11 untreated cases. The platelet values given for each trimester are the lowest values recorded. Those of most patients were above 50 000. Case 10 was referred to our hospital because of fetal death and had not been diagnosed as having ITP. We considered the possibility of DIC and fetal death syndrome, but the laboratory data, including bone marrow aspiration, showed only ITP. Case 8 was referred to us due to the onset of premature labor, and after hospitalization we diagnosed ITP.

Table 3 shows the treated group. Cases 1 and 2 are the same patient, who had the additional complication of systemic lupuserythematosus (SLE), so under stricter definition, she should not be classified under ITP. PSL was administered for treatment of SLE. Case 3 was the most severe case. Platelet values ranged

Table 4. Treatment for delivery (untreated cases)

Case	Age (years)	Pregnancy history	Platelet count 3rd trimester	Before delivery	After delivery	Blood loss (ml)
7	39	3 − 0 − 1 = 3	202 000	202 000	158 000	170
9	25	0 − 0 − 0 = 0	140 000	140 000	165 000	150
12	33	1 − 0 − 1 = 1	185 000	185 000	285 000	312

from 5 000 to 50 000 during the first and second trimesters but did not increase above 7 000 during the third. Case 14 was referred to us at 38 weeks.

Delivery

Next we investigated management during delivery. Table 4 depicts the untreated group. All patients have platelet values above 100 000, and intrapartum bleeding was slight. In the PSL-treated group (Table 5), PSL was administered for the first time in cases of 4, 5, 8, 10, and 13. Case 10 was referred to us because of fetal death and very low platelet counts. Efforts to increase platelet count rapidly by administration of PSL and γ-globulin could not be completed before labor pains started. Case 8 was similar in that, before we could complete our schedule, fetal distress such as late deceleration appeared, and we had to perform a cesarean section. Case 3 was particularly difficult. No increase in platelet count could be effected even though we raised the amount of PSL and adrenocorticotropic hormone (ACTH-Z) administered; finally, we were forced to transfuse 2 000 ml of fresh whole blood and 11 IU of concentrated platelets. At that time, γ-globulin injection therapy had not yet been developed. Except for cases 3, 8, and 10, the results were satisfying. Cases involving γ-globulin treatment are shown in Table 6. We believe that if we are able to complete therapy, the platelet value count will increase sufficiently for delivery.

In general in the 16 deliveries studied, intrapartum blood losses were within normal volumes (150–466 ml). Two perinatal deaths occurred: one fetal death at 29 weeks pregnancy (case 10) and another following fetal distress at 33 weeks pregnancy (case 8). One infant with a platelet count of 35 000 (case 15) had congenital thrombocytopenia. The cause was estimated to be the transfer of maternal antiplatelet antibody (Table 1).

Discussion

Treatments given for ITP ordinarily include pharmacotherapy, surgical therapy, and simple platelet substitution therapy (Table 7). However, when pregnancy is a complicating factor, immunosuppressants and anabolic steroids, splenectomy, and transfusion are not always viable choices because their effects are uncertain and their safety is not established. We believe PSL is the most effective choice to maintain a good platelet count during pregnancy. For delivery, when we adopt

Table 5. Prednisolone (PSL) treatment for delivery

Case	Age (years)	Pregnancy history	Treatment for delivery	Platelet count 3rd trimester	Before delivery	After delivery	Blood loss (ml)	Other
1	26	1 – 0 – 2 = 1	PSL 10 mg/d	264 000	260 000	221 000	190	+ SLE
2	33	2 – 0 – 2 = 2	PSL 20 mg/d	281 000	281 000	278 000	230	+ SLE
3	27	0 – 0 – 0 = 0	PSL 60 mg/d ACTH-Z 1 m/d Fresh blood 2000 ml Platelets 11 IU	7 000	108 000	25 000	412	
4	22	0 – 0 – 0 = 0	PSL 30 mg/d	48 000	118 000	40 000	292	Referral
5	26	1 – 0 – 1 = 1	PSL 20 mg/d	84 000	97 000	129 000	260	
8	27	0 – 0 – 1 = 0	PSL 10 mg/d	24 000	29 000	29 000	408	Referral Fetal distress
10	25	0 – 0 – 0 = 0	PSL 60 mg/d γ-gl. 25 g × 2	2 000	6 000	20 000	380	Referral Fetal death
13	21	0 – 0 – 0 = 0	PSL 20 mg/d	63 000	59 000	110 000	168	Referral
14	22	0 – 0 – 0 = 0	PSL 20 mg/d γ-gl. 12.5g × 3	33 000	101 000	138 000	466	Referral

ACTH-Z, adrenocortico tropic hormone; γ-gl., γ-globulin; SLE, systemic lupus erythematosus; d, day

Table 6. γ-Globulin (γ-gl.) treatment for delivery

Case	Age (years)	Pregnancy history	Treatment for delivery	Platelet count 3rd trimester	Before delivery	After delivery	Blood loss (ml)	Other
6	36	3 – 0 – 8 = 3	γ-gl. 15 g × 6	79 000	101 000	137 000	422	Fetal distress
10	25	0 – 0 – 0 = 0	PSL 60 mg/d γ-gl. 25 g × 2	2 000	6 000	20 000	380	Referral Fetal death
11	29	0 – 1 – 0 = 0	γ-gl. 25 g × 5	51 000	93 000	103 000	156	
14	22	0 – 0 – 0 = 0	PSL 20 mg/d γ-gl. 12.5 g × 3	33 000	101 000	138 000	466	Referral
15	35	2 – 0 – 0 = 2	γ-gl. 50 g × 1	81 000	162 000	137 000	454	Infant's platelet count 35 000
16	28	0 – 0 – 0 = 0	γ-gl. 50 g × 1	61 000	76 000	94 000	424	

Table 7. Treatment for idiopathic thrombocytopenic purpura

Treatment
Pharmacological
Corticosteroids
Immunosuppressant
Anabolic steroids
Immunoglobulin
Surgical therapy
Splenectomy
Platelet substitution therapy
Platelet suspension
Fresh blood
Concentrated platelets

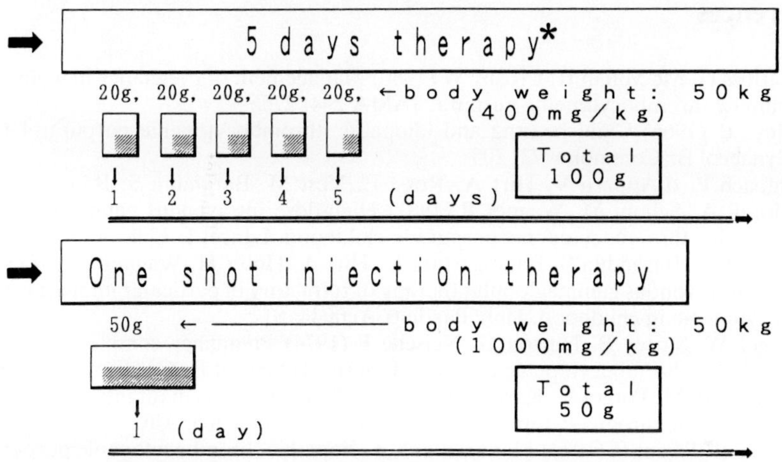

Fig. 1. Treatment of idiopathic thrombocytopenic purpura by γ-globulin. *Method reported by Imbach et al. [3,4]

corticosteroids, we must increase the doses to at least 1 mg/kg, and it takes at least 7–10 days for results.

Recently, high-dose γ-globulin injection has been reported effective in increasing platelet count rapidly (Fig. 1) [3,4]. According to Imbach et al. [3,4], 400 mg/kg daily is usually administered for 3–5 days. This treatment also takes several days to complete. In our first attempts with this method, we used 3–5 days of continuous injection therapy. Recently, however, we choose to inject a 1000 mg/kg dose within a single day (cases 15,16), because one-shot therapy demands only half the volume and half the cost, and we get satisfactory results. Three days after the treatment, because the platelet count has reached its peak, delivery is attempted. We believe immunoglobulin therapy to be the most effective for rapid treatment, and one-shot injection therapy in particular to be the best modern method in every respect.

Summary. Sixteen pregnancies complicated with idiopathic thrombocytopenic purpura (ITP) were referred to our hospital from 1977 to 1988. Five patients were treated during pregnancy with oral prednisolone (PSL) because of low platelet counts. Platelet or fresh whole blood transfusions were needed for deliveries in the past, but, recently, gross amounts of γ-globulin are given to increase platelet count. We infuse 20 g of γ-globulin daily for 3–5 days or 50 g of γ-globulin in a single day then attempt the delivery 3 days after the treatment. The course of each pregnancy we treated resulted in favorable conditions except for one case of intrauterine fetal death (IUFD). Vaginal deliveries accounted for 12 cases, while cesarean section was performed in 4 cases because of cephalopelvic disproportion (CPD) or fetal distress. The newborns had a tendency to be lighter than average, and one case of congenital ITP was found.

References

1. Carloss H, Mc Millan R, Crosby W (1980) Management of pregnancy in women with immune thrombocytopenic purpura. JAMA 244: 2756
2. Heys R (1966) Child bearing and idiopathic thrombocytopenic purpura. J Obstet Gynaecol Br Commonw 73: 205
3. Imbach P, d'Apuzzo V, Hirt A, Rossi E, Vest M, Barandun S, Baumgartner C, Morell A, Schoni M, Wagner P (1981) High-dose intravenous gammaglobulin for idiopathic thrombocytopenic purpura in childhood. Lancet I: 1228
4. Imbach P, Barandun S, Baumgartner C, Hirt A, Hofer H, Wagner P (1981) High-dose intravenous gammaglobulin therapy of refractory in particular idiopathic thrombocytopenia in childhood. Helv Paediatr Acta 44: 81
5. Jones W, Storey B, Norton G, Neische F (1974) Pregnancy complicated by acute idiopathic thrombocytopenic purpura. J Obstet Gynaecol Br Commonw 81: 330
6. Karpatkin M, Porges R, Karpatkin S (1981) Platelet counts in infants of women with autoimmune thrombocytopenic purpura. N Engl J Med 305: 936
7. Laros R, Sweet R (1973) Management of idiopathic thrombocytopenic purpura during pregnancy. Am J Obstet Gynecol 122: 182
8. Murray J, Major U, Harris R (1976) The management of the pregnant patient with idiopathic thrombocytopenic purpura. Am J Obstet Gynecol 126: 449
9. Robson HM, Davidson LSP (1950) Purpura in pregnancy with special reference to idiopathic thrombocytopenic purpura. Lancet II: 164
10. Schenker J, Polishuk W (1968) Idiopathic thrombocytopenic purpura in pregnancy. Gynecologia 165: 271

2.7 The Management of Immunologic Thrombocytopenic Purpura (ITP) During Pregnancy

M. Nakabayashi, K. Takagi, T. Mimuro, S. Mushiaki, Y. Takeda, and S. Sakamoto[1]

Introduction

Immunologic thrombocytopenic purpura (ITP), in which both mother and fetus are affected by an antibody which acts against platelets, is one of the major complications of pregnancy. The resultant thrombocytopenia may cause hemorrhage, not only in the mother but also in her fetus, because in some cases the antibody crosses the placenta which leads to fetal intracranial hemorrhage on vaginal delivery. The management of ITP during pregnancy has been controversial for the following reasons: Firstly, it is not clear whether pregnancy affects the natural course of ITP. Therefore, there is no clear-cut criteria for determining whether or not to terminate the pregnancy with the hope that ITP may be improved by this measure. Secondly, one has to consider the mode of delivery, because in the presence of maternal thrombocytopenia vaginal delivery is preferred, since this minimizes maternal blood loss and is thus less traumatic for the mother than cesarean section. In contrast, in the presence of fetal thrombocytopenia, although the incidence of severe fetal thrombocytopenia has been reported to be low, cesarean section is better. However it has been reported that there is not a strong correlation between fetal and maternal platelet counts [1]. This evidence makes the problem more complicated.

In 1985, Daffos et al. [2] reported direct umbilical blood sampling for the diagnosis of fetal thrombocytopenia. They also showed that platelet transfusion to the fetus via the umbilical cord could be effective in improving fetal condition. Although there is an increasing amount of literature reporting the successful outcome of pregnancy with ITP, managed by cordocentesis, the major problem seems to be that cordocentesis itself carries the risk of potential bleeding for both mother and fetus. Another recent advance in the treatment of ITP is high dose

[1]Maternal and Perinatal Center, Tokyo Women's Medical College, 8-1, Kawada-cho, Shinjuku-ku, Tokyo 162, Japan

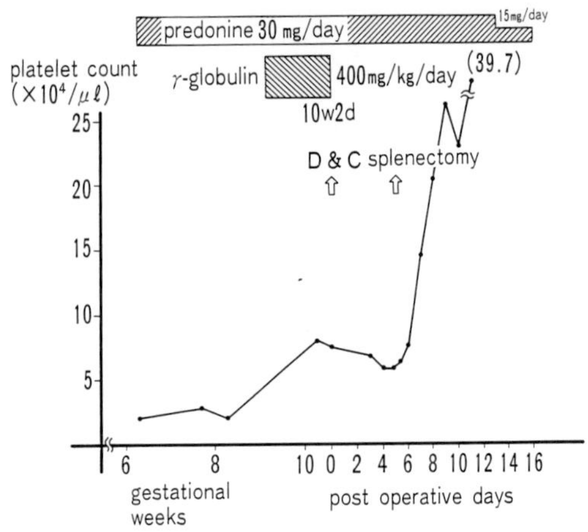

Fig. 1. Case 1, Termination of pregnancy with ITP successfully managed with high dose γ-globlin therapy followed by splenectomy

immunoglobulin therapy. But again, there is a limitation with this treatment because the effects of immunoglobulin therapy are usually transient. Therefore we would like to focus on the management of ITP during pregnancy, showing two representative cases in detail and then reviewing the cases we have had during the last 4 years.

Case 1. The patient was a 23-year-old primigravida, with a past history of hyperthyroidism at the age of 9 years. Thyroidectomy had been performed when she was 17 years old. Insulin dependent diabetes had been diagnosed when she was 16 years old. She had had continuous vaginal bleeding since being aware of her pregnancy. At 6 weeks of gestation, when she first visited our clinic, her platelet count was 20 000/μl. Serological testing revealed positive antiplatelet antibody. Predonine administration was started at 6 weeks of gestation and was continued for 2 weeks. At this point, there was no improvement in either the amount of vaginal bleeding or the platelet count. Therefore, since steroid therapy had not been effective, therapeutic abortion by dilatation and curettage (D & C) was performed at 10 weeks of gestation, after high dose immunoglobulin therapy (Fig. 1). Seven days after the initiation of this therapy, her platelet count increased to 79 000/μl. The D&C was uneventful; a splenectomy was performed 5 days after the D&C. The platelet count was 400 000/μl after the splenectomy.

Case 2. The patient was a 29-year-old primigravida, primipara. She was referred to our clinic because of thrombocytopenia which had been found on routine complete blood count examination in the third trimester. Her platelet count was 16 000/μl at 29 weeks of gestation. At 30 weeks of gestation, she was hospitalized for further examination and treatment. On admission, hematologic examinations showed anemia (Hb 7.0 g/dl) and thrombocytopenia, with a platelet count of 24 000/μl and an increased number of megakaryocytes in the bone marrow. Serological tests showed negative anti-platelet antibody. However, the level of platelet associated IgG (PAIgG) was elevated to 67.3 ng/10 cells. From 34 weeks-

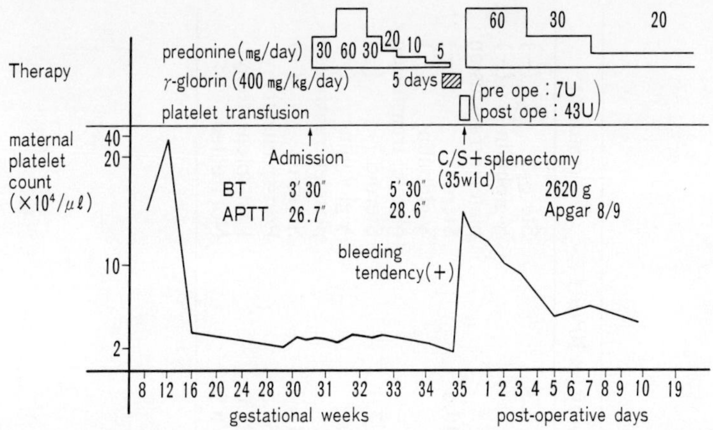

Fig. 2. Case 2, Cesarean delivery managed with combination of steroid, γ-globulin and platelet transfusion. Splenectomy was performed at the time of c/s. BT, bleeding time; APTT, activated partial thromboplastin time

of gestation, gingival bleeding began and petechia appeared on the lower extremities. At this point, we decided to deliver her. Prior to the delivery, high dose immunoglobulin therapy was employed (Fig. 2). However, there was no improvement in her platelet count. After platelet transfusion, her platelet count went up to 70 000/μl. Cesarean section and splenectomy were then performed. There were no neonatal complications. Prophylactic platelet transfusion was continued after these operations. Seven days after the cesarean section and splenectomy, her platelet count reached a level of 50 000/μl. In this case, neither steroid nor high dose immunoglobulin was effective. Only platelet transfusion and splenectomy were effective in increasing her platelets.

Table 1 shows the outcome of pregnancies with ITP treated in our perinatal unit during 1986–1989. In 3 074 deliveries during this period we had 7 cases with ITP. The first 3 cases did not respond to steroid therapy or high dose immunoglobulin therapy. In all of these cases the lowest platelet counts were below 50 000/μl. Thus, in order to perform cesarean sections and splenectomies, platelet transfusion was necessary. With successful platelet transfusion, the platelet counts at delivery were more than 50 000/μl in each of these patients and the blood loss at delivery was less than 500 ml for each of them. The rationale for performing cesarean sections is as follows: In cases with severe thrombocytopenia, laparotomy for cesarean section enables us to perform concomitant splenectomy, which would be necessary in any case for the future management of ITP with reasonable risk to the patient [3,4]. Also, one can thus avoid the risk of bleeding from umbilical cord blood sampling. In cases 4–7, the lowest platelet counts were above 50 000/μl either with or without steroid therapy. It is noteworthy that in cases 5 and 6 splenectomy had been performed prior to their pregnancies. Of these 4 cases, three delivered vaginally without complication. The only exception was case 4, in which cesarean section was performed due to cephalopelvic disproportion, despite the fact that there was no thrombo-

Table 1. Cases of pregnancy with ITP

Case	Obs.H.	Mode of delivery	Blood loss (ml)	Lowest plt. ($\times 10^4/\mu l$)	Plt. at delivery ($\times 10^4/\mu l$)	Treatment
1	G1P1	C/S	440	1.4	6.3	Steroid (−) γ-globulin (−) platelet transfusion
2	G2P2	C/S*	450	3.7	10.6	Steroid (−) γ-globulin (−) platelet transfusion
3	G0P0	C/S*	400	1.0	7.0	Steroid (−) γ-globulin (−) platelet transfusion
4	G1P1	C/S(CPD)	300	9.2	11.7	Steroid (+)
5	G0P0	Vaginal	135	29.9	36.5	Post-splenectomy
6	G3P1	Vaginal	230	26.0	28.0	Post-splenectomy
7	G1P0	Vaginal	740	6.0	6.9	Not treated

CS, Cesarean section; plt, Platelet count; ITP, Immunologic thrombocytopenic purpura
*Splenectomy was performed at the time of c/s No neonatal thrombocytopenia in any cases
(−). . . . . . Not effective
(+). . . . . . effective

cytopenia. There was no neonatal thrombocytopenia in any of the 4 cases. As mentioned above, there is poor correlation between maternal and neonatal platelet counts; it is therefore desirable to measure fetal platelet count prior to delivery, either by fetal scalp puncture when the cervix is dilated adequately, or by skillful cord centesis.

Conclusion

In the management of ITP during pregnancy, responsiveness to corticosteroids is crucial when the maternal platelet count is below 50 000/μl and/or when bleeding is present.

When steroids are effective, pregnancy may be continued, with frequent measurements of maternal platelet count and PAIgG. Termination of pregnancy is recommended if steroids are not effective.

In the management of ITP of delivery, vaginal delivery is considered when the maternal platelet count is more than 50 000/μl. Fetal blood sampling by puncture of the umbilical vein is desirable. When the maternal platelet count is less than 50 000/μl, high dose immunoglobulin therapy is indicated.

If this therapy is effective, vaginal delivery is considered for the cases with adequate fetal platelet count. If the therapy is not effective, cesarean section and splenectomy are recommended, after prior platelet transfusion.

Summary. In the management of pregnant women with immunologic thrombocytopenic purpura (ITP) it is important to control maternal bleeding tendencies and prevent fetal intracranial bleeding. Because of the difficulty of predicting fetal thrombocytopenia from maternal laboratory findings, fetal blood sampling is recommended in order to decide the method of delivery; however, its clinical usefulness in ITP during pregnancy is still controversial. In this paper, we report on two cases of pregnant women with ITP and propose a regimen for the management of ITP during pregnancy.

Regimen for the Management of ITP During Pregnancy
Corticosteroids are administered when the maternal platelet count decreases below 50 000/μl or bleeding tendency is recognized in an early stage of pregnancy. When steroid therapy is effective, term vaginal delivery is considered, with frequent measurement of maternal platelet count and platelet associated IgG (PAIgG). When steroid therapy is not effective, termination of pregnancy is recommended. Administration of high dose γ-globulin is recommended as additional theray when steroids become ineffective in advanced stages of pregnancy. When γ-globulin therapy is effective, fetal blood sampling by puncture of the umbilical vein is recommended. Vaginal delivery is preferred if the fetal platelet count is above 50 000/μl. When γ-globulin globulin therapy is ineffective, cesarean section and splenectomy are recommended, after prior platelet transfusion.

References

1. Scott JR, Rote NS, Cruikshank DP (1983) Antiplatelet antibodies and platelet counts in pregnancies complicated by autoimmune thrombocytopenic purpura. Am J Obstet Gynecol 145(8): 932–9
2. Daffos F, Capella-Pavlovsky M, Forestier F (1983) Fetal blood sampling via the umbilical cord using a needle guided by ultrasound. Report of 66 cases. Prenat Diagn 3(4): 271–7
3. Besa EC, MacNab MW, Solan AJ, Lapes M, Marfatia U (1985) High-dose intravenous IgG in the management of pregnancy in women with idiopathic thrombocytopenic purpura. Am J Hematol 18(4): 373–9
4. Cunningham FG, MacDonald PC, Gant NF (eds) (1989) Williams obstetrics 18th edn. Appleton, Norwalk p 791

2.8 Thrombocytopenia in Pregnancy

JOHN BONNAR[1]

Introduction

In obstetric practice a low platelet count is most often found in association with pregnancy complications associated with disseminated intravascular coagulation. The various causes of thrombocytopenia which may be encountered during pregnancy are listed in Table 1. When thrombocytopenia occurs as an isolated defect the commonest cause is auto-immune thrombocytopenia (AITP). The adult type of AITP is frequently a chronic disorder and is commonly found in women of childbearing age. This condition will be reviewed in relation to obstetric management.

Table 1. Thrombocytopenia in pregnancy

Obstetrical complications with DIC	Immune mechanisms
e.g. abruptio placentae;	Auto immune thrombocytopenic AITP
fetal death; pre-eclampsia.	Systemic lupus erythematosis
Massive blood transfusion	Anti phospholipid syndrome
Infections: bacterial, viral	Thryotoxicosis
Drugs: heparin, alcohol, quinine,	Allo-immune thrombocytopenia
sulphonamides, isoniazrol	Lymphoproliferative diseases
Megaloblastic anemia	Thrombotic thrombocytopenic purpura
Bone marrow malignant disease.	Hemolytic-uremic syndrome

Auto-Immune Thrombocytopenia

AITP is an acquired disorder of increased platelet destruction, which is caused by production of platelet auto antibodies. These can be measured as platelet-

[1]Trinity College Department of Obstetrics and Gynaecology, St James's Hospital and Coombe Hospital, Dublin, Ireland

associated immunoglobulins of the GorM class, ie., PAIgG or PAIgM. The antibody is directed against and coats the platelet which is then rapidly removed from the circulation, most likely by the reticuloendothelial system. The levels of the antibodies correlate with decreased platelet survival and the degree of thrombocytopenia. PAIgG crosses the placenta and produces thrombocytopenia in the fetus. Tests are available which distinguish between the PAIgG antibodies which cross the placenta and the PAIgM antibodies which do not and which identify platelet bound antibody and the free PAIgG antibody in the maternal plasma [1]. These tests are not widely available and their reliability is still in question.

In a review of the literature published between 1950 and 1983, Hegde reported an overall prevalence of neonatal thrombocytopenia of 52% with significant morbidity is 12% [2]. The probability of fetal thrombocytopenia increases with the severity of maternal thrombocytopenia; where maternal platelet counts are less than 100,000/μL at term, the incidence of neonatal thrombocytopenia is 70%. Where the mother has a platelet count in excess of 100,000/μL, the incidence of thrombocytopenia is approximately 20% in the newborn. If the mother has had a splenectomy the incidence of neonatal thrombocytopenia and morbidity is increased, even where the mother has a normal platelet count. The maternal platelet count at the time of the delivery does not correlate with the infant's cord blood platelet count [3].

Because of the rapid turnover and increased function of new platelets, spontaneous bleeding rarely occurs until the platelet count is less than 25,000/μL. Platelet counts of 50,000 μL–100,000μL provide adequate protection against bleeding from trauma and surgical procedures such as cesarean section and splenectomy. Maternal morbidity and mortality due to AITP is now very low. The main concern lies with assessing the effects on the fetus and deciding the mode of delivery for the infant who is at risk to significant thrombocytopenia. In this respect it should be emphasised that an easy vaginal delivery in a term baby should present no more risk of intracranial bleeding than a cesarean section. In the presence of maternal thrombocytopenia, a cesarean section will also carry increased risk of hemorrhage in the surgical incision of the abdominal wall and the uterus. Fatal intracranial hemorrhage can also occur in thrombocytopenic infants even during cesarean section [4].

In 1980, Carloss and colleagues, based on a literature review, recommended that pregnant women with AITP and a platelet count of less than 100,000/μL or a history of splenectomy should have a cesarean section regardless of their platelet count [5]. This recommendation would result in many unnecessary cesarean sections. The existence of PAIgG in mothers with AITP is predictive of infants who will be thrombocytopenic although it is not predictive of the severity of the thrombocytopenia [3]. Others have demonstrated that the IgG antibody in the maternal plasma correlates with thrombocytopenia in the infant [6].

Scott et al. [7] confirmed that maternal PAIgG was helpful but not conclusive and recommended the use of fetal scalp sampling, where feasible, in the first stage of labor to guide the method of delivery. If the scalp blood platelet count was less than 50,000/μL, cesarean section was performed immediately, otherwise vaginal delivery was allowed. In 25 infants none had intracranial bleeding.

In a series in which cesarean section was performed for obstetric reasons only and corticosteroids were given to all thrombocytopenic mothers (platelet counts less than 100,000/μL) no babies in 19 pregnancies suffered hemorrhagic complications [8]. This report suggests that scalp sampling to guide the mode of delivery does not determine whether cesarean section is really protective. Fetal scalp sampling is not without difficulty and Wahbeh et al. [9] found that the procedure was often not feasible or useful. They reported an excellent outcome in 13 pregnancies and urged that cesarean sections should be reserved for patients with numerous risk factors such as nulliparity, unfavorable cervix, large fetus, low maternal platelet count, and elevated anti-platelet antibodies.

In summary, therefore, neither maternal platelet counts, maternal steroid therapy nor maternal PAIgG is predictive of the level of the infant platelet count and hence the risks of different modes of delivery. Further controlled studies of the efficacy of predictive factors in maternal ITP are required. Management will also depend on whether there is access to reliable and reproducible platelet antibody tests. Where these are available and are performed throughout the antenatal period, the decision concerning the need for cesarean section and its timing can be based on an assessment of the disease activity and the risk to the mother and the fetus.

Immunoglobulin Therapy

The introduction of intravenous immunoglobulin in the management of AITP has proved to be an important advance in the management of pregnancy complicated by severe AITP. The intravenous administration of human IgG prolongs the clearance time of immune complexes by the reticuloendothelial system and this may be the mechanism whereby the number of circulated platelets is increased in patients with AITP. The effective use of high dose intravenous immunoglobulin in the treatment of acute and chronic ITP in children and adults who were refractory to steroid therapy led to its use in severe cases of maternal AITP in pregnancy. High dose intravenous immunoglobulin can also cross the placenta and should therefore have a protective effect on the fetus. The other possibility is that maternal immunoglobulin therapy may reduce the transplacental transfer of the antibodies. Several reports have claimed a successful outcome with high dose i.v. immunoglobulin [10,11]. The treatment is expensive, £2,500 or more for one five day course. There is need for a multicenter study to establish whether or not the treatment has beneficial effects for the fetus. While there is no doubt about the value of intravenous IgG in patients with severe thrombocytopenia not responding to steroid therapy, doubt remains as to the transplacental effect of intravenous IgG and its efficacy in protecting the fetus [12].

Management of AITP in Pregnancy

The following program is suggested for the pregnant patient with AITP and is based on the recommendations of Hathaway and Bonnar [13]. The supervision of the pregnancy and planning for delivery should be a team effort with close collaboration between the obstetrician, hematologist and neonatologist. Attention to the following is recommended:

1. A precise diagnosis will usually require bone marrow examination and platelet antibody studies.
2. Any drugs, such as aspirin or heparin, which could affect platelet function should be avoided.
3. No treatment is necessary unless the platelet count falls below 25,000/μL and/or a bleeding tendency occurs. Prednisolone at a dosage of 1.0 mg/kg/day given in two doses should be used; after two weeks the dosage should be tapered to the lowest possible level to maintain the platelet count above 50,000/μL. This level is adequate for hemostasis if operative delivery is required. A complete or partial remission in about 70% of patients will usually result from prednisolone therapy.
4. Patients who do not respond to cortico-steroids should be given intravenous immunoglobulin therapy. The immunoglobulin should be administered in doses of 400 mgs/kg during a period of several hours each day for five days. Responses are usually rapid, with the platelets beginning to rise on about the fourth day of the infusion and peaking about five days following infusion. A response occurs in over 80% of patients and the remission usually lasts for about 3 or 4 weeks. A maintenance dose (a single day's dose) can be given at monthly intervals.
5. Patients who do not respond to prednisolone or immunoglobulin may be considered for splenectomy. Splenectomy in pregnancy should only be carried out as a last resort as it has a significant mortality which will increase the risk of abortion or premature labor.
6. Even if the mother's platelet count is adequate, the baby may have thrombocytopenia, particularly where the mother has had a splenectomy. Unless contraindicated, a course of prednisone should be given to the mother over a two-week period prior to the date of estimated delivery with the aim of improving the baby's platelet count. If the maternal thrombocytopenia is refractory to steroid therapy, then high dose intravenous immunoglobulin therapy should be given one to two weeks before the estimated date of delivery.
7. Careful planning by the obstetrician, hematologist and neonatologist is required for the delivery. They should take into consideration the obstetrical history and the severity of the thrombocytopenia in the baby in any previous pregnancies. Platelet antibody titers in the maternal serum and the mother's hemostatic condition are important. The aim should be an easy vaginal delivery without trauma to the infant or the mother. When obstetric factors indicate that this is unlikely, then a cesarean section is advisable. In patients having a vaginal delivery a fetal blood scalp sample should be obtained in early labor, using EDTA anticoagulant in the capillary tube and not heparin. If the platelet count is less than 50,000 μL, the infant should be delivered by cesarean section.
8. Following delivery, the platelet count in the cord blood should be checked; the platelet count in the baby should be checked daily. In infants with severely depressed platelet counts (persistently below 10,000/μL) or significant

hemorrhage, exchange transfusion should be considered to remove the antibody; followed by platelet transfusions. Alternatively a course of intravenous immunoglobulin may be useful. Infants with petechiae or puncture wound bleeding in association with a platelet count of 50,000/μL or less may be given a short course of prednisone (2mgs/Kg/day) until the platelet count remains above 50,000/μL, which is usually after one to two weeks. Most babies show no evidence of any hemorrhage and in mild cases no treatment is required unless surgery is necessary. The platelet count in the newborn decreases in the first few days of life and usually rises to normal levels within the first month of life, but occasionally thrombocytopenia can persist for up to 16 weeks.

We can conclude that the risk to the mother and the baby in AITP have been dramatically reduced. This condition, which once had a maternal death rate of 8%–9%, should now with appropriate care have virtually no mortality. Likewise, the outlook for the fetus, which previously had a death rate of up to 26%, has been transformed to a very low mortality and morbidity. Further studies are, however, required to determine the effects of AITP on the fetus and to determine the most effective ways of preventing and treating thrombocytopenia in the baby before delivery.

Summary. This disorder is caused by the production of platelet auto-antibodies which can be measured as platelet associated immunoglobulins of the G or M class, i.e., PAIgG or PAIgM. The level of the antibodies usually correlates with decreased platelet survival and the degree of thrombocytopenia. PAIgG crosses the placenta and produces thrombocytopenia in the fetus. Spontaneous bleeding usually does not occur until the platelet count is less than 25,000/μl. Platelet counts above 50,000/μl usually provide adequate protection against bleeding from trauma and surgical procedures such as cesarean section. The maternal morbidity and mortality due to ITP is very low. The usual management is to use steroids during pregnancy to treat ITP if the platelet count falls below 50,000. In refractory patients, intravenous immunoglobulin (IGIV) is usually effective. Splenectomy in pregnancy has a sigificant mortality and should be avoided as it

To improve the baby's platelet count prior to delivery, maternal treatment with prednisone for 10–14 days before delivery is recommended. In early labor, platelet count on a fetal scalp sample is recommended and if the count is less than 50,000/μl in the baby, delivery by cesarean section should be considered unless a short labor and easy delivery are anticipated. The platelet count should be checked in the cord blood and subsequently on a heel prick. Platelet counts can remain low in the infant for several weeks after birth.

References

1. Hedge UM, Bowes A, Powell DK, Joyner MV (1981) Detection of platelet bound and serum antibodies in thrombocytopenia by enzyme linked assay. Vox Sang 41: 306–312

2. Hedge UM (1985) Immune thrombocytopenia in pregnancy and the newborn. Br J Obstet Gynaecol 92: 657–659
3. Kelton JC, Inwood MJ, Barr RM, Effer SB, Hunter D, Wilson WE, Ginsburg DA, Powers PJ (1982) The prenatal prediction of thrombocytopenia in mothers with clinically diagnosed immune thrombocytopenia. Am J Obstet Gynecol 144: 449–454
4. Laros RK Jr, Sweet RL (1975) Management of idiopathic thrombocytopenic purpura during pregnancy. Am J Obstet Gynecol 122: 182
5. Carloss HW, McMillan R, Crosby WH (1980) Management of pregnancy in women with immune thrombocytopenia purpura. J Am Med Assoc 244: 2756–2758
6. Cines DB, Dusak B, Tomaski A, Mennuti M, Schreiber AD (1982) Immune thrombocytopenic purpura and pregnancy. N Engl J Med 306: 826–831
7. Scott JR, Rote NS, Cruikshank DP, (1983) Antiplatelet antibodies and platelet counts in pregnancies complicated by autoimmune thrombocytopenic purpura. Am J Obstet Gynecol 145: 932–939
8. Laros RK Jr, Kagan R (1982) Route of delivery for patients with immune thrombocytopenic purpura. Am J Obstet Gynecol 148: 901–908
9. Wahbeh CJ, Eden RD, Killam AP, Gall SA (1984) Pregnancy and immune thrombocytopenic purpura. Am J Obstet Gynecol 149: 238
10. Lavery JP, Koontz WL, Liu YK, Howell R, (1985) Immunologic thrombocytopenia in pregnancy: use of antenatal immunoglobulin therapy: case report and review. Obstet Gynecol 66: 41S–43S
11. Morgenstern GR, Measday B, Hegde UM, (1983) Auto-immune thrombocytopenia in pregnancy. New approach to management. Br Med J 287: 584
12. Davies SV, Murray JA, Gee H, Giles H (1986) Transplacental effect of high-dose immunoglobulin in idiopathic thrombocytopenia (ITP) Lancet I: 1098–1099
13. Hathaway W, Bonnar J (1987) Hemostatic disorders of the pregnant woman and newborn infant. Elsevier, New York p. 87

Part 3. Brain Hemorrhage (Including Vitamin K Deficiency)

Basic Research of Hemostasis During the Perinatal Period

3.1 Absorption, Metabolism, and Storage of K Vitamins in the Newborn

MARTIN J. SHEARER[1]

Introduction

The fetal and neonatal physiology and biochemistry of vitamin K is probably the least understood of all the fat-soluble vitamins. Major questions surround the transplacental transfer, intestinal absorption, intermediary metabolism, plasma transport, bioavailability, storage, and turnover of the K vitamins. Such questions include the relative importance to fetal and neonatal requirements of phylloquinone (vitamin K_1), the plant synthesized form of vitamin K, and the menaquinones (vitamin K_2), which are of bacterial origin. For example, the establishment of an intestinal flora which synthesize menaquinones is known to occur in the first few days of life, but the role of enteric menaquinones as a potential source of vitamin K in neonates remains as controversial a question as it does in adults.

In the last decade or so, sophisticated techniques have been developed which can detect amounts of K vitamins in the low picogram range, thus making possible their measurement for the first time in various tissues. One problem is the time-consuming and technically demanding nature of current assay methods. The continuing development and critical assessment of tissue assays for K vitamins and their metabolites will ultimately provide the basis to answer many of the above questions. Attention should, however, be drawn to present limitations, e.g., the fact that only phylloquinone can be reliably detected in plasma and the problem of lack of agreement in published values between different centers. Such variations in plasma values are often so great that they can only be explained on the basis of assay differences. As will become evident later, the lack of agreement between laboratories has generated its own controversy not only over the absolute values of phylloquinone in cord plasma but also on the values relative to maternal plasma. This cord-maternal ratio is an important parameter

[1]Haematology Research Laboratory, Clinical Science Laboratories, Guys Tower (18th Floor), Guys Hospital, London SE1 9RT, United Kingdom

in trying to assess the efficiency of placental transfer of phylloquinone in the newborn.

Assays for K Vitamins

All assays for the measurement of tissue K vitamins are based on high performance liquid chromatography (HPLC) using different detection methods with varying degrees of sensitivity and selectivity. Because of the low concentrations in tissues, most methods employ an extensive multi-stage purification procedure (also by chromatography) to remove interfering lipids. To date, most emphasis has been placed on the measurement of plasma levels of phylloquinone. The earliest methods were based on HPLC with UV detection [1–3], but these have now been largely superseded by more sensitive and selective detection methods either by electrochemical detection [4,5] or by fluorescence detection of the quinol [6–8].

While the measurement of endogenous plasma levels by electrochemical or fluorescence detection normally requires a volume of 1–2 ml of plasma to be extracted, in the author's experience this is not sufficient to measure the low levels in cord plasma. On the other hand, the measurement of plasma levels after pharmacological doses is readily achieved on a few microliters, thus facilitating studies on the disposition of K vitamins after their administration by different routes. Such studies are assuming greater importance in evaluating the efficacy of various prophylactic regimes for the prevention of hemorrhagic disease of the newborn (HDN).

Intestinal Absorption of K Vitamins

Theoretical Principles

The intestinal absorption of vitamin K is thought to be governed by the same principles established for other fat-soluble vitamins and highly lipid-soluble nutrients [9,10]. In the intraluminal phase of absorption, this involves the solubilization of vitamin K into mixed micelles composed of bile salts and the products of pancreatic lipolysis. Consistent with this model is the striking impairment of absorption shown in adult patients with extrahepatic cholestasis (obstructive jaundice) and severe pancreatic insufficiency [9]. Patients with biliary obstruction lack the detergent component of micelles, and the degree of absorption depends on the severity of the bile salt deficiency. In some patients, no absorption of an isotopically labelled form of phylloquinone could be demonstrated [9]. In patients with chronic pancreatitis, the primary disturbance is a reduced generation of the solutes of mixed micelles, namely, 2-monoglycerides and fatty acids. This also impairs the absorption of phylloquinone, though this is less severe than in bile salt deficiency. Whether the greater absorption efficiency in patients with pancreatic insufficiency is due to the limited absorption of vitamin K from pure bile salt micelles or from a low but significant production of mixed micelles is unclear. Certainly, lipolysis is rarely completely absent in patients with chronic pancreatitis [11], and clinically significant vitamin K deficiency is also rare in patients with this disease [12].

Recent in vitro work has shown that phylloquinone is appreciably solubilized by bile salts below their critical miceller concentration and that the solubilizing power of dihydroxy bile salts is greater than trihydroxy bile salts [13]. The same authors also showed a dramatic increase in the solubility of phylloquinone when mixed micelles were produced by the addition of phosphatidylcholine to bile salt solutions.

Experimental Studies in Neonates

Few studies of the intestinal absorption of K vitamins have been undertaken in the newborn. This is in part due to ethical and practical considerations but also to the technical difficulties associated with the assay of K vitamins in biological samples. No balance studies equating dietary input with fecal output have been performed or seem likely, considering the practical problems of stool collection and the difficulties in the experimental design of balance studies in babies.

The data which are available derive from "tolerance" tests in which plasma levels alone have been measured after the administration of a pharmacological test dose. Again, for ethical reasons, it is not generally feasible to obtain serial blood samples in the same baby; therefore, the shape of the absorption time-curve is usually a composite one obtained by pooling the data from single sampling points taken at different time intervals from a large series of babies [14,15]. Both publications [14,15] also contain some serial data from a few babies in whom multiple sampling was possible.

Our study with McNinch et al. [14] was designed to test the efficacy of oral versus intramuscular administration of 1-mg doses of phylloquinone, with the oral dose given either at birth or with the first feed. In the oral group of 72 babies sampled at either 2, 4, 8, 12, or 24 h, the composite absorption curve suggested that the peak plasma level was attained at 4 h. Thereafter the levels gradually declined, although there was little difference in the median values at 8, 12, and 24 h (Fig. 1). In contrast, plasma levels after intramuscular injection rose up to 12 h but were lower at 24 h (Fig. 2). The effectiveness of these prophylactic regimes is probably best determined by comparing plasma levels at 24 h when interindividual differences in the rate of diffusion from the injection site should have equalized and intestinal absorption should be complete. In our study, the median plasma concentration 24 h after intramuscular injection was 10–20 times higher than the median levels in either of the two groups given phylloquinone orally [14]. These results point to the inefficient absorption of pharmacological doses, while the widely ranging plasma values suggest a wide interindividual variation in the degree of absorption. More detailed pharmacokinetic studies in adults [16] have also shown a marked interindividual variation in the availability of phylloquinone from doses (10–50 mg) which, when expressed as μg/kg body weight (approximately 150–750 μg/kg), are within the same range (approximately 350 μg/kg) as those administered to babies in our study.

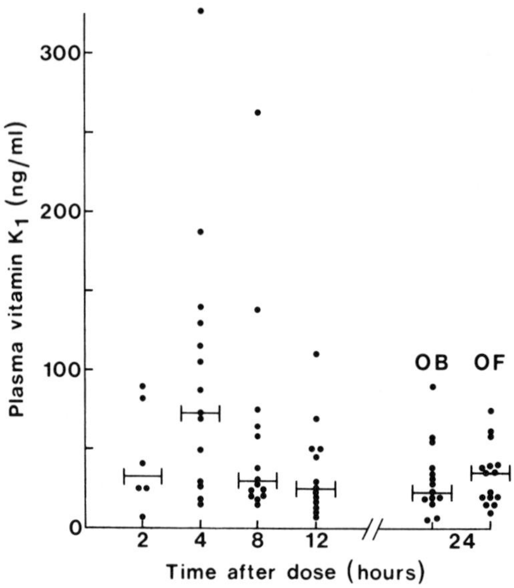

Fig. 1. Individual plasma phylloquinone concentrations and median values (*horizontal bars*) after the oral administration of 1 mg of phylloquinone to 72 newborns. Phylloquinone was given at birth (group *OB*) to all newborns except for a group of 15 newborns studied at 24 h to whom the vitamin was given with the first feed (group *OF*). (From [14])

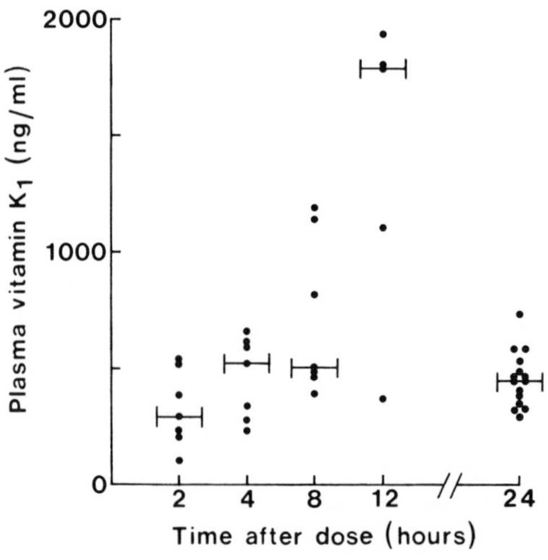

Fig. 2. Individual plasma phylloquinone concentrations and median values (*horizontal bars*) after the intramuscular injection of 1 mg of phylloquinone to 35 newborns. (From [14])

In Japan, in contrast to most other countries throughout the world, an oral syrup of menaquinone-4 is widely used for oral vitamin K prophylaxis instead of phylloquinone. In a large study of 194 infants on the 5th day of life, Shinzawa et al. [15] made plasma measurements 3 h after the oral administration of a 4-mg dose of menaquinone-4. As with phylloquinone [14], plasma concentrations and, by implication, the intestinal absorption of menaquinone-4 varied widely between individual babies. When plasma menaquinone-4 concentrations were corrected for weight, a significant negative correlation was found between the absorption index and the plasma concentration of PIVKA-II (protein induced by vitamin K absence or antagonist) measured by sensitive enzyme immunoassay. These results suggest an association of impaired vitamin absorption with the appearance of subclinical vitamin K deficiency, indicating that malabsorption may be a causative factor in the subsequent development of overt neonatal vitamin K deficiency. Indeed, experimental evidence of a temporary malabsorption of phylloquinone in a baby with late onset hemorrhagic disease of the newborn (HDN) had been reported previously by von Kries et al. [17]. The evidence obtained in the case report [17] suggested that the malabsorption of vitamin K, which dramatically improved 4 months later, may have been caused by a transient cholestasis which critically reduced the intraluminal concentration of bile salts. Further evidence of a relationship between mild liver dysfunction and late onset HDN has been gathered in a series of babies with late onset HDN by Matsuda et al. [18]. Such mild abnormalities in liver function tests, which, in the study of Matsuda and co-workers, were largely indicated by elevated serum alkaline phosphatase and bile acid levels, may quite easily go unrecognized. A significant finding in this study was the finding of reduced serum levels of 25-hydroxyvitamin D. This further supports the concept of an impairment of intestinal absorption caused by subclinical cholestasis.

Metabolism and Storage of K Vitamins

Maternal-Cord Plasma Concentrations

The first direct indication that there may be a placental barrier to the transport of vitamin K to the human fetus was the finding of a large maternal-fetal gradient in plasma concentrations for phylloquinone [1]. The concentrations of the other fat-soluble vitamins also tend to be lower in cord plasma than in the maternal circulation, but the magnitude of the maternal-fetal gradient predicated from this early study was much greater than previously found for retinol, 25-hydroxyvitamin D, and α-tocopherol. At the time of our study with vitamin K, the cord plasma concentrations, hence the maternal-fetal gradient, could not be accurately measured because of the limited sensitivity of the assay technique (HPLC with UV detection). Our inability to detect phylloquinone in some 50 ml of pooled cord plasma suggested, however, that the endogenous cord plasma concentrations of phylloquinone were at least one-tenth lower than the mean maternal concentration [1]. Evidence for a limited and poor equilibration of phylloquinone across the placenta was obtained by the even greater concentration gradient when the vitamin was administered to mothers shortly before delivery. However, there was some indication that this procedure could raise cord plasma phylloquinone to levels similar to those found endogenously in adults, including mothers at delivery. The conclusions reached in this early study have recently been confirmed using a more sensitive fluorimetric assay for phylloquinone [19].

Since our study in 1982, several other groups have reported on the endogenous concentrations in paired samples of maternal and cord plasma. The values obtained have varied enormously, but the greatest differences are found for cord plasma concentrations. At the most extreme, cord levels of phylloquinone have been reported to differ by several 1000-fold, ranging from levels in the ng/ml range [20–22] to the undetectable or levels in the low pg/ml range [19,23–25]. Although there is a tendency for the less sensitive and less selective techniques using HPLC with UV detection to yield higher values, this is not always the case [1], and the high values reported by Greer et al. [22] were obtained with a sensitive fluorescence detection method. Another tendency is for groups reporting high cord plasma concentrations to find slightly higher maternal concentrations. In our laboratory we have analyzed cord plasma using HPLC with UV detection and with electrochemical detection, and both yield very low values for phylloquinone in cord plasma. Using our current method of electrochemical detection, we have reported values ranging from 4–45 pg/ml (median 16 pg/ml) in 20 babies compared to values of 0.14–2.42 ng/ml (median 0.47 ng/ml) in their mothers [26]. The most recently published values using fluorescence detection [25] agree very closely with our own for maternal phylloquinone levels, and the cord plasma levels obtained for premature infants were even lower than those we have found in term infants. In this author's opinion, the high values obtained for cord plasma are due to a failure to completely resolve phylloquinone from interfering lipids. The fact that laboratories previously reporting high plasma levels in adults [3], or new borns [21] have found lower levels [19,27] on changing to more selective detection methods supports this view.

Infant Plasma Concentrations

There is little information on plasma levels in neonates after birth. One study, however, has shown that plasma phylloquinone rises rapidly in the first few days after birth; in breast fed infants to levels similar to those found in adults but to much higher levels in formula-fed infants [24]. Such high values reflect the much higher concentrations of phylloquinone in formula feeds compared to breast milk. An interesting finding was that at 1 month of age there was no difference between the plasma levels of breast-fed infants who received 1 mg of phylloquinone by intramuscular injection and those who were not given any prophylaxis [24].

Fetal and Neonatal Liver Stores of Vitamin K

Whatever the method of detection used, the measurement of K vitamins in liver is technically more difficult than in plasma. Consequently, little is known about human vitamin K stores, including those in the fetus and neonate.

Phylloquinone Stores. In a study conducted in our laboratory [26], phylloquinone was detected in the liver of the human fetus as early as 10 weeks at levels of 1–2 ng/g. Similar concentrations (median 1.3 ng/g) were measured in older fetuses with gestational ages ranging from 19–27 weeks. Further analyses of postmortem material at delivery also showed similar median levels in preterm (1.4 ng/g) and term (1.0 ng/g) infants. All these hepatic stores of phylloquinone were significantly less than adult stores, the median values being about one-fifth the median value in adults.

Vitamin K prophylaxis by intramuscular injection raises liver stores dramatically [26]. At birth, endogenous hepatic stores are around 0.1 μg, corresponding to a concentration of around 1 ng/g. At 10 h after vitamin K prophylaxis, values for hepatic stores were mostly around 20 μg and after 20–100 h were in the range of 50–200 μg. An important question which remains to be answered is the extent to which hepatic stores from various prophylactic regimes decine after the first week of life. Clinical evidence supports the view that intramuscular prophylaxis protects against late onset HDN, but there is increasing evidence that the protection afforded by oral prophylaxis may be less.

Menaquinone Stores. A surprising finding of our fetal and neonatal studies was our inability to positively identify any menaquinones in the livers from fetuses or stillborn neonates, regardless of gestatinal age; neither could we detect menaquinones in three neonates who survived for 3, 4 and 7 days [26]. These findings were in complete contrast to adults in whom a wide spectrum of menaquinones, which accounted for some 75%–97% (median 92%) of total hepatic stores of vitamin K, was readily detectable. The earliest time at which menaquinones could be confidently identified was 13 days after birth. Even higher levels were found in two infants of 28 and 42 days survival. The results suggested a gradual build-up of hepatic stores of menaquinones after birth. Similar observations suggesting a gradual increase in hepatic menaquinones after birth have also been made by Kayata et al. [28]. If correct, the clear implication of these findings is that the needs of the human fetus and newborn for vitamin K are met largely by phylloquinone. Whether this relative deficit of hepatic menaquinones in the newborn accounts for their increased susceptibility to vitamin K deficiency remains to be established. It is also not known whether these menaquinones derive from the diet, gut flora, or a combination of both sources. A gradual increase in hepatic concentrations of menaquinones after birth would of course be consistent with the gradual colonization of the gut by enteric microflora. Lipophilic menaquinones probably have a greater affinity for liver membranes and turn over more slowly than phylloquinone. If this is true, then the gradually increasing hepatic concentrations could be also explained by quite low dietary intakes of menaquinones.

If there is a message to the reader, it is that the answers to many of the outstanding problems in this rather specialized field will not be easy to obtain. Nevertheless, the introduction of the new assay methods for K vitamins has meant that significant advances have already been made and have provided researchers with at least some insights into the metabolism and stores of vitamin K in the newborn, where none previously existed.

Summary. The fetal and neonatal physiology of vitamin K is the least understood one of all the fat-soluble vitamins. Major questions surround the transplacental transfer, intestinal absorption, bioavailability, storage, and turnover. With the development, however, of sophisticated methods for sensitive tissue measurements of vitamin K_1 and menaquinones (MKs), some important concepts are being established. One of these is the very low plasma levels at birth (K_1 being barely detectable and long chain MKs undetectable) and the large maternal-fetal concentration gradient which reflects, at least in part, the inefficient placental transport of K vitamins. For vitamin K_1, the magnitude of this plasma gradient (median 30: 1) is not mirrored in the liver, where neonatal stores at birth, though reduced, are about one-fifth of adult stores (1 ng/g vs 5 ng/g). In contrast, the adult and presumably the maternal liver stores of MKs (comprising about 90% of total K) are largely unavailable to the fetus because of the low circulating levels in maternal plasma and poor placental transport.

After birth, plasma K_1 levels rapidly increase to adult values in newborns fed on breast milk and to even higher levels in newborns fed on supplemented infant formulas. Hepatic stores of MKs gradually increase during the first weeks of life, though whether they derive from the diet or intestinal synthesis is still unclear. Recent research has also cast doubt on the bioavailability of hepatic MKs.

Although there is little quantitative information on the intestinal absorption of vitamin K, clinical and laboratory evidence suggests that even mild cholestatic syndromes may impair absorption sufficiently to cause depleted liver stores and that when combined with a low dietary supply (as in entirely breast-fed infants) this reduced absorptive capacity may be a significant cause of late onset hemorrhagic disease.

References

1. Shearer MJ, Rahim S, Barkhan P, Stimmler L (1982) Plasma vitamin K_1 in mothers and their newborn babies. Lancet II: 460–463
2. Shearer MJ (1983) High-performance liquid chromatography of K vitamins and their antagonists. Adv Chromatogr 21: 243–301
3. Lefevere MF, De Leenheer AP, Claeys AE, Claeys IV, Steyaert H (1982) Multidimensional liquid chromatography: a breakthrough in the assessment of physiological vitamin K levels. J Lipid Res 23: 1068–1072
4. Haroon Y, Schubert CAW, Hauschka PV (1984) Liquid chromatographic dual electrode detection system for vitamin K compounds. J Chromatogr Sci 22: 89–93
5. Hart JP, Shearer MJ, McCarthy PT (1985) Enhanced sensitivity for the determination of endogenous phylloquinone (vitamin K_1) in plasma using high-performance liquid chromatography with dual-electrode electrochemical detection. Analyst 110: 1181–1184
6. Langenberg JP, Tjaden UR (1984) Determination of (endogenous) vitamin K_1 in human plasma by reversed-phase high performance liquid chromatography using fluorometric detection after post-column electrochemical reduction: comparison with ultraviolet, single and dual electrochemical detection. J Chromatogr 305: 61–72
7. Lambert WE, De Leenheer AP, Lefevere MF (1986) Determination of vitamin K in serum using HPLC with post-column reaction and fluorescence detection. J Chromatogr Sci 24: 76–79
8. Haroon Y, Bacon DS, Sadowski JA (1986) Liquid-chromatographic determination of vitamin K_1 in plasma with fluorometric detection. Clin Chem 32: 1925–1929
9. Shearer MJ, McBurney A, Barkhan P (1974) Studies on the absorption and metabolism of phylloquinone (vitamin K_1) in man. Vitam Horm 32: 513–542
10. Hollander D (1981) Intestinal absorption of vitamins A, E, D and K. J Lab Clin Med 97: 449–462
11. Hofmann AF (1966) A physicochemical approach to the intraluminal phase of fat absorption. Gastroenterology 50: 56–64

12. Evans WB, Wollaeger EE (1966) Incidence and severity of nutritional deficiency states in chronic exocrine pancreatic insufficiency: comparison with nontropical sprue. Am J Dig Dis 11: 594–606
13. Nagata M, Yotsuyanagi T, Ikeda K (1988) Solubilization of vitamin K_1 by bile salts and phosphatidylcholine-bile salt mixed micelles. J Pharm Pharmacol 40: 85–88
14. McNinch AW, Upton C, Samuels M, Shearer MJ, McCarthy P, Tripp JH, Orme RL'E (1985) Plasma concentrations after oral or intramuscular vitamin K_1 in neonates. Arch Dis Child 60: 814–818
15. Shinzawa T, Mura T, Tsunei M, Shiraki K (1989) Vitamin K absorption capacity and its association with vitamin K deficiency. Am J Dis Child 143: 686–689
16. Park BK, Scott AK, Wilson AC, Haynes BP, Breckenridge AM (1984) Plasma disposition of vitamin K_1 in relation to anticoagulant poisoning. Br J Clin Pharmacol 18: 655–662
17. Von Kries R, Reifenhäuser A, Göbel U, McCarthy P, Shearer MJ, Barkhan P (1985) Late onset haemorrhagic disease of newborn with temporary malabsorption of vitamin K_1. Lancet I: 1035
18. Matsuda I, Nishiyama S, Motohara K, Endo F, Ogata T, Futagoishi Y (1989) Late neonatal vitamin K deficiency associated with subclinical liver dysfunction in human milk-fed infants. J Pediatr 114: 602–605
19. Mandelbrot L, Guillaumont M, Leclercq M, Lefrère JJ, Gozin D, Daffos F, Forestier F (1988) Placental transfer of vitamin K_1 and its implications in fetal hemostasis. Thromb Haemost 60: 39–43
20. Pietersma-de Bruyn ALJM, Van Haard PMM (1985) Vitamin K_1 in the newborn. Clin Chim Acta 150: 95–101
21. Sann L, Leclercq M, Guillaumont M, Trouyez R, Bethenod M, Bourgeay-Causse M (1985) Serum vitamin K_1 concentrations after oral administration of vitamin K_1 in low birth weight infants. J Pediatr 107: 608–611
22. Greer FR, Mummah-Schendel LL, Marshall S, Suttie JW (1988) Vitamin K_1 (phylloquinone) and vitamin K_2 (menaquinone) status in newborns during the first week of life. Pediatrics 81: 137–140
23. Hiraike H, Kimura M, Itokawa Y (1988) Distribution of K vitamins (phylloquinone and menaquinones) in human placenta and maternal and umbilical cord plasma. Am J Obstet Gynecol 158: 564–569
24. Widdershoven J, Lambert W, Motohara K, Monnens L, De Leenheer A, Matsuda I, Endo F (1988) Plasma concentrations of vitamin K_1 and PIVKA-II in bottle-fed and breast-fed infants with and without vitamin K prophylaxis at birth. Eur J Pediatr 148: 139–142
25. Yang Y-M, Simon N, Maertens P, Brigham S, Liu P (1989) Maternal-fetal transport of vitamin K_1 and its effects on coagulation in premature infants. J Pediatr 115: 1009–1013
26. Shearer MJ, McCarthy PT, Crampton OE, Mattock MB (1988) The assessment of human vitamin K status from tissue measurements. In: Suttie JW (ed) Current advances in vitamin K research. Elsevier, New York, pp 437–452
27. De Leenheer AP, Nelis HJ, Lambert WE, Bauwens RM (1988) Chromatography of fat-soluble vitamins in clinical chemistry. J Chromatogr 429: 3–58
28. Kayata S, Kindberg C, Greer FR, Suttie JW (1989) Vitamin K_1 and K_2 in infant human liver. J Pediatr Gastroenterol Nutr 8: 304–307

3.2 Vitamin K_1 and K_2 Contents in Blood, Stool, and Liver Tissues of Neonates and Young Infants

AKIRA SHIRAHATA, TOSHO NAKAMURA, and NOBUAKI ARIYOSHI[1]

Introduction

Vitamin deficiency is only rarely seen in Japan at present. However, one exception is vitamin K deficiency. In fact, the deficiency of this vitamin is a serious problem in Japan [1].

Vitamin K deficiency is often seen in the neonatal period and early infancy [2]. Various explanations have been given as to why vitamin K deficiency is more likely to occur at these stages than at later stages of life, but those reasons have not yet been proven fully because of a lack of suitable methods for measuring vitamin K [3,4].

Several years ago, we succeeded in developing a singificantly effective method for measuring vitamin K (Fig. 1) [5]. By using this method, each vitamin K family can be measured individually with high specificity and sensitivity. The recovery of our method is more than 95%, and the sensitivity is more than 10 pg for phylloquinone and 50 pg for menaquinone families. Therefore, in order to demonstrate the etiology of neonatal and infantile vitamin K deficiency, we studied the pharmacokinetics of vitamin K in neonates and young infants by using our method for measuring vitamin K.

Vitamin K Concentration in Umbilical Cord Blood

We determined vitamin K concentrations in umbilical cord blood to estimate the extent to which vitamin K is transferred to the fetus via the placenta under physiological conditions. As shown in Fig. 2, both vitamin K_1 and menaquinone-7 concentrations in umbilical cord blood were significantly lower than those in adult blood. No menaquinone families except menaquinone-7 were detected

[1] Department of Pediatrics, School of Medicine, University of Occupational and Environmental Health Japan, 1-1 Iseigaoka, Yahatanishi-ku, Kitakyushu City, Fukuoka, 807 Japan

Serum 1.0 ml
- Isopropyl alcohol 4 ml
- H_2O 2 ml
- N-hexane 10 ml

Extracted and collected upper layer 8 ml
(3000 rpm, 5 min)

Evaporated
- N-hexane 200 µl x 2 times

Silica gel column (200 x 5 mm i.d.)
- Washed with N-hexane-Benzene (3:2) 15 ml
- Eluted with N-hexane-Benzene (1:2) 10 ml

Evaporated
- N-hexane 200 µl x 2 times

Alumina short column (50 x 5 mm i.d.)
- Washed with N-hexane-Benzene (6:1) 3 ml
- Eluted with N-hexane-Benzene (3:1) 5 ml

Evaporated
- Ethanol 200 µl

HPLC analysis
Column: Cosmosil $5C_{18}$, 250 x 4.6 mm i.d.
Post column: PtO_2 50 x 4.6 mm i.d.
Solvent: Methanol (1:2)
containing 2 % H_2O and saturated H_2-gas
0.5 ml/min

Fig. 1 Detector: Ex 254 nm, Em 430 nm

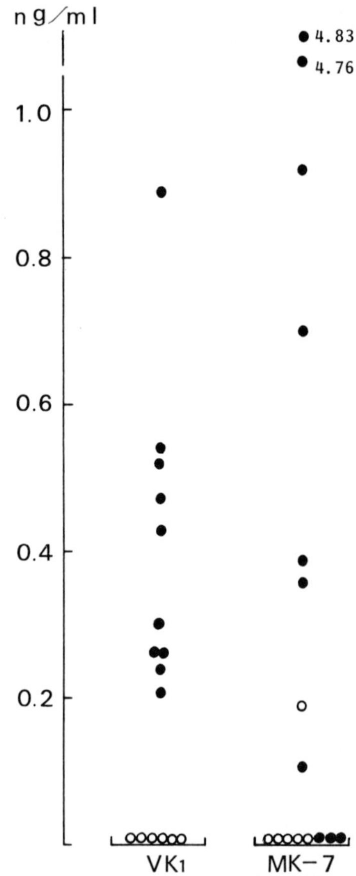

Fig. 2

Fig. 1. Method of measuring vitamin K (phylloquinone and menaquinone families)

Fig. 2. Serum vitamin K (phylloquinone and menaquinone-7) levels in normal adults (*closed circles*) and neonates (*open circles*)

in the umbilical cord blood. This result suggests that vitamin K crosses the placental barrier only to a very slight extent and that this vitamin is transferred from maternal blood to the fetus in only very small amounts.

Vitamin K Contents in Liver Tissues of Neonates

Data obtained in adults have shown that vitamin K can be stored in the liver tissues. Although vitamin K is transferred from maternal blood to the fetus in only a very small amount, this small amount of vitamin K might be accumulated in fetal liver tissues. To resolve this question, we examined liver tissues of neonates for vitamin K content.

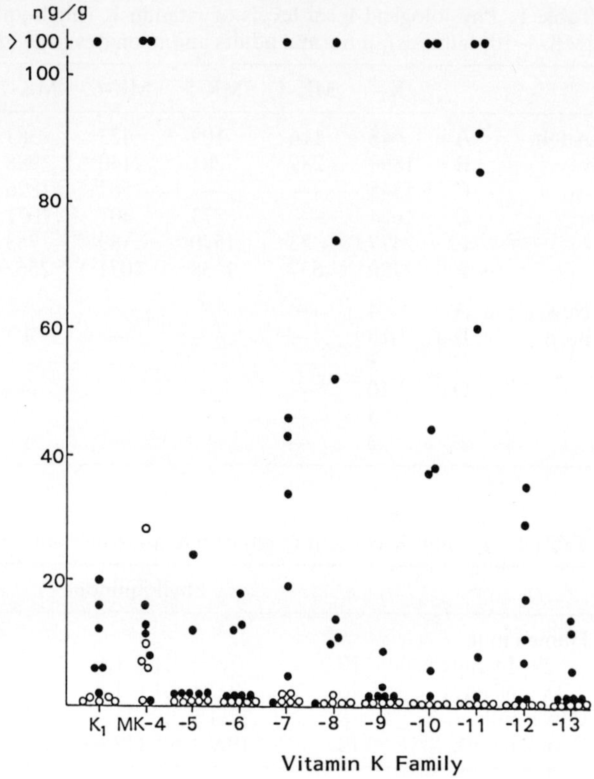

Fig. 3. Vitamin K (phylloquinone and menaquinone families) contents of liver tissues in adults (*closed circles*) and neonates (*open circles*) without definite liver dysfunction

Liver tissues were obtained from 5 neonates who died within 24 h of birth. Their gestational ages ranged from 28 weeks to 38 weeks. They did not receive any additional vitamin K, antibiotics, or blood preparations, and they showed no liver injuries. As shown in Fig. 3, vitamin K content other than menaquinone-4 was very low in the neonatal liver tissues examined and did not vary significantly according to gestational ages. Although the sample size is small, the finding suggests that neonates have little vitamin K reserve upon birth regardless of their gestational ages.

Vitamin K Contents in Meconium

We also determined vitamin K_2 which derives from intestinal bacteria, a major source of vitamin K supply. Table 1 shows the vitamin K content in adult stool and in meconium obtained from neonates within 3 days after birth. In addition to vitamin K_1, adult stools contain a very large amount of vitamin K_2 family. On the other hand, meconium contains a very small amount of vitamín K, indicating that it is impossible to expect a supply of vitamin K in a meaningful amount from bacteria in neonates.

Table 1. Physiological fecal levels of vitamin K (phylloquinone [K_1] and menaquinone [MK-4–10] families) in normal adults and neonates (ng/g dry weight)

		K_1	MK-4	MK-5	MK-6	MK-7	MK-8	MK-9	MK-10
Adult	A	648	116	109	422	387	910	2054	11854
	B	1898	289	281	2140	1988	511	3080	15662
	C	5345	—	—	507	1826	2476	2702	7085
	D	1634	—	273	407	1071	525	—	5167
	E	2477	73	1570	189	753	389	1411	5745
	F	2220	537	1138	2071	2562	1273	2548	9585
Newborn	A	4	—	—	—	—	—	—	—
	B	18	—	—	—	1	—	—	—
	C	3	—	—	—	—	—	—	—
	D	10	—	—	—	—	—	—	—
	E	3	—	—	—	—	—	—	—
	F	2	—	—	—	1	—	—	—

Table 2. Vitamin K content (μg/l) of human, cow's and formula milk

	n	Phylloquinone	Menaquinone-4
Human milk			
2 ~ 14 days	29	7.7 ± 4.1 (1.6 ~ 17.1)	2.7 ± 2.8 (<0.4 ~ 13.2)
15 ~ 60 days	76	9.2 ± 6.1 (1.6 ~ 33.9)	2.5 ± 3.0 (<0.4 ~ 16.2)
Cow's milk	8	17.4 ± 3.0 (11.3 ~ 20.2)	4.5 ± 4.7 (<0.4 ~ 15.2)
Formula milk	12	19.9 ± 6.5 (12.6 ~ 32.0)	5.4 ± 4.6 (1.2 ~ 13.2)

Mean ± SD.
Numbers in parentheses indicate range.

Vitamin K Contents in Breast, Cow's and Formula Milk

An alternative source for vitamin K could be from breast milk. However, as shown in Table 2, the vitamin K content in breast milk is about one half of that in formula milk and varies greatly from one individual to another. This explains the high prevalence of vitamin K deficiency among breast-fed neonates.

Time Dependence of Blood Vitamin K Concentration after Oral Administration of Vitamin K in Neonates

It is difficult to determine whether or not the rate of vitamin K metabolism is different in adults and newborn infants. In order to indirectly compare the metabolism, we examined the changes in blood vitamin K concentration with time by administering vitamin K to adults and neonates.

Figure 4 shows the time course changes in blood menaquinone-4 levels after oral administration of 1 mg/kg of menaquinone-4 preparation (Keytwo, Eisai Co.). Menaquinone-4 remained in the blood over a longer period in neonates

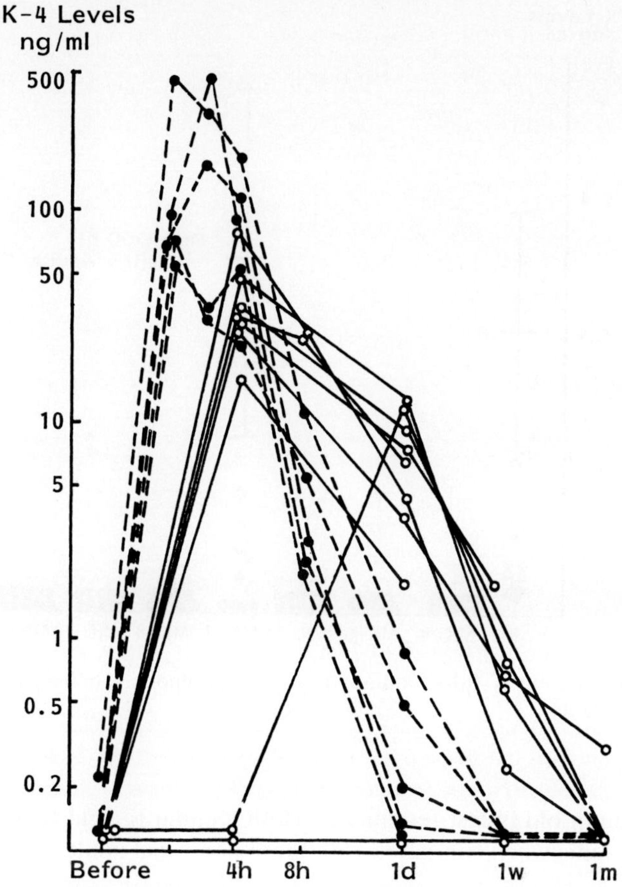

Fig. 4. Time dependence of serum menaquinone-4 (*MK-4*) levels after oral administration of vitamin K (menaquinone-4) syrup in normal adults (*closed circles*) and neonates (*open circles*)

than in adults. The half life of menaquinone-4 seems to be longer in neonates than in adults. The mean concentration of peak menaquinone-4 in premature neonates, mature neonates, and adults were 33.2 ± 25.5 ng/ml, 23.1 ± 6.3 ng/ml, and 285.9 ± 212.9 ng/ml, respectively.

This result suggests that vitamin K is only poorly absorbed in neonates. Although the number of neonates was limited in our study, there was no apparent difference in absorption between mature and premature newborn infants.

Vitamin K Concentration in Blood of 1-Month-Old Infants

We studied whether or not physiological vitamin K deficiency is also present in 1-month old infants. Figure 5 shows the serum vitamin K concentration in

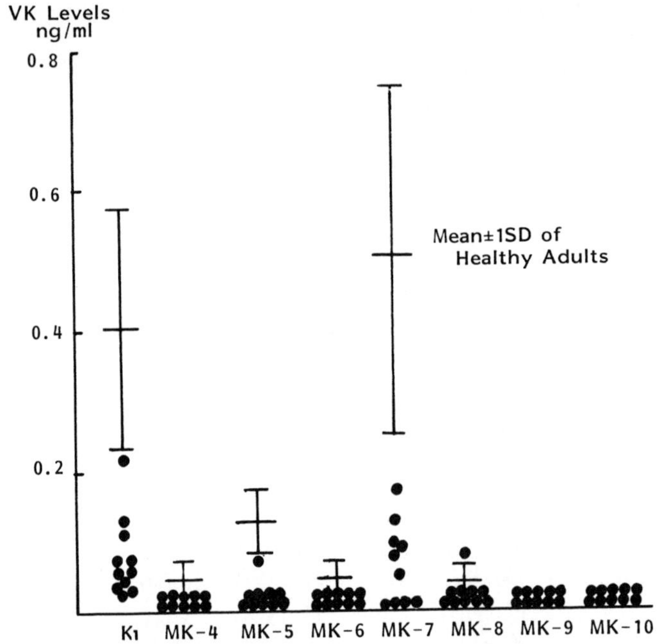

Fig. 5. Serum vitamin K (phylloquinone and menaquinone families) levels in normal 1-month-old infants

normal 1-month-old breast-fed infants. Both vitamin K_1 and K_2 concentrations are low in infants when compared with those in normal adults.

Vitamin K Contents in Liver Tissues of Young Infants

We determined vitamin K content in liver tissues obtained from two young infants who died from sudden infant death syndrome. Both patients were otherwise very healthy until the sudden death. In the liver tissue of the 1-month-old infant, vitamin K_1 and menaquinone-4, -7, and -8 were detected at levels of 7.0, 2.0, 20.8, and 0.9 ng/g dry weight, respectively. On the other hand, the liver tissues of the 4-month-old infant showed menaquinone-4, -7, -9, and -10 with respective levels 1.6, 54.6, 6.2, 9.2, and 15.7 ng/g dry weight. Both sets of data were lower than the normal adult control, as shown in Fig. 3. The results suggest that young infants are physiologically in a state of vitamin K deficiency, although to a lesser extent than newborn infants.

Infants who received menaquinone-4 upon birth and who died 2 days, 3 days, 11 days, and 83 days after birth had 558, 822, 764, and 3.8 ng/g of menaquinone-4 in their liver tissues, respectively. This result shows that vitamin K is not retained in the liver throughout infancy.

Vitamin K Epoxide Reductase Activity in 1-Month-Old Infants

Vitamin K is needed for the conversion of glutamic acid into γ-carboxy-glutamic acid. Carboxylase, which is present in hepatic microsome, fixes CO_2 to the glutamic acid of vitamin K dependent factors using vitamin K as a cofactor, resulting in the conversion of glutamic acid into γ-carboxy-glutamic acid. Reducing type vitamin K (vitamin K hydroquinone) is oxidized into vitamin K 2,3-epoxide in this process. Vitamin K epoxide is reduced by vitamin K 2,3-epoxide reductase into vitamin K. Vitamin K is then reduced by vitamin K reductase into vitamin K hydroquinone and reused. Warfarin and dicumarol show their anticoagulant effects by inhibition of vitamin K epoxide reductase. If the activity of vitamin K epoxide reductase is decreased, vitamin K 2,3-epoxide should accumulate in the liver tissues after vitamin K loading.

Recently, Nishimura et al. [6] reported that a strongly significant correlation between levels of vitamin K 2,3-epoxide in blood and in liver tissues was seen. Therefore, we administered a menaquinone-4 preparation intravenously to adults and 1-month-old infants and measured the plasma levels of menaquinone-4 and menaquinone-4 2,3-epoxide after 30 min of infusion. The menaquinone-4, 2,3-epoxide/menaquinone-4 ratio was higher in young infants than in adults (Fig. 6). These results indicate that the vitamin K epoxide reductase activity level of 1-month-old infants is physiologically lower than that of adults.

Most patients with idiopathic vitamin K deficiency were breast-fed, and this disease is more common in boys than in girls. Therefore, we compared the activity of vitamin K epoxide reductase between types of feeding and between sexes. There was no significant difference in vitamin K epoxide reductase activity between sexes or in types of feeding.

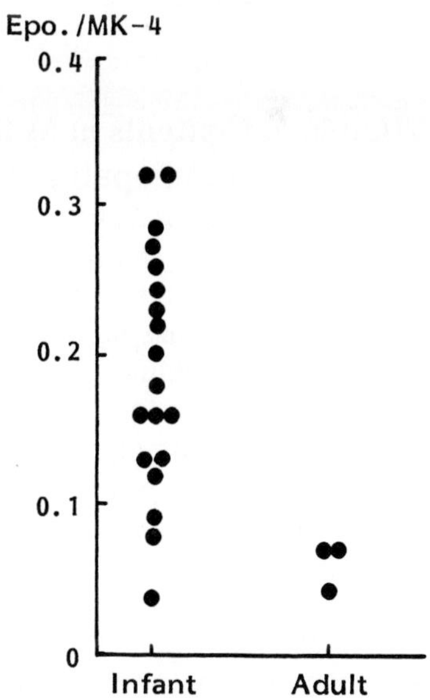

Fig. 6. Menaquinone-4 2,3-epoxide/menaquinone-4 ratio after loading of vitamin K (menaquinone-4) in normal adults and 1-month-old infants

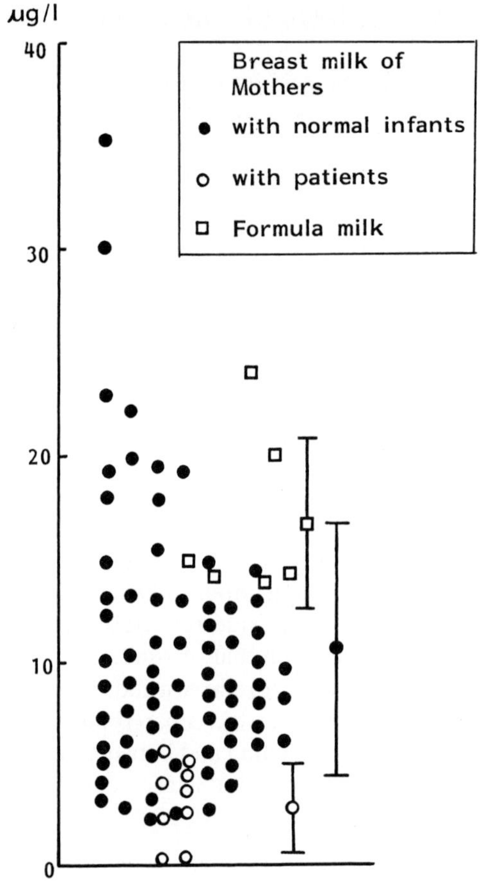

Fig. 7. Vitamin K (phylloquinone plus menaquinone-4) contents in breast and formula milk

Vitamin K Contents in Milk Obtained from Mothers Whose Babies Suffered from Idiopathic Vitamin K Deficiency in Infancy

The results shown in the previous section suggest that young infants are physiologically in a vitamin K deficient state. However, this does not necessarily mean that all young infants show clinical symptoms of vitamin K deficiency. Figure 7 shows vitamin K content in breast milk. Vitamin K content is significantly lower in the breast milk taken by vitamin K deficient infants than in that taken by normal infants. However, the vitamin K content in milk taken by some vitamin K deficient infants may even be a little high. These results suggest that the etiology of vitamin K deficiency cannot be explained by low vitamin K content in breast milk alone, although low vitamin K content in some mother's milk is a very important cause of this disease.

One possible explanation of why vitamin K content in breast milk is low in some mothers could be poor transfer of this vitamin to breast milk. Accordingly, we administered a vitamin K_1 preparation to three mothers whose babies had

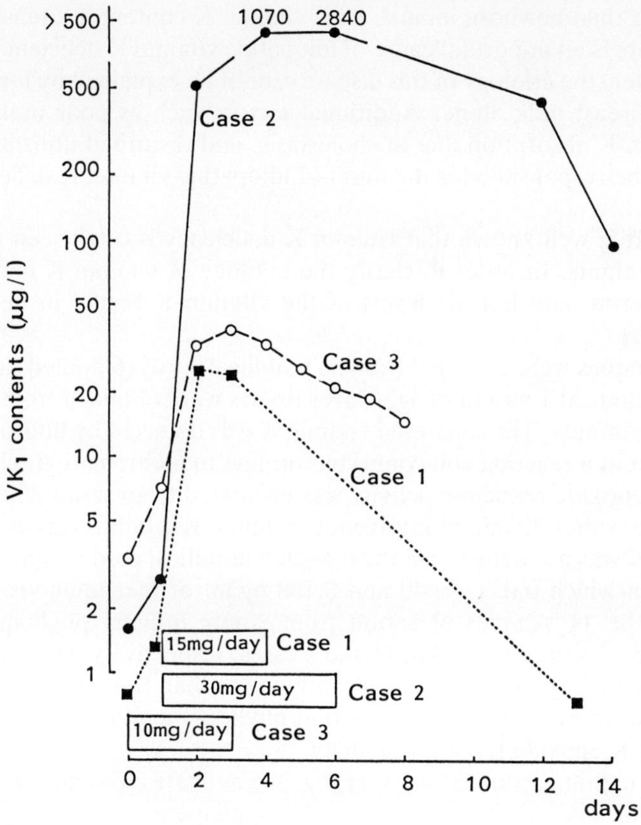

Fig. 8. Time dependence of phylloquinone contents in milk obtained from mothers treated with vitamin K (phylloquinone)

vitamin K deficiency and determined the vitamin K_1 content in their breast milk over time. Case 1, 2, and 3 received 15, 30 and 10 mg of vitamin K_1, respectively. Vitamin K_1 contents in breast milk from all mothers markedly increased after oral administration of vitamin K_1 (Fig. 8). Therefore, poor transfer of vitamin K to breast milk is unlikely as the cause of idiopathic vitamin K deficiency in infancy.

Conclusion

Newborn infants have very limited vitamin K reserve upon birth and depend largely on milk for its supply as the supply from intestinal bacteria is limited [7–11]. Furthermore, since vitamin K is absorbed only poorly from the intestine [12,13], vitamin K deficiency is often caused due to a decrease in milk ingestion and/or a decrease in the vitamin K content of the breast milk [14,15]. Young infants are also physiologically in a state of vitamin K deficiency, although to a lesser extent than newborn infants. Low vitamin K content in breast milk from some mothers is an important cause of idiopathic vitamin K deficiency in infancy [16]. However, the etiology of this disease cannot be explained by low vitamin K content in breast milk alone. Additional factors such as poor milk ingestion, poor vitamin K absorption due to cholestasis, and disturbed utilization of vitamin K may be responsible for the onset of idiopathic vitamin K deficiency.

Summary. It is well known that vitamin K deficiency is often seen in newborn and young infants. In order to clarify the etiology of vitamin K deficiency, we measured serum and hepatic levels of the vitamin K family in neonates and young infants.

Serum samples were obtained from 56 umbilical cords (6 pooled samples) and 11 young infants at 1 month of age. Liver tissues were obtained from 8 neonates and 3 young infants. The separated vitamin K was detected by fluorometry after its reduction in a reaction coil connected on-line to a chromatographic column. Vitamin K epoxide reductase activity was estimated from serum vitamin K 2,3-epoxide levels after 30 min of intravenous vitamin K administration.

Vitamin K was not detected in the 6 pooled umbilical cord samples, excluding 3 samples in which 0.039, 0.040 and 0.188 ng/ml of menaquinone-7 were detected. In the 11 samples of serum from young infants, phylloquinone and menaquinone-7 were detected in 11 and 6 cases, respectively. However, vitamin K levels in young infants were significantly lower than those in adults. A significant correlation was seen between serum phylloquinone level in young infants and vitamin K epoxide reductase activity.

Hepatic vitamin K content was very low in 5 neonates who died within 24 h of birth and who had received no vitamin K supplements, blood transfusions, or antibiotics. In comparison with adults, vitamin K content was also low in liver tissue from young infants who died from sudden infant death syndrome, although vitamin K content in young infants was higher than that in neonates.

The results suggest the poor supply of vitamin K from mother to fetus, the poor storage of vitamin K in liver tissues of neonates, and the low activity of vitamin K epoxide reductase in young infants are responsible for the vitamin K deficiency of newborn and young infants.

References

1. Hanawa Y, Maki M, Murata B, Matsuzawa E, Yamamoto Y, Nagao T, Yamada K, Ikeda I, Terao T, Mikami S, Shiraki K, Komazawa M, Shirahata A, Tsuji Y, Motohara K, Tsukimoto I, Sawada K (1988) The second nation-wide survey in Japan of vitamin K deficiency in infancy, Eur J Pediatr 147: 472–477
2. Lane PA, Hathaway Wm E (1985) Vitamin K in infancy. J Pediatr 106: 351–359
3. Savage D, Lindenbaum J (1983) Clinical and experimental human vitamin K deficiency. In: Lindenbaum J (ed) Nutrition in hematology. Churchill Livingstone, New York, pp 271–320
4. Tripp JH, McNinch AW (1987) Haemorrhagic disease and vitamin K. Arch Dis Child 62: 436–437
5. Shirahata A, Nakamura T (1985) Studies on contents of phylloquinone and menaquinones family in native serum and feces from human adults and newborn infants. Blood Vessels 16: 395–401

6. Nishimura N, Usui Y, Kobayashi N (1989) Menaquinone-4, vitamin K_1 and epoxide levels in blood after intravenous administration of menaquinone and vitamin K_1. Proceeding of 5th seminar of vitamin K function. Eisai, Tokyo, pp 155–162
7. Shearer MJ, Rahim S, Barkhan P, Stimmler L (1982) Plasma vitamin K_1 in mothers and their newborn babies. Lancet I: 460–463
8. Hamulyak K, De Doer-Van Den Berg MAG, Thijssen HHW (1987) The placental transport of (^{3}H) vitamin K_1. Br J Haematol 65: 335–338
9. Mandlblot L, Guillaumont M, Leclercq M (1988) Placental transfer of vitamin K_1 and implications in fetal hemostasis. Thromb Haemost 60: 39–43
10. Shearer MJ, McCarthy PT, Crampton OH (1988) The assessment of human vitamin K status from tissue measurements. In: Suttie JW (ed) Current advance in vitamin K research. Elsevier, New York, pp 437–452
11. Kayata S, Kindberg C, Greer FR, Suttie JW (1989) Vitamin K_1 and K_2 in infant human liver. J Pediatr Gastroenterol Nutr 8: 304–307
12. Shinzawa A, Tsunei M, Shiraki K (1989) Absorption of vitamin K in newborn infants. J Jpn Pediatr Soc 93: 144–145
13. Shirahata A, Nakamura T, Ariyoshi N, Komatsu K, Kayashima N (1988) Hemorrhage due to vitamin K deficiency with special reference to the etiology of vitamin K deficiency. Vitamin 62: 417–424
14. Endo F, Motohara I (1988) Vitamin K deficiency in the newborn—milk intake and plasma PIVKA-II. In: Suttie JW (ed) Current advances in vitamin K research. Elsevier, New York, pp 505–507
15. von Kries R, Shearer MJ, Haug M, Harzer G, Göbel U (1988) Vitamin K deficiency and vitamin K intake in infants. In: Suttie JW (ed) Current advances in vitamin K research. Elsevier, New York, pp 515–523
16. Shirahata A, Nakamura T, Komatsu K, Shiiki M, Kayashima N, Yamada K, Miyaji Y (1985) Clinical aspects of vitamin K deficiency in infancy. Vitamin 59: 387–394

3.3 The Role of Hemostasis in Neonatal Intracranial Hemorrhage

W.E. HATHAWAY[1]

The Role of Hemostasis in Neonatal Intracranial Hemorrhage

The causes of intracranial hemorrhage in the newborn infant include congenital bleeding disorders (hemophilia), thrombocytopenia, disseminated intravascular coagulation (DIC), asphyxia, infection, trauma, hemorrhagic disease of the newborn (vitamin K deficiency), and those of unknown etiology. The last category occurs primarily in the premature infant and is usually termed subependymal hemorrhage-intraventricular hemorrhage (SEH-IVH). The role of hemostatic defects in IVH has been reviewed previously by Hathaway and Bonnar [1,2]. The purpose of this communication is to review and update these discussions and to emphasize an hypothesis relating abnormal hemostasis to the etiology of neonatal IVH.

Early anatomic studies of intracranial bleeding in the preterm infant indicated that thrombosis of small venules [3] and subependymal infarction were lesions which were prominently associated with IVH [4]. Hambelton and Wigglesworth [5] first pointed out that the initial site of hemorrhage in the preterm infant was within the capillary bed of the germinal matrix. Subsequent studies [6–8] have indicated that this lesion as well as more extensive periventricular lesions are hemorrhagic infarcts with an ischemic or microthrombotic component and are closely related to IVH. Perfusion and vascular pressure changes which are major components in the ultimate bleeding have been recently reviewed [9]. Thus, alterations of the coagulation system could have a more direct etiologic role, i.e., the initial infarct may be in part related to hypercoagulability and the hemorrhagic extension may be secondary to a concomitant hemostatic impairment.

The following studies bear on these hypotheses. In a prospective study of 50 newborn infants of less than 33 weeks of gestation and therefore, of great risk for IVH, the prevalence of coagulopathy (defined as low fibrinogen or platelet

[1]University of Colorado, Health Sciences Center, Campus Box C222, 4200 East Ninth Ave., Denver, Colorado 80262, U.S.A.

count, decreased micro whole blood clotting time, increased bleeding time (BT) or decreased AT-III level) in the first few hours of life before demonstrable IVH was 32%. The incidence of significant bleeding complication (mostly IVH) was correlated with the abnormal hemostasis [10]. These findings are in agreement with the results of Hope et al. [11] who found increased partial thromboplastin times (PPTs) and prothrombin times (PTs) to be an independent variable preceeding the development of IVH. A significant correlation was found between the severity of IVH and the degree of hemostatic abnormality (reduced factors II, VII, X activity) in the study of Beverley and others [12]. In another prospective study [13], even though lower platelet counts and factor V levels were noted in infants with IVH, the conclusion was that hypocoagulability does not play an important etiological role in IVH.

The possible contribution of platelet-vessel interaction to neonatal IVH was supported by the findings of thrombocytopenia [14] and prolonged BT's [15] in infants with more severe grades of IVH. Others [16] did not find a positive correlation with low platelet counts. Other reports have shown defective fibrinolysis [17], decreased AT-III [18] and low protein C [19] in groups of infants at high risk for IVH.

Table 1 lists intervention or treatments which were used in an attempt to maintain normal hemostasis or to prevent hypercoagulability and thus to affect the incidence or severity of IVH. All of these studies were performed using sensitive methods (computerized tomography or ultrasonography) to detect the IVH. Both enhancement of coagulation factor levels and anticoagulation (heparin or the platelet inhibitor, indomethacin) had a positive effect on the incidence of IVH. Other recent studies [26,27] have confirmed the findings of Ment and others using indomethacin. An older study [17] using only autopsy incidence of IVH has demonstrated the beneficial effect of therapeutic heparinization on reduction of severe IVH. However, a recent retrospective review [28] of adverse clinical events in preterm infants noted an association between

Table 1. Hemostatic treatment used to decrease incidence or severity of neonatal intraventricular hemorrhage (IVH)

Reference	Treatment	Percent IVH *treatment* (control)	Possible mechanism
Beverley et al. [20]	Fresh frozen plasma	*14* (41)	Replace clotting factors
Benson et al. [21]	Ethamsylate	*18.5* (29.8)	Strengthen capillaries
Hensey et al. [22]	Tranexamic acid	*44* (40)	Antifibrinolysis
Ment et al. [23]	Indomethacin	*10.5* (47)	Decrease prostacyclin, anti-platelet agent
Pomerance et al. [24]	Maternal vitamin K	*5* (30)	Increase clotting factors
Manco-Johnson et al. [25]		*0* (28)	Anticoagulant

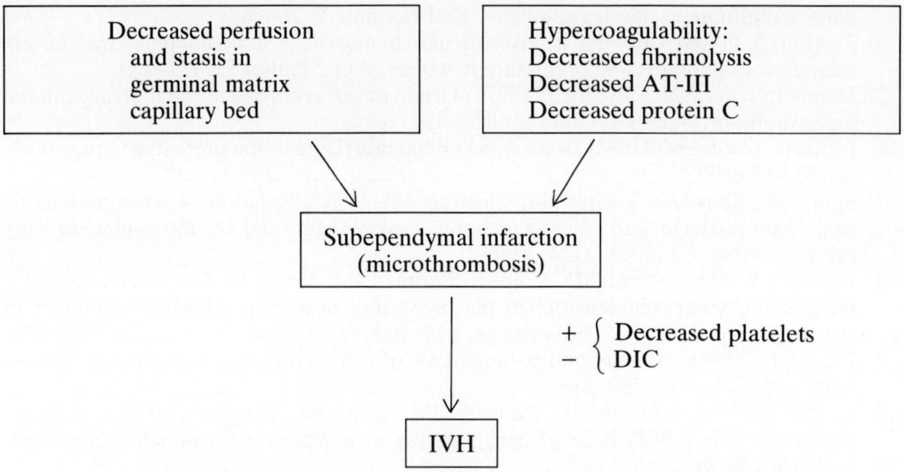

Fig. 1. The role of hemostasis in nenatal intraventricular hemorrhage

germinal matrix IVH and the use of low dose heparin (1–2 units/kg/h) and concluded that use of heparin in the umbilical artery catheter (UAC) may increase the risk of IVH.

The etiology of neonatal IVH is obviously multifactorial [6,9]. This discussion of published studies concerning the role of hemostasis suggests that the associated early hypercoagulability of the preterm infant (low AT-III, low protein C, defective fibrinolysis) at risk for IVH may be a factor in the early subependymal matrix lesion (microthrombosis, infarct). The hemorrhagic extension of this lesion may be influenced by the subsequent hypocoagulability (DIC, decreased platelets and function). This hypothesis is outlined in Fig. 1 and forms the basis for further study.

Summary. Although neonatal intracranial hemorrhage may have many causes (hemophilia, thrombocytopenia, DIC, trauma, vitamin K deficiency), the etiology of the most common type, intraventricular (IVH), is unknown. IVH, a disorder of the preterm infant, is frequently associated with alterations in the coagulation system. Recent information demonstrating that the initial lesson is due to hemorrhagic infarction raises the possibility that hypercoagulability may have an etiologic role. Studies showing low AT-III and protein C with defective fibrinolysis in the premature infant and improvement with anticoagulation (heparin, indomethacin) support this concept.

References

1. Hathaway WE, Bonnar J (1978) Perinatal coagulation. Grune and Stratton, New York
2. Hathaway WE, Bonnar J (1987) Hemostatic disorders of the pregnant woman and newborn infant. Elsevier, New York, pp 130–132
3. Larroche JC (1964) Hemorragies cerebrales intraventriculaires chez le premature Ie

partie: anatomie et physiopathologie. Biol Neonate 7: 26–56
4. Towbin A (1968) Cerebral intraventricular hemorrhage and subependymal matrix infarction in the fetus and premature newborn. Am J Pathol 52: 121–139
5. Hambelton G, Wigglesworth JS (1976) Origin of intraventricular haemorrhage in the preterm infant. Arch Dis Child 51: 651–659
6. Editorial comments (1984) Ischaemia and haemorrhage in the premature brain. Lancet II: 847–848
7. Sinha SK, Sims DG, Davies JM, Chiswick ML (1985) Relation between periventricular haemorrhage and ischaemic brain lesions diagnosed by ultrasound in very pre-term infants. Lancet: 1154–1155
8. Guzzetta F, Shackelford GD, Volpe S, Perlman JM, Volpe JJ (1986) Periventricular intraparenchymal echodensities in the premature newborn: critical determinant of the neurologic outcome. Pediatrics 78: 995–1006
9. Pape KE (1989) Etiology and pathogenesis of intraventricular hemorrhage in newborns. Pediatrics 84: 382–385
10. McDonald MM, Johnson ML, Rumack CM, Koops BL, Guggenheim MA, Babb C, Hathaway WE (1984) Role of coagulopathy in newborn intracranial hemorrhage. Pediatrics 74: 26–31
11. Hope RL, Thorburn RJ, Stewart AL, Reynolds EOR (1982) Timing and antecedents of periventricular haemorrhage in very preterm infants. Ross Laboratories conference on perinatal intracranial hemorrhage, Washington DC. Syllabus I: 78–101
12. Beverley DW, Chance GW, Inwood MJ, Schaus M, O'Keefe B (1984) Intraventricular haemorrhage and hemostasis defects. Arch Dis Child 59: 444–448
13. Van De Bor M, Briet E, Van Bel F, Ruys JH (1986) Hemostasis and periventricular-intraventricular hemorrhage of the newborn. Am J Dis Child 140: 1131–1134
14. Andrew M, Castle V, Saigail S, Carter C, Kelton JG (1987) Clinical impact of neonatal thrombocytopenia. J Pediatr 110: 457–464
15. Setzer ES, Webb IB, Wassenaar JW, Reeder JD, Mehta PS, Eitzman DV (1982) Platelet dysfunction and coagulopathy in intraventricular hemorrhage in the premature infant. J Pediatr 100: 599–605
16. Lupton BA, Hill A, Whitfield MJ, Carter CJ, Wadsworth LD, Roland EH (1988) Reduced platelet count as a risk factor for intraventricular hemorrhage. Am J Dis Child 142: 1222–1224
17. Markarian M, Lubchenco LO, Rosenblut E, Fernandez F, Lang D, Jackson JJ, Bannon AE, Lindley A, Githens JH, Martorell R (1971) Hypercoagulability in premature infants with special reference to the respiratory distress syndrome and hemorrhage II. The effect of heparin. Biol Neonate 17: 98–111
18. Peters M, ten Cate JW, Breederveld C, de Leeuw R, Emeis J, Koppe J (1984) Low anithrombin III levels in neonates with idiopathic respiratory distress syndrome: poor prognosis. Pediatr Res 18: 273–276
19. Manco-Johnson MJ, Marlar RA, Jacobson LJ, Hays T, Warady BA (1988) Severe protein C deficiency in newborn infants. J Pediatr 113: 359–363
20. Beverley DW, Pitts-Tucker TJ, Congdon PJ, Arthur RJ, Tate G (1985) Prevention of intraventricular haemorrhage by fresh frozen plasma. Arch Dis Child 60: 710–713
21. Benson JWT, Hayward C, Oschborne JP, Schulte JF, Drayton MR, Murphy JF, Rennie JM, Speidel BD, Cooke RWI (1986) Multicentre trial of ethamsylate for prevention of periventricular haemorrhage in very low birthweight infants. Lancet II: 1297–1300
22. Hensey OJ, Morgan MEI, Cooke RWI (1984) Tranexamic acid in the prevention of periventricular haemorrhage. Arch Dis Child 59: 719–721
23. Ment LR, Duncan CC, Ehrenkranz RA, Kleinman CS, Pitt BR, Taylor KJW, Scott DT, Stewart WB, Gettner P (1985) Randomized indomethacin trial for prevention of intraventricular hemorrhage in very low birth weight infants. J Pediatr 107: 937–943
24. Pomerance JJ, Teal JG, Gogolok JF, Brown S, Stewart ME (1987) Maternally administered antenatal vitamin K1: effect on neonatal prothrombin activity, partial thromboplasin time, and intraventricular hemorrhage. Obstet Gynecol 70: 235–241

25. Manco-Johnson MJ, Manco-Johnson ML, Rumack CM, Marlar RA, Hay W, Hathaway WE (to be published) Prophylactic heparinization of low birth weight infants: reduction of catheter related thromboses and decreased incidence of severe intracranial hemorrhage.
26. Bandstra ES, Montalvo BM, Goldberg RN, Pacheco I, Ferrer PL, Flynn J, Gregorios JB, Bancalari E (1988) Prophylactic indomethacin for prevention of intraventricular hemorrhage in premature infants. Pediatrics 82: 533–542
27. Hanigan WC, Kennedy G, Roemisch F, Anderson R, Cusack T, Powers W (1988) Administration of indomethacin for the prevention of periventricular-intraventricular hemorrhage in high-risk neonates. J Pediatr 112: 941–947
28. Lesko SM, Mitchell AA, Epstein MF, Louik C, Giacoia GP, Shapiro S (1986) Heparin use as a risk factor for intraventricular hemorrhage in low-birth-weight infants. N Engl J Med 314: 1156–1160

3.4 Vitamin K Prophylaxis and Late Onset Hemorrhagic Disease of the Newborn in West Germany During 1988

ULRICH GÖBEL, RÜDIGER VON KRIES, and CHRISTIAN PETRICH[1]

Introduction

Since 1980, an increased incidence of late onset hemorrhagic disease of the newborn has been noted in the Federal Republic of Germany. Details of these cases have been collected and the clinical data thoroughly analyzed by Sutor et al. [1,2]. The initially mysterious vitamin K deficient bleedings affected fully breast-fed infants who seemed in good health during the first three to seven weeks of life. In 1985 we described decreased absorption of vitamin K in an infant with late vitamin K deficiency and were able to relate this—as in some other cases—to minimal cholestasis as an underlying pathogenetic mechanism [3,4].

Due to the worrying increase in late onset vitamin K deficiency bleedings, in 1986 vitamin K prophylaxis for all newborns was again generally recommended in West Germany. The mode of administration of vitamin K: per os; intramuscularly; subcutaneously; once or repeated was discussed with great controversy [5] leading to two different recommendations. Sutor [6] recommended a single oral administration of vitamin K for healthy newborns and intramuscular injection for newborns at risk. This recommendation was based on Japanese experience, and on the concern that injuries from intramuscular injections could be considered malpractice. The committee of nutrition of the German Society of Pediatrics, [5] however, has preferred parenteral vitamin K prophylaxis for all newborns. If this was not permitted by the parents, the alternative of oral administration of vitamin K, 1 mg twice weekly for three months, was recommended. This recommendation takes into account decreased intestinal vitamin K absorption as the pathogenesis of late onset bleedings due to vitamin K deficiency [3,4].

In order to obtain detailed information about current practices of vitamin K prophylaxis and about whether the incidence of vitamin K deficiency associated

[1]Abt. für Hämatologie und Onkologie, Kinderklinik der Heinrich-Heine-Universität, Moorenstraße 5, 4000 Düsseldorf 1, Federal Republic of Germany

Table 1. Survey 1988: vitamin K_1 prophylaxis

Prophylaxis	☐ in all newborns ☐ in newborns at risk only ☐ in breast-fed newborns only ☐ none
Mode of administration of vitamin K_1	☐ p.o. 1 mg ☐ p.o. 2mg ☐ i.m. ☐ s.c.
Time of vitamin K prophylaxis	☐ 1st day of life ☐ 2nd day of life ☐ 3rd–5th day of life ☐ repeated application

Table 2. Survey 1989: late onset haemorrhagic disease of newborns

Occurence of hemorrhagic disease of newborns observed in 1988 and 1989:
yes ☐ no ☐

Age of infants at bleeding: ____________

Administration of vitamin K: yes ☐ no ☐ unknown ☐

Mode of prophylaxis: ____________

Other abnormalities: ____________

Side effects of vitamin K prophylaxis: yes ☐ no ☐

Mode of administration of vitamin K: ____________

bleedings has decreased following these recommendations, two surveys were conducted.

Material and Methods

The first survey was conducted in 1988 and was directed to all obstetric hospitals in the Federal Republic of Germany (Table 1). This questionnaire focused on the following items: which newborns receive vitamin K; how vitamin K is administered; and when vitamin K is given. The questionnaire did not address the question of preferences for particular recommendations on the type of vitamin K prophylaxis.

The second survey referred to the incidence of late onset hemorrhagic disease of the newborn, the mode of administration of vitamin K, and side effects of vitamin K prophylaxis; this survey was directed to all childrens hospitals in the Federal Republic of Germany (Table 2). Of each reported case of late onset hemorrhagic disease of the newborn, an anonymous report was requested to

Table 3. Survey 1988: use of vitamin K_1 prophylaxis in German obstetric hospitals

Hospital characteristics	Number of inquiries	Number of responses	Percentage
University hospitals	31	19	61
Large community hospitals	141	140	100
Small departments	969	472	49
Total	1 141	631	55

differentiate whether bleedings were definitely or only possibly, due to vitamin K deficiency, and to identify cases unrelated to vitamin K deficiency.

Bleeding was considered to be a definite result of vitamin K deficiency when Quick's prothrombin time was below 15% at the time of bleeding and returned to normal within 24 hours following vitamin K administration. Hemorrhage was considered to be possibly due to vitamin K deficiency if the results of coagulation tests prior to or after vitamin K administration were not available. Vitamin K deficiency was excluded when the bleeding episodes were not the result of a hypoprothrombinemia, or if, following vitamin K administration, no return to normal was seen.

Results

Survey 1988

The questionnaires were sent to 1141 obstetric hospitals; 631 responses were received (Table 3). The responses were analyzed and categorized, according to the size of the institution, into university hospitals, large community hospitals, and smaller obstetric departments. Since no major differences were seen between institutions, the results are presented together.

Figure 1 shows which newborns receive vitamin K. In 500 of the 637 responding institutions a general vitamin K prophylaxis is administered to all newborns; in 107 hospitals vitamin K is given only to infants at risk; in five hospitals to breast-fed newborns only; in 18 institutions to breast-fed and newborns at risk only, and seven institutions did not use any vitamin K prophylaxis.

Figure 2 shows how, and how often, vitamin K is administered when general vitamin K prophylaxis is used. In the majority of hospitals, vitamin K is given via the intramuscular route; approximatley 20% of institutions prefer subcutaneous administration. Approximately 57% of all institutions use the parenteral route of administration. Oral administration of vitamin K and parenteral use in newborns at risk is used in 9% institutions; oral prophylaxis exclusively in only 7%. In the great majority of institutions vitamin K is given only once following birth. Only 1% of all hospitals use sequential doses for prophylaxis.

With vitamin K prophylaxis given to two-thirds of all newborns and elective prophylaxis to the remaining third of newborns, a definite decrease in late onset vitamin K deficiency bleedings was to be expected. To examine this hypothesis,

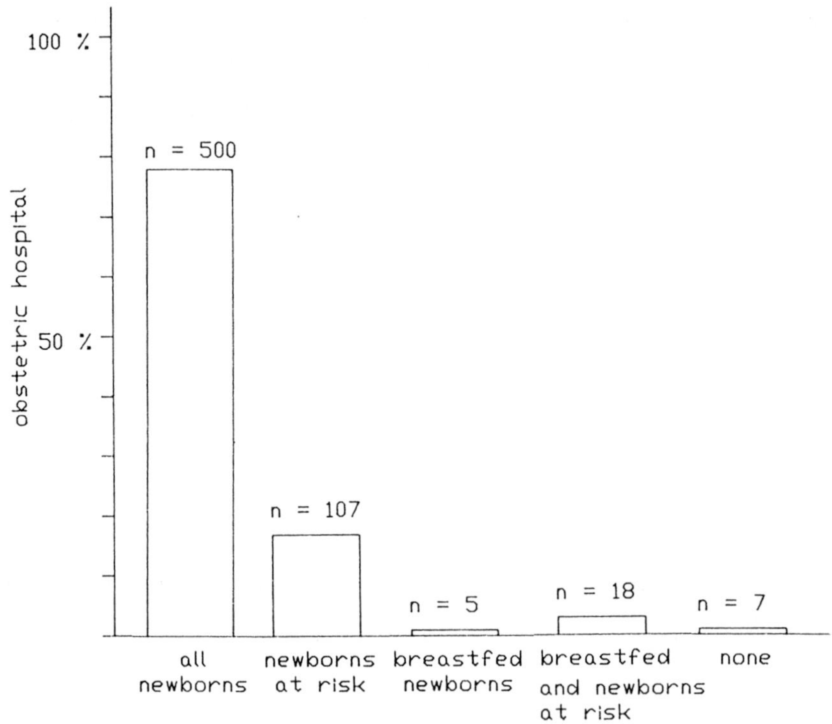

Fig. 1. Survey 1988: use of vitamin K_1 prophylaxis in 637 German obstetric hospitals

pediatric hospitals were surveyed in 1988 and 1989. The results of the 1989 survey are presented in Tables 4 and 5.

Survey 1989

Of 225 pediatric hospitals, 191 or 85% replied to the survey (Table 4). The proportion of replies did not differ according to the size of the institution.

Of 18 reported cases with hemorrhagic disease, 14 had proven evidence of vitamin K deficiency (Table 5). Ten of the infants reported were born in 1988 and four in the first three months of 1989. Vitamin K prophylaxis was given intramuscularly in one case; orally in three cases; and no prophylaxis was administered in the nine remaining infants. In one infant it remained unclear whether vitamin K had been given or not.

All infants but one with bleeding were exclusively breast-fed; one infant had been supplemented with a soy-based formula. Liver function test results were available for seven of the 14 infants with proven Vitamin K deficiency; in five of these infants there was laboratory evidence of cholestasis with increased direct serum bilirubin. In case number ten the serum alkaline phosphatase was in-

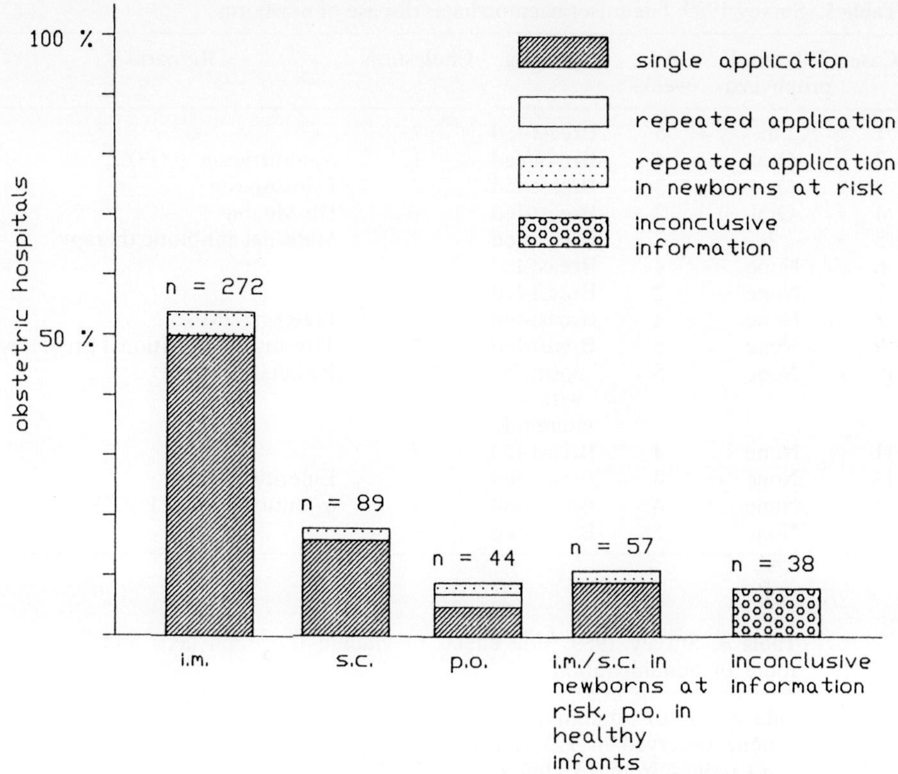

Fig. 2. Survey 1988: administration of vitamin K_1 in 500 German obstetric hospitals using vitamin K prophylaxis

Table 4. Survey 1989: late haemorrhagic disease of newborns in German pediatric hospitals

Hospital characteristics	Number of inquiries	Number of responses	Percentage
University hospitals	22	20	91
Large community hospitals	148	122	82
Small departments	65	60	78
Total	225	192	85

creased, with clinical evidence of rickets despite vitamin D prophylaxis. Nutritional problems existed in cases 3, 9, and 12. In two cases there was evidence of homozygous α_1-antitrypsin deficiency. Side effects of vitamin K injection were observed in only four cases reported by four different pediatric hospitals (Table 6).

Table 5. Survey 1989: late onset haemorrhagic disease of newborns

Case	Vitamin K prophylaxis	Age weeks	Feeding	Cholestasis	Remarks
1	i.m.	5	Breast-fed	?	
2	Oral	4	Breast-fed	+	α_1-antitrypsin ↓ (PiZZ)
3	Oral	3	Breast-fed	?	Pylorospasm
4	Oral	2	Breast-fed	+	Hb-Moabit
5	?	7	Breast-fed	?	Maternal antibiotic therapy
6	None	4	Breast-fed	+	
7	None	2	Breast-fed	?	
8	None	4	Breast-fed	+	Preterm, HMS
9	None	5	Breast-fed	?	Trisomy 21, nutritional problems
10	None	5	Formula without vitamin K	+	Rickets
11	None	4	Breast-fed	?	
12	None	4	Breast-fed	?	Enteritis (1 day)
13	None	4	Breast-fed	+	α_1-antitrypsin ↓ (PiZZ)
14	None	5	Breast-fed	–	

Table 6. Survey 1989: side effects of vitamin K_1 prophylaxis and route of administration

Side effects of vitamin K_1:	
none observed in 175 clinics	
no replies from 13 clinics	
observed reactions: 3 cases of transient reddening	
1 case of generalized urticaria	
Route of prophylaxis (110 clinics replied):	
	Percentage
i.m./s.c.	85
p.o. in healthy, i.m. in babies at risk	12
p.o.	4

Discussion

The rate of replies from obstetric hospitals was 55%. These questionnaires came mainly from larger hospitals with a high number of deliveries. Further replies were returned to Scharbau and Sutor [7], who also described very similar results concerning the practice of vitamin K prophylaxis in West Germany. Adding the number of questionnaires returned to us together with those returned to Scharbau and Sutor [7], the rate of replies increased to 70%. Although vitamin K prophylaxis did not differ between the three categories of obstetric hospitals, the results are not necessarily representative of all hospitals.

Even with this survey, it is not possible to state how many of the 600 000 babies born per year in West Germany receive which kind of vitamin K prophylaxis. Seventy-eight% of the replying obstetricians use general vitamin K prophylaxis, which is predominately given parenterally (i.m./s.c.). Elective prophylaxis for newborns at risk or those with difficult deliveries is used in about 20% of hospitals. The definition of newborns at risk does not include breast-feeding as a potential risk factor for late hemorrhagic disease [8,9]. Elective prophylaxis for breast-fed newborns in given only in 3%–4% of the hospitals.

With vitamin K prophylaxis for all newborns preferred by nearly 80% of all responding obstetricans and elective prophylaxis given by approximately 20%, a definite decrease in late onset vitamin K deficiency bleeding was to be expected. To examine this hypothesis a survey was directed to all pediatric hospitals one year later.

In this survey ten cases of hemorrhagic disease were reported for 1988; four were reported for the first three months of 1989. Compared to previous years, particularly the 26 cases reported in 1986, these data can only indicate a decrease in the incidence of late hemorrhagic disease. Since 1 case only was observed following parenteral vitamin K prophylaxis, this form of vitamin K prophylaxis has to be considered particularly effective. Side effects of parenteral vitamin K prophylaxis (i.m./s.c.) were minimal; only three cases of temporary rash were observed. Following three parenteral administrations of vitamin K to one baby urticaria was observed, suggesting rapid sensitisation.

Three failures following single dose oral vitamin K prophylaxis were observed, suggesting that this form of vitamin K prophylaxis is less effective than the parenteral. These observations correspond to the observations noted by Tönz [10]. In Switzerland, about half of the obstetrical hospitals give vitamin K orally, and the other half give vitamin K parenterally. Follwing oral vitamin K prophylaxis eight failures were reported; compared to none following parenteral vitamin K prophylaxis. The large number of cases of bleeding in babies who had not received any form of vitamin K prophylaxis is a strong argument to encourage vitamin K prophylaxis for all babies.

Coagulation data of the babies with late vitamin K deficiency hemorrhage show that the marginal vitamin K supply from maternal milk is a major factor in this hemorrhagic disease. The low dietary supply, however, does not lead to late hemorrhagic disease [11] unless additional factors are present [3,4].

The high proportion of children in this series with cholestasis further supports the concept of impaired vitamin K absorption in a large proportion of the affected babies [3,4]. This factor is also relevant for the fat soluble vitamin D [12].

Summary. In 1988 a survey of obstetric hospitals, concerning vitamin K prophylaxis, resulted in 78% of the responding hospitals showing a preference for general vitamin K prophylaxis, mainly given parenterally, (i.m./s.c.). About 20% of infants received vitamin K—2 mg orally on the first day of life. In about 20% of obstetric hospitals elective prophylaxis was given to newborns with eventful gestational histories or deliveries.

The parenteral mode of vitamin K prophylaxis seems to be more effective than the oral one, as shown by a 1989 survey of pediatric hospitals. Fourteen infants with late vitamin K deficiency were registered, of whom nine had no vitamin K prophylaxis, three had oral and one had parenteral vitamin K prophylaxis (one unknown). Signs of mild cholestasis were detected in six of seven infants.

Side effects after parenteral vitamin K prophylaxis consisted of redening of the skin and one case of generalized urticaria after the third dose had been given.

References

1. Sutor AH, Pancochar H, Niederhoff H, Pollmann H, Hilgenberg F, Palm D, Künzer W (1983) Vitamin K-Mangelblutungen bei vier vollgestillten Säuglingen im Alter von 4–6 Lebenswochen. Dtsch Med Wochenschr 108: 1635–1639
2. Sutor AH, Pollmann H, Von Kries R, Brückmann C, Jörres H, Künzer W (1988) Spätform der Vitamin K-Mangelblutung. Sozialpädiatrie 10: 557–560
3. Von Kries R, McCarthy P, Shearer M, Göbel U (1985) Late onset haemorrhagic disease of newborn with temporary malabsorption of vitamin K_1. Lancet I: 1035
4. Von Kries R, Kreppel S, Becker A, Tangermann R, Göbel U (1987) Acarboxy-prothrombin detectability after oral prophylactic vitamin K. Arch Dis Child 62: 938–940
5. Bergmann KH, Bremer HJ, Droese W, Grüttner R, Kübler W, Schmidt E, Schöch G (1986) Empfehlungen der Ernährungskommission der Deutschen Gesellschaft für Kinderheilkunde zur Vitamin K-Prophylaxe bei Neugeborenen. Monatsschr Kinderheilkd 134: 824–824
6. Sutor AH (1986) Spätmanifestation der Vitamin K-Mangelblutung bei vollgestillten Säuglingen. Kinderarzt 9: 1246′–1250
7. Scharbau A, Sutor AH (1988) Ergebnisse der Freiburger Auswertung. In: Sutor AH, Göbel U (eds) Gegenwärtiger Stand der Vitamin K-Prophylaxe in Deutschland. Arbeitstagung Freiburg 10–11 July 1988. "Roche", Basel, p 21
8. Von Kries R, Becker A, Göbel U (1987) Vitamin K in the newborn: influence of nutritional factors on acarboxy-prothrombin detectability and factor II and VII clotting activity. Eur J Pediatr 146: 123–127
9. Motohara K, Matsukane I, Endo F, Kiyota Y, Matsuda I (1989) Relationship of milk intake and vitamin K-status in newborns. Pediatrics 84: 90–93
10. Tönz O (1988) Erfahrungen mit der Vitamin K-Prophylaxe in der Schweiz. In: Sutor AH, Göbel U (eds) Gegenwärtiger Stand der Vitamin K-Prophylaxe in Deutschland. Arbeitstagung Freiburg 10–11 July 1988. "Roche" Basel, pp 151–159
11. Göbel U, Bewersdorff S, Henninghausen B, Schmidt E (1986) Erniedrigte Prothrombin-Gerinnungsaktivitäten bei gestillten Kindern? Klin Padiatr 198: 13–16
12. Matsuda I, Nishiyama S, Motohara K, Endo P, Ogata T, Futagoishi Y (1989) Late neonatal vitamin K deficiency associated with subclinical liver dysfunction in human milk-fed infants. J Pediatr 114: 602–605

3.5 Vitamin K Deficiency and Breast-Feeding

RÜDIGER VON KRIES[1]

Introduction

A dietary component which is essential for hemostasis was detected some fifty years ago and was called vitamin K. The clinical relevance of this vitamin in pediatrics was studied during this period [1]. Classical hemorrhagic disease of the newborn characteristically presents with gastrointestinal, nasal, skin and circumcision bleeding during the first 7 days of life [2,3]. For many years vitamin K deficiency bleeding beyond the neonatal period appeared to be related to malabsorption and cholestasis syndromes, such as celiac disease [2], bile duct atresia, [4] and cystic fibrosis [5] only. Bleeding in these cases may be observed at any time during the course of the underlying disease unless sufficient vitamin K supplements are given [6]. An early infantile hemorrhagic syndrome due to vitamin K deficiency, was not recognized until 1970 [7,8]. This hemorrhagic syndrome is characterized by intracranial hemorrhage which accounts for more than 50% of cases and is observed mainly in the fourth to sixth week of life [2,3].

A potential etiologic role for breast-feeding in classical hemorrhagic disease was postulated in the 1940s and prompted the analysis of the vitamin K content of both human milk and cows' milk [9]. The lower vitamin K concentrations in human milk compared to cows' milk appeared to be the explanation for the higher incidence of classical hemorrhagic disease in breast-fed babies. A higher incidence of classical hemorrhagic disease in breast-fed babies has been found in a number of studies [10–12] and has always been attributed to the low vitamin K content of human milk. If a low concentration of vitamin K_1 in human milk is the only explanation for classical hemorrhagic disease, why is the vitamin K supply sufficient for the vast majority by breast-fed babies? Why should human milk, the only milk designed for human beings which has proved its benefits during

[1] Abt. für Neonatologie, Universitäts-Kinderklinik, Moorenstraße 5, 4000 Düsseldorf 1, Federal Republic of Germany

evolution, be insufficient in this one vitamin? Conclusive answers to these questions have emerged from recent studies, which we now review.

The late form of vitamin K deficiency hemorrhage like classical hemorrhagic disease of the newborn (HDN), is virtually confined to breast-fed infants. The relation of breast-feeding to late hemorrhagic disease has been the subject of studies performed in Japan and West Germany [13,19]. Current concepts of the role of breast-feeding in late hemorrhagic disease are presented.

Sources of Dietary Vitamin K of Newborns and Young Infants

During the neonatal period and in early infancy milk is the only diet for babies. In 1942 Dam et al. reported the first estimates of vitamin K in human and in cows milk [9]. These estimates were based on bioassays. These assays allow a rough estimation of total vitamin K activity in a sample. The studies showed that vitamin K is detectable both in cows' milk and in most human milk samples. The vitamin K concentrations in the cows' milk samples were three to fourfold higher than those in human milk. For decades these estimates were the only available information for the assessment of babies' vitamin K supplies from human or cows' milk feeds. In the late 1970s more specific and sensitive techniques for vitamin K determination were developed.

In 1982 Haroon et al. demonstrated that vitamin K_1 is the main K vitamin in human and cows' milk [20]. Several investigators have shown that vitamin K_1 concentrations in mature human milk are lower than the total vitamin K activity reported by Dam et al. in 1942 [9]. The data from different groups, however, has varied considerably, as reviewed in a recent paper [21]. Several factors may account for these differences: Different methods for the determination of vitamin K were used, the milk sampling techniques were not standardized, and the lipid extraction methods varied. Standardized milk sampling is particularly important. The lipid concentration in human milk increases during the course of expression of the breast [22]. A similar increase of vitamin K concentrations during the course of breast-expression has been demonstrated recently [23].

Even with standardized milk sampling, lipid extraction and vitamin K determination techniques, however, vitamin K_1 concentrations in different mature milk samples from one mother were found to vary considerably (Fig. 1). The maternal dietary intake of vitamin K was found to influence the vitamin K concentration in mature human milk. A substantial increase in the concentration of vitamin K_1 could be obtained with supplements given to the mother, or with a vitamin K rich diet [23,24]. Although vitamin K_1 concentrations in human milk may vary widely, they are almost always lower than those in cows' milk or in infant formulas. The composition of cows' milk, however, is not uniform in vitamin K content either. Higher vitamin K_1 concentrations were observed in samples collected in summer and autumn compared to samples collected in the winter and spring months [9].

No baby, however, is fed pure cows' milk. Infant formula prepared by the parent or commercially is made by diluting of cows' milk and adding fat and carbohydrates. The vitamin K_1 concentration in all cows' milk based formulas

Fig. 1. Variability of vitamin K content in mature human milk. Fifteen samples from one mother collected under standardized conditions on days 22–36 of lactation

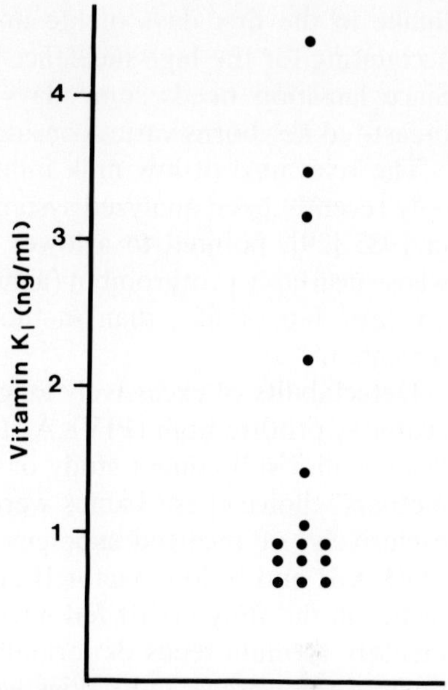

therefore, is usually lower than in cows' milk, unless vitamin K supplements are added. There may be considerable variation between different producers, depending on raw materials and losses in the production process. Most commercial infant formulas, however, are supplemented with vitamin K_1 in order to guarantee a vitamin K concentration of 30–70 μg/l [25]. Since most non-breast-fed babies in Germany are given commercial formulas, their dietary vitamin K_1 intake is much higher than that in exclusively breast-fed babies.

Classical Hemorrhagic Disease of Newborns and Breastfeeding

Shearer et al. were the first to demonstrate vitamin K deficiency in newborns by showing excessively low vitamin K concentrations in cord blood [26]. These studies have subsequently been extended to determinations of vitamin K concentrations in fetal, neonatal, and adult livers, and have shown that the vitamin K_1 stores in neonatal livers are much lower than those in adults [27]. A rapid and continuous vitamin K supply, therefore, is essential during the first week of life. The only definitely proven source of vitamin K in man is the diet [2].

The pathogenetic role of breast-feeding in classical hemorrhagic disease was recognized in 1940, when Salomonsen reported "... prevention of hemorrhagic disease of the newborn by readministration of cows' milk during the first two days of life" [11]. In their classical 1942 paper, Dam and coworkers explained these findings by showing low vitamin K concentrations in human milk compared to cows' milk [9]. The data appeared so convincing that the authors' reluctance to attribute the high incidence of classical HDN in breastfed newborns to the low vitamin K concentrations in human milk alone was forgotten. Dam and coworkers [9] had, in addition, introduced the hypothesis that a low milk intake in the first days of life in breast fed babies could be a further factor accounting for the high incidence of vitamin K deficiency in breast-fed infants. Since lactation needs some days to become established, the milk intake in breast-fed newborns varies considerably during the first days of life [28].

The relevance of low milk intakes in vitamin K deficiency in newborns has only recently been analyzed systematically. The first of these studies, published in 1985 [29], pointed to a lower human milk intake in the breast-fed babies whose acarboxy prothrombin (a marker for vitamin K deficiency) was detectable on days 5–6 of life, than in those babies without detectable acarboxy prothrombin.

Detectability of excessively long factor II and factor VII clotting times and of acarboxy prothrombin (PIVKA II) was used for the definition of vitamin K deficiency in a subsequent study of healthy five day old newborns [30]. At their mothers' choice these babies were fully breast-fed, or received formula feeds exclusively, or received supplementary formula feeds. The detection rates of PIVKA II and of long factor II and factor VII clotting times were significantly higher in the fully breast-fed newborns than in the babies given either supplementary formula feeds or formula feeds exclusively. The PIVKA II detection rates in fully breast-fed babies were only 50%, however, suggesting that low vitamin K concentrations in human milk could not be the only pathogenetic factor for vitamin K deficiency in these breast-fed babies.

Analysis of the babies' milk intakes revealed that vitamin K deficiency in breast-fed newborns was almost always confined to babies receiving small amounts of milk during the first days of life.

The same was found to be true in the rare cases of vitamin K deficiency in formula fed newborns; these were babies whose mothers' lactation was insufficient, but for whom supplementary formula feeds were not introduced before the second or third day of life. These results were confirmed by Motohara and coworkers in 1989 [31].

In summary, these studies demonstrate that a sufficient milk intake of 100 ml to 200 ml of human milk per day is essential for an adequate vitamin K supply during the first week of life. Since lactation may need some days to become fully established, vitamin K deficiency, which accounts for classical HDN, may be a major problem in fully breast-fed babies. Vitamin K deficiency, however, may occur in formula fed newborns as well, if the total milk intake is low or if the formula milk feeds are not introduced on the first or second day of life.

Some of the confusion as to the incidence of vitamin K deficiency in healthy newborns can be explained in the light of these new findings and in the light of changing feeding practices in neonates during recent decades. One of the classical papers that seemed to exclude vitamin K deficiency in newborns was based on clotting analysis in breast-fed newborns, who had been given supplementary formula feeds on the first days of life if lactation had been insufficient [32]. No evidence for vitamin K deficiency was detected on the third or fourth days of life in any of these children, irrespective of whether they had been breast- or formula fed. Ten years later a paper from the same institution reported a significantly higher incidence of long factor II clotting times in 5 and 6 day old breast-fed newborns compared to those receiving exclusive or supplementary formula feeds [13]. At that time none of the breast-fed babies was given supplementary formula feeds during the first days of life, even if the mothers' milk supply was low. From recent studies [29–31], it is now evident that the failure to detect vitamin K deficiency in the earlier study was a consequence of supplementary formula feeds having been given to babies irrespective of their mothers' intent to breast-feed.

Because the early introduction of supplementary cows' milk based formula in breast-fed infants seems to be a major risk factor for cows' milk protein intolerance, the practice of giving supplementary cows milk formula on the first days of life has been abandoned in many nurseries. As a consequence of this practice there is again a population of fully breast-fed newborns at risk for classical HDN, and the recurrance of HDN has been reported in parts of England where vitamin K prophylaxis had been abandoned [33].

Late Hemorrhagic Disease of the Newborn (HDN)

Late HDN occurs in the period when lactation is fully established. Most of these babies are 4–8 weeks old and appear healthy before bleeding occurs. Still the disease is virtually confined to breast-fed babies [2,3]. Breast-fed babies obtain much less vitamin K_1 from their diet than those babies fed commercial formulas, and lower plasma vitamin K_1 in breast-fed infants, compared to those fed infant formula, has been reported [34]. The clinical relevance of the relatively low plasma vitamin K_1 in breast-fed infants has been analyzed in different studies in Europe and Japan. In the first European study the factor II clotting times in 4–6 week old healthy infants were analyzed. They revealed identical distribution patterns in fully breastfed babies and in babies receiving supplementary formula feeds or formula feeds exclusively.

Since clotting analysis permits the detection of overt vitamin K deficiency only [35] a subsequent study, using more sensitive tests for the detection of the vitamin K deficiency state, was performed. The subjects were 202 healthy newborns [15]. Acarboxy prothrombin (PIVKA II) detection rates were determined on day 5 or 6 and during week 5 or 6 in all 202 babies and the factor II clotting times were determined in 100 of the 202 babies. Table 1 shows the PIVKA II detection rates in relation to feeding in the neonatal period and in early infancy. On days 5 and 6 PIVKA II was detected in 109 out of 167 breast-fed babies. During weeks five and six 113 of these babies were still exclusively breast-fed. PIVKA II was detectable in only one of these 113 breast-fed babies.

Table 1. PIVKA II detectability in healthy babies in relation to feeding and age, day 5 + 6, week 5 + 6

Breast only	109/167	1/113
Breast and formula	5/28	0/67
Formula only	2/7	0/22

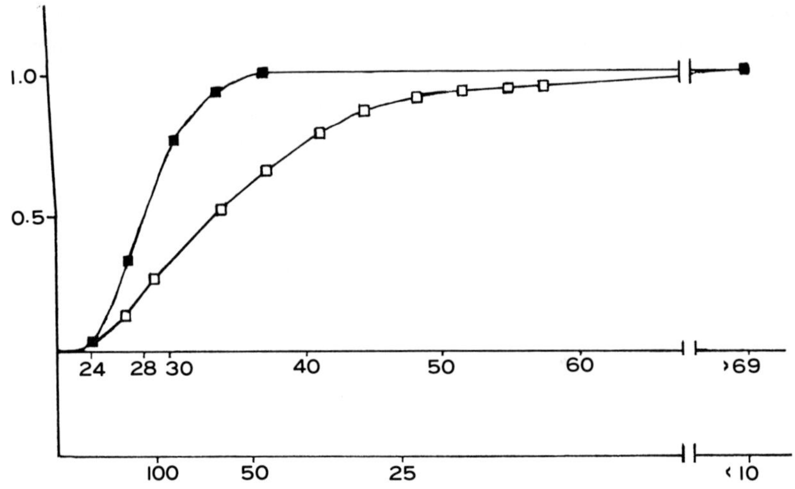

Fig. 2. Cumulative distribution of factor II clotting activity in healthy babies aged 5 or 6 days □ and 5 or 6 weeks ■

The cumulative distribution of the factor II clotting times on days 5 and 6 and in weeks 5 and 6 is shown in 100 of the 202 babies (Fig. 2). Hypoprothombinemia was common in these babies on days 5 and 6. Although no vitamin K supplements had been given, none of these babies had hypothrombinemia in weeks 5 and 6.

Similar results have been obtained in other studies on populations in Europe and Japan [19,36]. These studies show that subclinical vitamin K deficiency is more common in early infancy than clinically manifest vitamin K deficiency bleeding. Subclinical vitamin K deficiency is observed mainly in breast-fed infants. The absolute incidences of PIVKA II detectability in breast-fed babies, however, varied with the sensitivities of the tests used. The highest detection rates were found with a monoclonal PIVKA II antibody [37,35].

The important message of these studies is that low vitamin K intake in breast-fed infants is a relevant risk factor for vitamin K deficiency. Subclinical vitamin K deficiency (PIVKA II detectability without clinical hemorrhage or hypoprothrombinemia) is more common than manifest vitamin K deficiency hemorrhage. The low dietary vitamin K intake in breast-fed infants, however, is sufficient to maintain normal hemostasis in the vast majority of infants. Several pathophysiological hypotheses for the insufficient vitamin K supply in breast-fed babies have been considered.

The vitamin K_1 concentrations in milk samples from different mothers varies considerably [38,23]. Since the maternal dietary vitamin K intake influences the vitamin K concentration in the milk [23,24], the vitamin K concentration in the milk of some mothers might be excessively low, and thereby could account for an insufficient vitamin K supply in their babies. Three studies of vitamin K_1 concentrations in milk samples from a total of 28 mothers of affected babies have been published [39,16,18]. Two of the 3 studies suggested lower mean concentrations of vitamin K_1 in the samples from mothers whose children had bleeding episodes. Vitamin K_1 concentrations below those for controls were reported in 5 of 9 cases from Thailand [39], 3 of 10 cases from Japan [2], and none of 9 cases from West Germany [16]. From these studies it must be assumed that an extremely low vitamin K intake might account for late HDN in some affected babies, but certainly not in all.

Impairment of vitamin K absorption can account for insufficient vitamin K supply in infants [2]. Vitamin K deficiency hemorrhage has been reported in babies with bile duct atresia, cystic fibrosis, celiac disease, and alpha 1 antitrypsinemia. Most of the babies with late hemorrhagic disease, however, appeared healthy; late hemorrhagic disease in these babies has therefore been considered to be idiopathic [40]. However, more detailed clinical and laboratory investigations of babies with idiopathic late hemorrhagic disease has demonstrated that a substantial proportion of these babies has slightly elevated direct bilirubin concentrations, suggestive of mild cholestasis [40]. Cholestasis can account for impaired vitamin K absorption, since bile salts are essential for the absorption of fat soluble vitamins [41]. In babies receiving only small amounts of vitamin K with their diets, even mild malabsorption might become a relevant factor in the insufficient supply of vitamin K.

Impaired vitamin K absorption in a baby with late HDN was first demonstrated in 1985 [14]. Vitamin K malabsorption in this baby was temporary and associated with mild cholestasis. Evidence supporting this concept was obtained in a recent paper from Japan, demonstrating low vitamin D plasma-concentrations in babies with late HDN and mild cholestasis [17]. Further studies are needed to assess the interdependecy between mild cholestasis and malabsorption of vitamin K, and the clinical relevance of these factors for breast-fed babies.

Summary. Breast-feeding is a major risk factor for classical and late hemorrhagic disease of the newborn. The assessment of this association has been the subject of a number of studies performed in West Germany and Japan. These studies suggest that low milk intakes on the first days of lactation, which occurs in a substantial number of breast-fed babies, must be considered as the main reason for the higher incidence of classical hemorrhagic disease of the newborn in breast-fed newborns as compared to the incidence in those fed infant formula. Late hemorrhagic disease of the newborn was found to be only rarely a consequence of insufficient vitamin K supply from excessively low vitamin K concentrations in the milk of mothers of affected babies, although subclinical vitamin K deficiency appears to be more common in exclusively breast-fed babies than vitamin K deficiency hemorrhage. The potential role of impaired vitamin K absorption due to subclinical cholestasis in addition to the low dietary vitamin K intake in exclusively breast-fed infants needs further study.

References

1. Dam H, Dyggve H, Larsen H, Plum P (1952) The relation of vitamin K deficiency to hemorrhagic disease of the newborn. Adv Pediatr 5: 129–153

2. Von Kries R, Shearer MJ, Göbel U (1988) Vitamin K in infancy. Eur J Pediatr 147: 106–112
3. Lane PA, Hathaway WE (1985) Vitamin K in infancy. J Pediatr 106: 351–59
4. Fujimura Y, Mimura Y, Kinoshita S, Yoshioka A, Kitawaki T, Yoshioka K, Takamiya O (1982) Studies on vitamin K-dependent factor deficiency during early childhood with special reference to prothrombin activity and antigen level. Haemostasis 11: 90–95
5. Torstensen OL, Humphrey GB, Edson JR, Warwick WJ (1970) Cystic fibrosis presenting with severe hemorrhage due to vitamin K malabsorption: a report of 3 cases. Pediatrics 45: 857–861
6. American Academy of Pediatrics, Committee on Nutrition (1971) Vitamin K supplementation for infants receiving milk substitute infant formulas and for those with fat malabsorption. Pediatrics 48: 483–487
7. Bhanchet P, Tuchinda S, Hathirat P, Visudhiphan P, Bhamaraphavati N, Bukkavesa S (1977) A bleeding syndrome in infants due to acquired prothrombin complex deficiency. Clin Pediatr 16: 992–998
8. Nammacher MA, Willemin M, Hartmann JR, Gaston LW (1970) Vitamin K deficiency in infants beyond the neonatal period. J Pediatr 76: 549–554
9. Dam H, Glavind J, Larsen EH, Plum P (1942) Investigations into the cause of the physiological hypoprothrombinemia in newborn children. IV. The vitamin K content of woman's milk and cow's milk. Acta Med Scand 112: 210–216
10. Keenan WJ, Jewett T, Glueck HI (1971) Role of feeding and vitamin K in hypoprothrombinemia of the newborn. Am J DIS Child 121: 271–277
11. Salomonsen L (1940) On the prevention of hemorrhagic disease of the newborn by the administration of cow's milk during the first two days of life. Acta Pediat 28: 1–7
12. Sutherland JM, Glueck HI, Gleser G (1967) Hemorrhagic disease of the newborn: breast-feeding as a necessary factor in the pathogenesis. Am J Dis Child 113: 524–533
13. Göbel U, Von Kries R, Bewersdorff S, Henninghausen B, Schmidt E (1986) Erniedrigte Prothrombin-Gerinnungsaktivitäten bei gestillten Kindern? Klin Padiatr 198: 13–16
14. Von Kries R, Reifenhäuser A, Göbel U, McCarthy PT, Shearer MJ, Barkhan P (1985) Late onset haemorrhagic disease of newborn with temporary malabsorption of vitamin K_1 (letter). Lancet I: 1035
15. Von Kries R, Maase B, Becker A, Göbel U (1985) Latent vitamin K deficiency in healthy infants (letter). Lancet II: 1421–1422
16. Von Kries R, Tangermann R, Shearer MJ, Göbel U (1987) Vitamin K deficiency in breast-fed infants. In: Goldman AS, Atkinson SA, Hanson LA (eds) Human Lactation 3. The effects of human milk on the recipient infant. Plenum, New York, pp 317–324
17. Matsuda I, Nishiyama S, Motohara K, Endo P, Ogata T, Futagoishi Y (1989) Late neonatal vitamin K deficiency associated with subclinical liver dysfunction in human milk-fed infants. J. Pediatr 114: 602–605
18. Motohara K, Matsukura M, Matsuda I, Iribe K, Ikeda T, Kondo Y, Yonekubo A, Yamamoto Y, Tsuchiya F (1984) Severe vitamin K deficiency in breast-fed infants. J Pediatr 105: 943–945
19. Motohara K, Endo, F, Matsuda I (1987) Screening for late neonatal vitamin K deficiency by acarboxy prothrombin in dried blood spots. Arch Dis Child 62: 370–375
20. Haroon Y, Shearer MJ, Rahim S, Gunn WG, McEnery G, Barkhan P (1982) The content of phylloquinone (vitamin K_1) in human milk, cow's milk and infant formula foods determined by high-performance liquid chromatography. J Nutr 112: 1105–1117
21. Canfield LM, Hopkinson JM (1989) State of the art vitamin K in human milk. J Ped Gastroenterol Nutr 8: 430–441
22. Harzer G, Haug M (1984) Abhängigkeit der Frauenmilchlipide von der Dauer der Stillperiode, der Tageszeit, dem Stillvorgang und der mütterlichen Ernährung. Z Ernährungswiss 23: 113–125

23. Von Kries R, Shearer M, McCarthy PT, Haug M, Harzer G, Göbel U (1987) Vitamin K_1 content of maternal milk: influence of the stage of lactation, lipid composition, and vitamin K_1 supplements given to the mother. Pediatr Res 22: 513–517
24. Sawada K, Hanawa Y (1988) Vitamin K_1 content of human milk various maternal nutritional states. In: Berger H (ed) Vitamins and minerals in pregnancy and lactation. Nestle nutrition workshop series, vol. 16 Nested, Vevey/Raven Press, New York, pp 389
25. American Academy of Pediatrics, Committee on Nutrition (1976) Commentary on breast-feeding and infant formulas, including proposed standards for formulas. Pediatrics 57: 278–285
26. Shearer MJ, Rahim S, Barkhan P, Stimmler L (1982) Plasma vitamin K_1 in mothers and their newborn babies. Lancet II: 460–463
27. McCarthy PT, Shearer MJ, Gau G, Crampton OE, Barkhan (1986) Vitamin K content of human liver at different ages (abstract). Haemostasis 16: 83–84
28. Rosegger H, Pürstner P (1985) Zufütterung von volladaptierter Kunstmilch oder kalorienlosem Tee in den ersten Lebenstagen. Wien Klin Wochenschr 97: 411–414
29. Von Kries R, Göbel U, Maase B (1985) Vitamin K deficiency in the newborn (letter). Lancet II: 728–729
30. Von Kries R, Becker A, Göbel U (1987) Vitamin K in the newborn: influence of nutritional factors on acarboxy-prothrombin detectability and factor II and VII clotting activity. Eur J Pediatr 146: 123–127
31. Motohara K, Matsukane I, Endo F, Kiyota Y, Matsuda I (1989) Relationship of vitamin K intake and vitamin K supplementation to vitamin K status in newborns. Pediatr 84: 90–94
32. Göbel U, Sonnenschein-Kosenow S, Petrich C, Von Voss H (1977) Vitamin K deficiency in the newborn (letter). Lancet II: 187–188
33. McNinch AW, L'Orme R, Tripp JH (1983) Haemorrhagic disease of the newborn returns. Lancet I: 1089–1090
34. Lambert WE, De Leenheer AP, Tassaneeyakul W, Widdershoven J (1987) Study of vitamin K in the newborn by HPLC with wet-chemical post-column reduction and fluorescence detection. In: Suttie JW (ed) Current advances in vitamin K research. Elsevier, New York, pp 437–452
35. Widdershoven J, Kollee L, van Munster P, Bosman AM, Monnens L (1986) Biochemical vitamin K deficiency in early infancy: diagnostic limitation of conventional coagulation tests. Helv Paediatr Acta 41: 195–201
36. Widdershoven J, Motohara K, Endo F, Matsuda I, Monnens L (1986) Influence of the type of feeding on the presence of PIVKA-II in infants. Helv Paediatr Acta 41: 25–29
37. Motohara K, Kuroki Y, Kan H, Endo F, Matsuda I (1985) Detection of vitamin K deficiency by the use of an enzyme-linked immunosorbent assay for circulating abnormal prothrombin. Pediatr Res 19: 354–357
38. Von Kries R, Göbel U, Shearer MS, McCarthey PT (1985) Vitamin K deficiency in breast-fed infants (letter). J Pediatr 650–651
39. Isarangkura PB, Mahadandana C, Panstienkul B, Nakayama K, Tsukimoto I, Yamamoto Y, Yonekubo A (1983) Vitaman K level in maternal breast milk of infants with acquired prothrombin complex deficiency. Southeast Asian J Trop Med Public Health 14: 275–276
40. Hanawa Y, Maki M, Murata B, Matsuyama E, Yamamoto Y, Nagao T, Yamada K (1988) The second nationwide survey in Japan of vitamin K deficiency in infancy. Eur J Pediatr 147: 472–477
41. Shearer MJ, McBurney A, Barkhan P (1974) Studies on the absorption and metabolism of phylloquinone (vitamin K_1) in man. Vitam Horm 32: 513–542

Vitamin K Deficiency 2

3.6 The Third Nationwide Survey on Vitamin K Deficiency in Infancy in Japan

TAKESHI NAGAO[1] and YOSHIYUKI HANAWA[2]

Methods

The Ministry of Health and Welfare of Japan has organized a research committee (chairmen: Kentaro Nakayama and Yoshiyuki Hanawa) on "Idiopathic Vitamin K Deficiency in Infancy since 1980." The Ministry has funded nationwide surveys on vitamin K deficiency in infancy three times, i.e., in 1980, 1985, and 1988 [1–5]. Questionnaires were sent to the pediatric departments of 1 011, 1 218, and 1 315 hospitals with 200 beds or more, respectively. Return rates were 42%, 40% and 59% respectively. On the surveys, we classified hemorrhage due to vitamin K deficiency as shown in Table 1 [6]. A secondary type is those infants with an apparent cause for vitamin K deficiency such as congenital biliary atresia, neonatal hepatitis, and so on. Infants without these apparent reasons are categorized as idiopathic.

Table 1. Vitamin K deficiency

Hemorrhagic disease of the newborn (melena neonatorum)
Vitamin K deficiency in infancy (late onset hemorrhagic disease of the newborn)
Secondary vitamin K deficiency in infancy
Congenital biliary atresia
Chronic diarrhea
Antibiotics
Idiopathic vitamin K deficiency in infancy

Results of the Surveys

Through the 1st survey, 334 idiopathic type infants and 91 secondary types were reported to have been seen between 1978 and 1980 (Table 2). In the 2nd survey

[1]Kanagawa Children's Medical Center, 2-138-4 Mutsukawa, Minami-ku, Yokohama, 232 Japan
[2]First Department of Pediatrics, Toho University, 6-11-1 Oomori-nishi, Oota-ku, Tokyo, 143 Japan

Table 2. Vitamin K deficiency in infancy

Survey	Period	Idiopathic	Secondary	Total
1st	Jan. 1, 1978–Dec. 31, 1980	334	91	425
2nd	Jan. 1, 1981–June 30, 1985	427	57	484
3rd	July 1, 1985–June 30, 1988	129	28	157
Total	Jan. 1, 1978–June 30, 1988	890	176	1066

(1981–1985), infants classified as idiopathic totalled 427 and secondary types totalled 57. In the 3rd survey, 129 idiopathic and 28 secondary types were found. Through the three surveys, 890 idiopathic and 176 secondary types (in total 1 066 infants) were reported during the 10-year period.

As for the type of feeding the infants with idiopathic vitamin K deficiency in infancy received, most of the infants were fed with breast milk only, namely 86% (1st survey), 91% (2nd survey), and 92% (3rd survey). In the general population about half of Japanese infants are fed with breast milk only. However, more than 90% of the idiopathic group are fed with breast milk only.

The age distribution of the idiopathic group is also characteristic. Most of the infants developed their bleeding episodes at the age of one month or a little bit earlier. In the 1st survey, 75% of the idiopathic type were a month old; in the 2nd, 62%; and in the 3rd, 70%. About one-fifth of the infants with the idiopathic type were between 2 and 4 weeks old when they were diagnosed, namely, 13% (1st survey), 28% (2nd survey), and 23% (3rd survey). In other words, bleeding episodes of idiopathic types are concentrated in the infants between 15 and 60 days old, i.e., 88% (1st survey), 90% (2nd survey), and 93% (3rd survey).

The site of bleeding in the idiopathic group of the 3rd survey also shows the same pattern seen in the previous two surveys. A high margin, 92% of the 129 infants, did have intracranial hemorrhage, whereas 87% were seen in the 1st survey and 83% in the 2nd survey. The characteristics of idiopathic vitamin K deficiency in infancy, i.e., intracranial hemorrhage in breast-fed infants around one month of age, are again confirmed through the third survey.

Prognosis of the 129 infants in the idiopathic group of the 3rd survey is as follows: 6% dead (1st, 14%; 2nd, 15%), 42% alive with sequellae (1st, 37%; 2nd, 40%), 49% alive without sequellae (1st, 44%; 2nd, 43%), and 3% unknown (1st, 5%; 2nd, 2%).

Prophylaxis

Although the prognosis is improving slightly , prevention of intracranial hemorrhage is preferable to early treatment. In the 1970s, most Japanese obstetricians abandoned giving prophylactic vitamin K at birth. They were probably influenced by cases of kernicterus after routine administration of water soluble synthesized vitamin K_3 and K_4 and by the statements of the Japanese Society

Table 3. Tentative recommendation of prophylactic administration of vitamin K

All full-term newborns without complication
A dose of 2 mg of vitamin K_2 syrup (1 ml) is to be given:
Within 24 h after birth (The syrup is to be diluted with 9 ml of water and given after one or two feedings.)
A week of age (at the time of discharge)
A month of age (at the time of routine checkup) (This dose can be omitted if screening tests are normal.)

of Pediatrics, i.e., intramuscular injections are to be avoided in infants because of shortening of the quadriceps muscles. In fact, most of the infants in the idiopathic group did not have received any type of prophylactic vitamin K administration.

In 1983, the committee made the recommendations shown in Table 3 [7,8]. We do not know the real cause of vitamin K deficiency in the idiopathic group. That is the reason we chose to call it "idiopathic." Although we were not sure whether prophylactic administration of vitamin K orally in such doses could prevent the intracranial hemorrhage at a month of age, we needed an active plan and wanted to see the results. By that time, we knew idiopathic vitamin K deficiency in infancy to be rare in European countries and the United States, where vitamin K was routinely given intramuscularly at birth. The committee's recommendations were followed by others widely after development of an oral syrup preparation of vitamin K_2 in 1985.

Through the three nationwide surveys, a decrease in the incidence of idiopathic vitamin K deficiency in infancy was observed. Between 1978 and 1980, the incidence was 18.0: 100 000 births. In 1982, it increased to 19.7: 100 000 births. Then, it gradually, but constantly, decreased to 4.3: 100 000 births in 1988. In 1987, the Japan Association for Maternal Welfare estimated that about 80% of full-term newborn babies received at least one dose of prophylactic vitamin K at birth or during the neonatal period according to its own survey.

Figure 1 shows the survey results in our prefecture (Kanagawa Prefecture, population 7.5 million) [9]. The *vertical bars* indicate the number of infants with intracranial hemorrhage. Most did not have any vitamin K prophylaxis. However, three patients (designated by asterisks) did have oral vitamin K once or twice. Two of the three were reported to have had liver dysfunction. In 1984, oral vitamin K was given to 26% of the newborn babies. The rate of prophylaxis has increased steadily, up to 92% in 1988. If we compare the incidence of intracranial hemorrhage between the two groups—the prophylaxis group and the non-prophylaxis group—based on the prevalence of vitamin K prophylaxis in Kanagawa Prefecture, the incidence of intracranial hemorrhage in the prophylaxis group is significantly lower than in the non-prophylaxis group (chi-squared test, $p < 0.05$).

In Nagasaki Prefecture, the number of infants suffering from intracranial hemorrhage has decreased sharply after the initiation of prophylactic vitamin K administration orally in 1981. Since 1982, more than 90% of the newborn babies

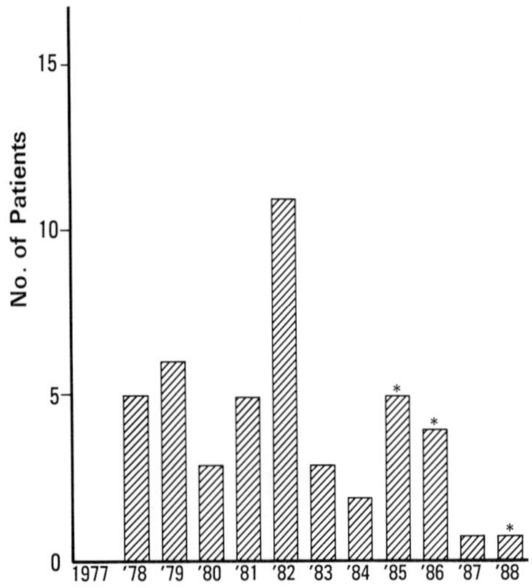

Fig. 1. Intracranial hemorrhage due to idiopathic vitamin K deficiency in infancy in Kanagawa Prefecture. *One of the patients was given prophylactic vitamin K

have received vitamin K. Intracranial hemorrhage was seen in 8 infants in 1980, 4 in 1981, 2 in both 1982 and 1983, 1 in 1985, and zero in 1984, 1986, 1987, and 1988. All but one of the 17 above-mentioned babies did not have prophylactic vitamin K. Incidence of intracranial hemorrhage was significantly lower in the prophylaxis group than in the non-prophylaxis group. Based on these data, oral vitamin K prophylaxis seems to be effective in decreasing the incidence of intracranial hemorrhage due to idiopathic vitamin K deficiency in infancy. However, this regimen may not be perfect, because there are still a few cases of intracranial hemorrhage even after vitamin K prophylaxis.

As to the history of the infants in the 3rd survey in regards to vitamin K administration, among the 129 infants in the idiopathic group, 110 did not have any vitamin K prophylaxis. However, 8 infants had oral vitamin K once before development of bleeding episodes, 6 infants had two administrations, and 2 infants had three. Although one of the infants in the last group may be too old (210 days) to be included into the idiopathic group and the other infant had other risk factors, about 10% of the 129 babies did have prophylaxis. Moreover, 3 of the 8 infants studied in detail had an increased level of ALT (or GPT).

Secondary Vitamin K Deficiency in Infancy

For the secondary group, the total number affected has also decreased recently. The age distribution tends to be similar to the idiopathic group's although the sharp peak at a month of age is not seen in the secondary group (Fig. 2).

The possible causes which might have induced vitamin K deficiency in these infants are as follows: (1) neonatal/infantile hepatitis, 9 infants (4 thought to be related to cytomegalovirus infection); (2) congenital biliary atresia and other hepatobiliary disorders, 11 infants; (3) severe diarrhea, 3 infants; and (4)

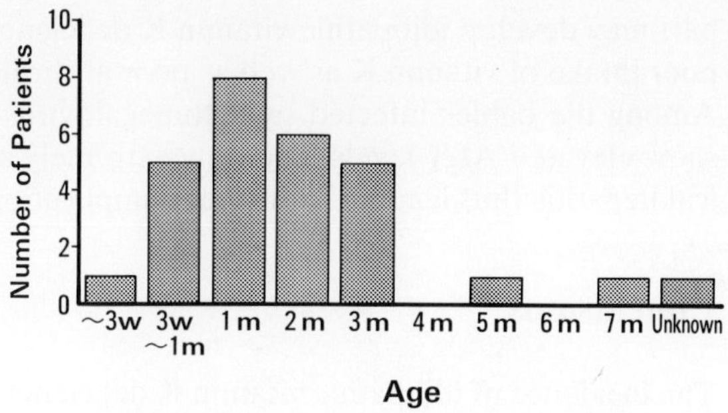

Fig. 2. Secondary vitamin K deficiency in infancy according to age distribution in the 3rd survey. *W*, week; *m*, month

others, 5 infants. Again, liver diseases are frequent. We have already reported that about half of our cases of the idiopathic type did have mild elevations of ALT sometime during their courses. This elevation, as previously noted, was also seen in the infants who developed bleeding after vitamin K prophylaxis.

Hypothesis

Our hypothesis on the pathogenesis of idiopathic vitamin K deficiency in infancy is shown in Table 4. When considering the pathogenesis of the idiopathic type, breast feeding and peak incidence at one month must be the keys. Relatively low intake of vitamin K through breast milk may be a partial cause. However, only an extremely small number of breast-fed infants develops intracranial hemorrhage even without vitamin K prophylaxis. There must be some other reason besides breast milk.

Our working hypothesis involves the contribution of mild and otherwise nonsymptomatic liver dysfunction, which is seen in about half of the infants extensively studied in the idiopathic group. Further, it could be that the mild liver dysfunction may be caused by vertical transmission of cytomegalovirus at the time of delivery or through breast milk. This may explain the peak incidence at one month and also explain why the incidence of the idiopathic type seems to be higher in the southern part of Japan and Southeast Asia [10].

Altogether, through infection of cytomegalovirus in the very early period of life (a rare occurrence even in Japan where the prevalence of cytomegalovirus infection is high [11]), a few babies may have subclinical liver dysfunction. Only

Table 4. Idiopathic vitamin K (VK) deficiency in infancy (hypothesis)

Poor intake of VK (breast milk)
Poor absorption of VK (liver dysfunction*)
Poor utilization of VK (liver dysfunction*)

*VK deficiency is not prevented in patients with severe liver dysfunction, and liver dysfunction could be caused by vertical transmission of cytomegalovirus (CMV).

part may develop idiopathic vitamin K deficiency in infancy in conjunction with poor intake of vitamin K as well as poor absorption and/or poor utilization of it. Among the babies infected by cytomegalovirus in early life, a few babies may show elevated ALT levels, and only extremely affected babies will develop clinical hepatitis thus leading to further complications.

Conclusions

The incidence of idiopathic vitamin K deficiency in infancy has decreased during the past 10 years in Japan. The low incidence was probably achieved by prophylactic oral administration of vitamin K. All cases could not be prevented even with prophylactic administration of oral vitamin K. Some of the infants who developed intracranial hemorrhage even after vitamin K prophylaxis did have liver dysfunction. Further research into the actual pathogenesis of "Idiopathic Vitamin K Deficiency in Infancy" is needed.

Summary. The Ministry of Health and Welfare of Japan organized a research committee on idiopathic vitamin K deficiency in infancy since 1980. The committee (chairman: Kentaro Nakayama, 1980–1982; Yoshiyuki Hayama, 1983–1988) has now performed nationwide surveys on vitamin K deficiency in infancy three times, i.e., in 1980, 1985, and 1988. After collecting information on infants with bleeding symptoms due to vitamin K deficiency, two groups were defined. The "secondary" group consists of those with well-known causes of vitamin K deficiency, i.e., congenital biliary atresia, prolonged administration of antibiotics, chronic diarrhea, etc. "Idiopathic" designates those without such obvious sources. The three surveys confirmed the characteristics of idiopathic vitamin K deficiency in infancy—intracranial hemorrhage in 1 to 2-month-old infants fed exclusively breast milk. In 1983, the committee made a recommendation of prophylactic administration of three doses of oral vitamin K_2 to all full-term newborns. Incidence of idiopathic cases has decreased from 19.7 to 4.3 out of 100 000 births during the past 10 years. Incidence of secondary cases has also decreased.

References

1. Nakayama K, Ikeda I, Shirahata S (1981) Hemorrhagic disease due to vitamin K deficiency in infancy. Nihon Iji Shinpo 2996: 22–28
2. Hanawa Y, Murata B, Maki M (1986) Hemorrhagic disease due to vitamin K deficiency in infancy; Second nation-wide survey. Nihon Iji Shinpo 3239: 26–29
3. Hanawa Y, Murata B, Maki M (1988) The second nation-wide survey in Japan of vitamin K deficiency in infancy. Eur J Pediatr 147: 472–477
4. Hanawa Y, Maki M, Matsuyama E (1989) Hemorrhagic disease due to vitamin K deficiency in infancy; Third nation-wide survey. Nihon Iji Shinpo 3397: 43–46
5. Hanawa Y, Maki M, Matsuyama E (1989) The third nation-wide survey in Japan of vitamin K deficiency in infancy. Acta Paediatr Jpn Overseas Ed (in press)
6. Nagao T, Iizuka A (1982) Idiopathic vitamin K deficiency in infancy; Its entity and enigmas. Acta Haematol Jpn 45: 849–859

7. Nakayama K, Nagao T, Ikeda I (1983) Prophylaxis of vitamin K deficiency in infancy with oral vitamin K_2. Nihon Iji Shinpo 3086: 19–21
8. Nagao T (1988) Vitamin K deficiency in infancy; Japanese experience with oral vitamin K to prevent early and late HDN. In: Suvatte V, Tuchinda M (eds) Proceedings of First International Congress of Tropical Pediatrics, 8–12 Nov 1987. Bangkok, Thailand
9. Nagao T, Adachi K, Kuwabara T (1988) Prophylaxis and incidence of idiopathic vitamin K deficiency in infancy in Kanagawa Prefecture. Kanagawa Children's Medical Center Igakusi 17: 125–128
10. Isarangkura PB (1988) Vitamin K deficiency in infancy; Historical background and experience with prevention of the late hemorrhagic disease of infant (APCD syndrome) in Thailand. In: Suvatte V, Tuchinda M (eds) Proceedings of First International Congress of Tropical Pediatrics, 8–12 Nov 1987, Bangkok, Thailand
11. Chiba S (1988) Vertical transmission of cytomegalovirus. Sanfujinka no Jissai 37: 35–39

3.7 Time Interval Between Vitamin K Administration and Effective Hemostasis

ANTOH H. SUTOR and WILHELM KÜNZER[1]

Introduction

In adults with vitamin K deficiency, correction of abnormal coagulation tests with vitamin K therapy cannot be expected for several hours; therefore, bleeding patients are given plasma concentrates to bridge the time before vitamin K becomes effective [1,2]. In newborns a time gap of several hours, in some instances up to 12 h, is reported [3,4]. The aim of the present study is to investigate the time interval between administration of vitamin K and, first, a significant increase of the PT value (in %) and, second, a demonstrable hemostatic effect to reverse the vitamin K deficiency bleeding with administration of vitamin K.

Patients and Methods

All patients had the late form of vitamin K-deficiency bleeding and have been described in detail elsewhere [5]. The diagnosis of vitamin K deficiency was established by a PT (expressed not as time but as percent, whereby normal values are between 70% and 100%) of < 10%, of vitamin K-dependent factors (one stage method) of < 15%, and a positive protein in vitamin K absence (PIVKA) value.

Results

Patient 1

This 22-day-old female presented with melena and multiple hematomas. She was breast-fed and did not receive vitamin K (VK) prophylaxis at birth. One

[1] Universitäts-Kinderklinik, D-7800 Freiburg, Federal Republic of Germany

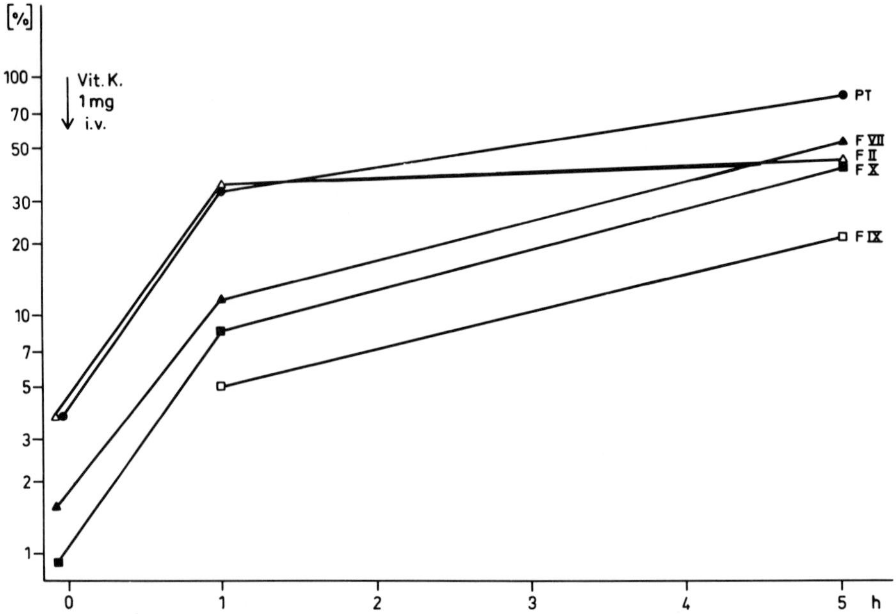

Fig. 1. Kinetics of prothrombin time (*PT*) and vitamin K-dependent coagulation factors in patient 1 after vitamin K

hour after intravenous vitamin K (1 mg), the PT value rose from 3.7% to 33% (Fig. 1). This increase was similar for factor II, whereas F VII, X, and especially F IX were lower after 1 h. After 1 h the increase in the PT value and the VK-dependent clotting factors was slower. The patient, who had a cytomegalovirus (CMV) infection, recovered without sequelae.

Patient 2

This 3.5-week-old breast-fed male, who did not receive VK prophylaxis at birth, was bleeding from the mouth. His PT value was unmeasurable (< 1%): F II, 1.5%; F VII, 6.3%; F IX, 2.3%; and F X, 3.8% (Fig. 2). Fifteen minutes after intravenous vitamin K (1 mg) was given, his mother noticed that the bleeding had stopped completely. Coagulation studies after 1.8 h revealed a concentration of the VK-dependent factors between 40% and 50%, PT value was 66%. Unfortunately, coagulation studies were not done when effective hemostasis was proven clinically.

Patient 3

This 27-day-old male had multiple bruises and bleeding from the umbilical stump. He was breast-fed and did not receive vitamin K prophylaxis at birth. Thirty minutes after intravenous vitamin K (1 mg), the PT value rose from < 1% to 51%; similar increases were noted for the VK-dependent factors (Fig. 3). The

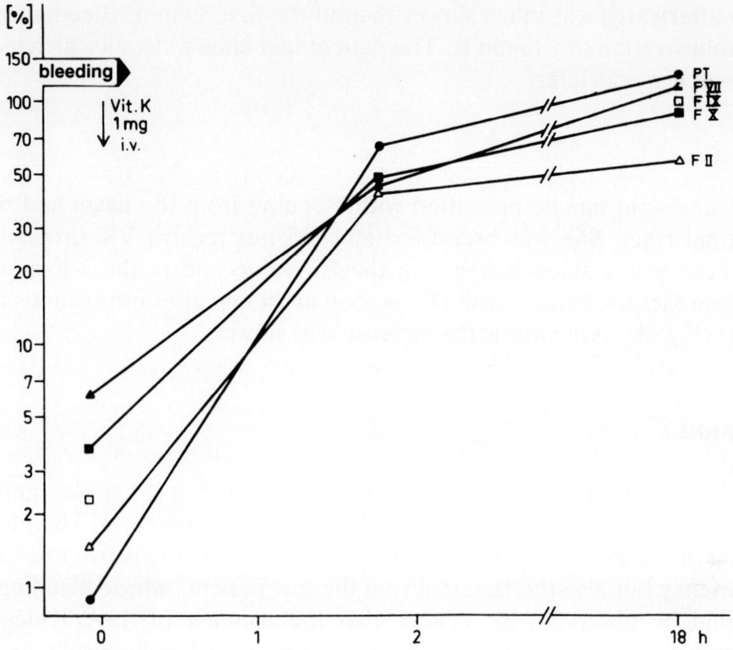

Fig. 2. Kinetics of prothrombin time (*PT*) and vitamin K-dependent coagulation factors in patient 2 after vitamin K

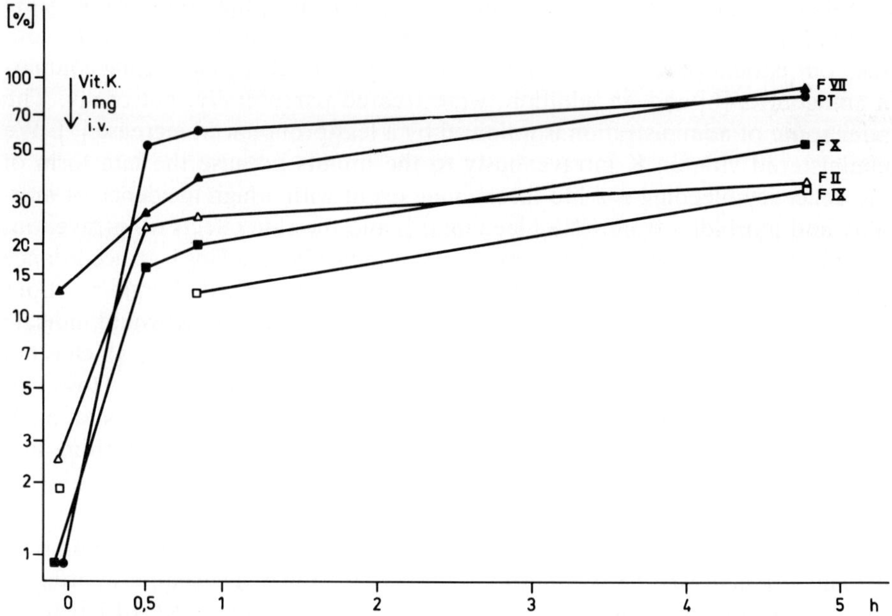

Fig. 3. Kinetics of prothrombin time (*PT*) and vitamin K-dependent coagulation factors in patient 3 after vitamin K

increase afterwards was much slower than in the first 30 min. Bleeding stopped after administration of vitamin K. The patient had biliary atresia which led to his death several weeks later.

Patient 4

This 2.5-week-old female presented with bleeding from the navel and the gastrointestinal tract. She was breast-fed and did not receive VK prophylaxis at birth. There was a steep increase in the PT value and in the VK-dependent coagulation factors, except for F IX, as soon as 20 min after intravenous vitamin K (3 mg) (Fig. 4). Afterwards the increase was slower.

Discussion

Our study indicates that VK-dependent coagulation factors increase significantly as soon as 20–30 min after intravenous vitamin K administration. Therefore, the repetition of the PT (KOLLER-test) is not only the most sensitive test to detect VK deficiency but also the fastest. From the few patients whose bleeding symptoms could be observed, we believe that the increase of the VK-dependent coagulation factors represents an effective hemostasis biochemically as well as clinically. This data contrasts with that from adult patients. In adults, it was shown in an randomized clinical trial that vitamin K did not show any great effect at 2 h in comparison with the rapid correction of the prothrombin time and the VK-dependent factors with prothrombin complex concentrate [1]. The reasons for this discrepancy may be explained by the fact that the adults were being treated for an overdose of coumarins and were given vitamin K orally. In contrast, our patients had pure vitamin K deficiency without any circulating coumarin antagonists [6] and, in addition, were treated parenterally, not orally. The latter route of administration is followed by a less-pronounced increase [7]. We administered vitamin K intravenously to the infants because the late form of VK-deficency bleeding is a life-threatening event with a high incidence of mortality and morbidity from CNS bleeding [5], and the side effects of intravenous VK injections [8] have not yet been observed in newborns. This is in accordance with the observation that anaphylactic shock and generalized allergic reactions are not seen in the newborn [9]. The fast response to vitamin K would indicate its use as an alternative to the treatment with prothrombin complex, which is not as readily available and is a potential transmitter of infectious agents. However, it has yet to be proven in an adequate sample of patients whether vitamin K would be as effective as prothrombin complex concentrates in controlling life-threatening bleeding.

Summary. According to reports, an effect of vitamin K on the prothrombin time (PT) and on hemostasis cannot be expected before 3–4 h. Therefore, in order to differentiate between vitamin K deficiency and liver disease (KOLLER-test), measurement of PT should be repeated after 6–8 h; and, when hemostasis is

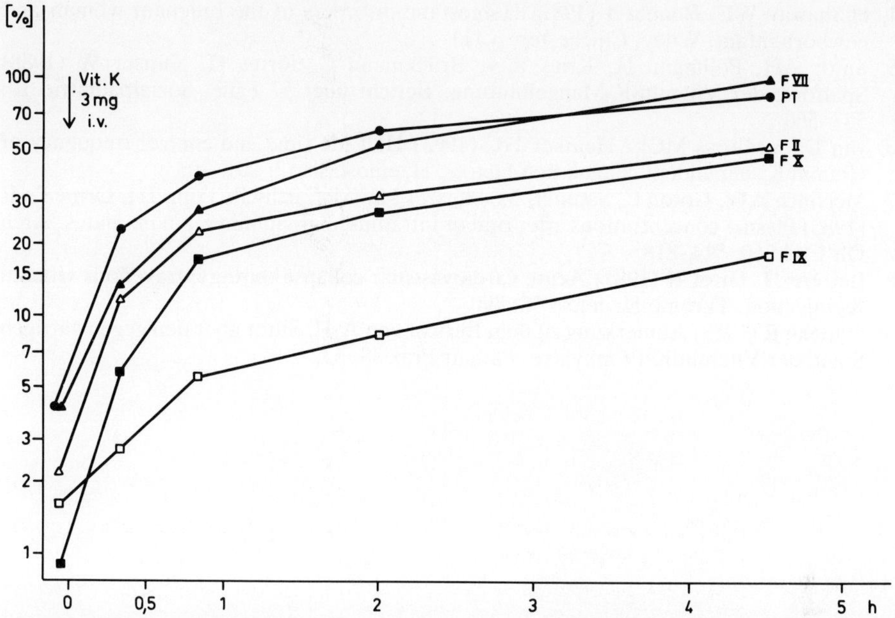

Fig. 4. Kinetics of prothrombin time (*PT*) and vitamin K-dependent coagulation factors in patient 4 after vitamin K

required, the application of prothrombin complex is advised to bridge the time between vitamin K administration and its efficacy. Our studies in infants suffering from the late form of vitamin K-deficiency bleeding, indicate however, that a significant shortening of the PT occurred as soon as 20 min after intravenous vitamin K (1–3 mg). Therefore, the KOLLER-test is not only the most sensitive but also the fastest test to detect vitamin K-deficiency. Kinetic studies revealed a rapid shortening of the PT within the first hour and a slower reduction within the next 8–16 h. Clinically, the hemostatic effect on a bleeding wound could be demonstrated as soon as 20 min after intravenous vitamin K injection. From our findings we conclude that the time interval between vitamin K administration and shortening of the PT and/or the hemostatic effect is much shorter than the widely published time of 3–4 h.

References

1. Taberner DA, Thomson JM, Poller L (1976) Comparison of prothrombin complex concentrate and vitamin K_1 in oral anticoagulant reversal. Br Med J II: 83–85
2. Barthels M, Poliwoda H (1987) Verminderung des Prothrombinkomplexes In: Barthels M, Poliwoda H (eds) Gerinnungsanalysen. Thieme, Stuttgart, pp 63–72
3. Furie B (1983) Disorders of the vitamin K-dependent coagulation factors. In: Williams WJ, Beutler E, Erslev AJ, Lichtman MA (eds) Hematology, 3rd edn. McGraw-Hill, New York, pp 1421–1424

4. Hathaway WE, Bonnar J (1987) Hemostatic disorders of the pregnant woman and newborn infant. Wiley, Chichester, p 111
5. Sutor AH, Pollmann H, Kries R v, Brückmann C, Jörres H, Künzer W (1988) Spätform der Vitamin-K-Mangelblutung. Bericht über 57 Fälle. Sozialpädiatrie 10: 557–560
6. van Dam-Mieras MCE, Hemker HC (1983) Half-life time and control frequency of vitamin K′-dependent coagulation factors. Haemostasis 13: 201–208
7. McNinch AW, Upton C, Samuels M, Shearer MJ, McCarthy P, Tripp JH, Orme l'e R (1985) Plasma concentrations after oral or intramuscular vitamin K_1 in neonates. Arch Dis Child 60: 814–818
8. Lefrère JJ, Girot R (1987) Acute cardiovascular collapse during intravenous vitamin K_1 injection. Thromb Haemost 58: 790
9. Gädeke R (1989) Anmerkung zu dem Bericht von A.H. Sutor über den gegenwärtigen Stand der Vitamin-K-Prophylaxe. Pädiatr Prax 38: 632

3.8 Effect of Vitamin K Prophylaxis on the Incidence of the Late Form of Vitamin Deficiency Bleeding

ANTON H. SUTOR and OTTO SCHARBAU[1]

Introduction

During the last 20 years routine vitamin K (VK) prophylaxis has been gradually abandoned in the Federal Republic of Germany. One reason for this tendency may be reservations towards all kinds of medication given to the newborn, especially if they are given by injection. In addition, Künzer [1] was able to show that reduced VK-dependent coagulation factors in newborns do not represent a deficiency state but a physiological condition, and prospective studies indicated that "vitamin K prophylaxis is unnecessary in healthy newborn babies" [2]. Indeed, the classic hemorrhagic disease of the newborn became rare in Germany. Published cases of four breast-fed male infants aged from 4 to 6 weeks who suffered from the late form of VK-deficiency bleeding [3] drew attention to VK-deficiency bleeding again. Since then an increasing number of new cases has become known [4]. However, there were doubts as to whether VK-prophylaxis at birth could prevent the late form due to the short half-life to vitamin K in blood [5]. In addition, in 1983 three cases with the late form of VK-deficiency bleeding in spite of intramuscular VK-prophylaxis at birth were reported [6]. Nevertheless, at the first Freiburg VK symposium, it was thought on the basis of clinical, epidemiological, and laboatory data that VK prophylaxis at birth may also prevent the late form of VK-deficiency bleeding [7]. Routine VK prophylaxis was consequently recommended by Künzer [8] and in many German medical journals in late 1986 [9]. Since 1980, we have learnt of 79 cases of the late form of VK-deficiency bleeding, and the results of a nationwide survey of the administration of VK prophylaxis in the Federal Republic of Germany have become available [10,11]. With the aid of these data we have attempted to estimate the efficacy of VK prophylaxis and to investigate whether the route of administration affects the results.

[1] Universitäts-Kinderklinik, D-7800 Freiburg, Federal Republic of Germany

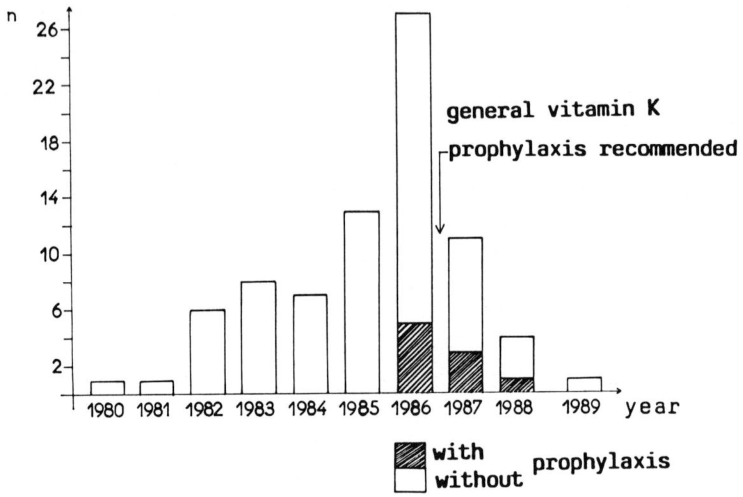

Fig. 1. Incidence of the late form of vitamin K-deficiency bleeding in the Federal Republic of Germany from 1980 to early 1989. The data up to 1987 include cases reported in a nationwide survey

Results

Changing Incidence of the Late Form of VK Deficiency Bleeding

Since 1980, cases with the late form of VK deficiency bleeding have been recorded with increasing frequency to a total of 79 (Fig. 1). Whereas in 1980 and 1981 we calculated an annual incidence of 0.2 per 100 000 births, this figure increased in 1983 to 1.4, in 1985 to 2.2, and reached a peak in 1986 with 4.3 per 100 000 (1 per 23 000) births. After routine VK prophylaxis had been recommended, the number of cases fell from 27 in 1986 to 11 in 1987. These results take into account the cases discovered in the course of a nationwide survey [10,11]. Since 1988, five more cases have come to our attention.

From the 38 cases of 1986 and 1987, 6 died; all of these had intracranial hemorrhage. Intracranial bleeding occurred in 20 (53%) cases, of which 7 (18%) had neurological sequelae. The male-female ratio was 2.2 to 1. Breast-fed infants accounted for 82%. The mean age was 5 weeks and 2 days; the youngest patient was 8 days old, and the oldest 13 weeks. Most cases (66%) occurred between the ages of 2 weeks 6 days and 7 weeks 5 days. This period represents the standard deviation from the mean. According to the criteria of Hanawa et al. [12], 55% had the secondary form of VK-deficiency bleeding manifested by hepatobiliary lesions, sustained diarrhea, or prolonged antibiotic therapy. 36 percent had the idiopathic form, where no underlying disease could be identified, and 8% were "near miss" cases which were diagnosed as a result of abnormal coagulation studies conducted, for example, in preparation for surgery.

VK Deficiency Bleeding After Recommendation of VK Prophylaxis

Of the 16 cases seen after the recommendation of VK prophylaxis, 12 did not receive VK prophylaxis at birth, 2 received oral, 1 received subcutaneous (s.c.), and 1 received intramuscular (i.m.) VK prophylaxis. The survey of the administration of VK-prophylaxis in the Federal Republic of Germany (68% response) revealed that 99% of obstetric departments give VK prophylaxis at birth, 20% only to newborns at risk, and 79% to all newborns [10,11]. The routine VK prophylaxis is given i.m. in 53%, s.c. in 17%, and orally in 21%. Although these data may change when more hospital have complied with the survey and all cases up to the present time have been included, they can serve to estimate the likelihood of acquiring the disease on the basis of 600 000 births per year in the Federal Republic of Germany.

Since 1987 the risk of suffering the late form of VK deficiency bleeding has been 38×10^{-6} (1: 27 000) for newborns not receiving VK prophylaxis at birth and 3.4×10^{-6} (1: 296 000) for newborns receiving VK prophylaxis. The risk of acquiring the disease is 2.4×10^{-6} (1: 417 000) for newborns receiving parenteral (i.m. or s.c.) VK prophylaxis: for i.m. injection the figures are 1.6×10^{-6} (1: 629 000), for s.c. injection 5.0×10^{-6} (1: 202 000), and for newborns receiving single oral VK prophylaxis, 8.0×10^{-6} (1: 125 000).

From these data it can be concluded that vitamin K prophylaxis is significantly more effective than no prophylaxis. Parenteral VK prophylaxis seems to be more efficient than oral prophylaxis. However, the difference is statistically not significant.

Of the 4 infants suffering from the late form of VK-deficiency bleeding in spite of having received VK prophylaxis at birth, two had factors considered to put them at risk for hemorrhagic disease of the newborn: one was premature and the other had a complicated delivery.

Discussion

Incidence, Symptoms, and Outcome of the Late Form of VK-Deficiency Bleeding

The annual incidence in Japan with 7.2 cases per 100 000 births (1981–1985) is 3.6 times higher than the incidence of German cases between 1982 and 1986 [12]. However, at its peak in 1986, the German incidence was 4.3 per 100 000 births. The incidence of the late form of VK-deficiency bleeding might be even higher when more hospitals have complied with the survey. In one district in England in the 17-month period up to March 1982, an incidence of 1 in 1 200 births was observed [13].

The prevalence of males is similar in Japan (1.8 to 1) and the Federal Republic of Germany (2.2 to 1). Mortality is comparable in Japan (14.5%) and the Federal Republic of Germany (16%); intracranial bleeding occurred more often in Japan (83%) than in the Federal Republic of Germany (53%). Sequelae of intracranial bleeding were higher in the Japanese cases (40%) than in the German cases (18%). Whereas in Japan the idiopathic cases were predominant (79%), we found, in 55% of the cases, an underlying disease which promotes the VK deficiency (secondary form).

Efficacy of K Prophylaxis

From our data we assume that VK prophylaxis reduces the late form of VK-deficiency bleeding. From local Japanese data from the Nagasaki and Shizuoka Prefectures, where prophylactic administration of vitamin K during the neonatal period had been carried out since 1981, a "remarkable decrease of vitamin K deficiency has been reported in these areas" [12]. These data are confirmed by the fact that the late form of VK-deficiency bleeding was more often reported in those countries where routine VK prophylaxis was not administered [4] and that the number of cases fell after VK prophylaxis was recommended [12,13]. This long-lasting effect of VK prophylaxis at birth in spite of the short half-life of vitamin K in the blood is probably due to the storage of vitamin in the liver [14].

Route of Administration of VK

Our data suggest a greater efficacy of parenteral vs single oral administration. In the literature the efficacy of a single oral dose has been judged variously; in Sweden among 50 000 infants [15] and in England among 120 000 infants [13] not a single case of the late form of VK-deficiency bleeding has been observed after single oral VK prophylaxis. In England, however, newborns at risk receive intramuscular prophylaxis. In Switzerland, where 99% of newborns receive VK prophylaxis (59% orally and 41% intramuscularly), 7 babies suffered from the late form of VK-deficiency bleeding in spite of single oral prophylaxis. Six of them had severe underlying disease, e.g., α_1-antitrypsin deficiency, liver disease, hemangioepithelioma of the liver cytomegalovirus, infection, diarrhea, and sepsis [16].

The advantage of parenteral over oral prophylaxis is that the parenteral prophylaxis is more reliably absorbed as is proven by vitamin K level determinations [5,17,18], and the incidence of failure is lower. This discrepancy might be diminished by repeating the oral dose, as has been proposed by Japanese studies [19] and recommended by [20]. In Japan the oral prophylaxis is given 2–3 times, i.e., optionally on the day of delivery and compulsorily on the day of discharge from hospital and after 4 weeks. With increasing acceptance of the routine repeated oral VK prophylaxis, a decrease in the number of cases with the late form of VK-deficiency bleeding has been reported in Japan, where this disease occurred frequently before [12].

The disadvantages of parenteral vitamin K prophylaxis are: (1) puncture wounds with risks of injury to the skin, vessels, and nerves, (2) abscesses, and (3) bleeding into muscles especially in newborns with bleeding diathesis [21,27]. In the Federal Republic of Germany local complications after intramuscular injections are very high on the list of law suits in adults [23]. There are several reports of accidental injection of Syntometrine or Methergin in adult dosage to newborn supposed to receive intramuscular vitamin K with ensuing severe sequelae including death [24,25]. In Japan intramuscular application of vitamin K has been discontinued because of concern about intramuscular injections (personal communication from Nagao, Yamada, and Yoshioka, cited in [26]. In addition to legal aspects to be considered by doctors [21,27], intramuscular injections are not as well accepted by parents as oral administration. After parenteral application of vitamin K, the VK level in the blood is ten times higher than after oral application, and the individual values differed considerably [5]. This is far above the physiological need of vitamin K for reducing protein in VK absence (PIVKA)-positive levels on the fifth day of life [28]. Several authors have pointed to the potential risks of high levels of vitamin K especially in premature infants [29,30] although side effects of overdosage have not yet been recorded. The daily oral administration of vitamin K in a low dose of 50–100 μg [31], which would solve the problems of the single oral prophylaxis as well as of the parenteral prophylaxis, is not at present practicable because of the lack of an appropriate vitamin K preparation.

Recommendation for VK Prophylaxis

At present neither the risk nor the benefit of repeated oral or single parenteral doses of vitamin K with regard to effect and side effects can yet be accurately assessed. Therefore, the Subcommittee on Hemostasis in the Newborn of the Gesellschaft für Thrombose und Hämostaseforschung (GTH) recommends the postpartum administration of vitamin K to prevent the late form of VK-deficiency bleeding in the following ways [32]: (1) VK prophylaxis is recommended for all *newborns* with either parenteral (1 mg) administration on the first day of life or repeated oral doses (2 mg) at each of the three routine postnatal examinations, i.e., immediately after delivery, between the third and the tenth day of life, and between the fourth and sixth week of life, preferably in the fourth week. (2) *Premature babies* should receive vitamin K parenterally (0.5–1.0 mg vitamin K). (3) *Babies with disturbed absorption of vitamin K*, i.e., cystic fibrosis, α_1-antitrypsin deficiency, hepatitis, biliary atresia, or chronic diarrhea, should have vitamin K administered according to prothrombin time (PT) values. Normally 1 mg per month administered parenterally should be sufficient.

Summary. Since 1980 we have recorded 79 cases of the late form of vitamin K (VK)-deficiency bleeding in the Federal Republic of Germany. From 1980 to 1986 the incidence rose from 0.2 to 4.3 cases per 100 000 births. In late 1986 recommendations for routine VK prophylaxis were published in many German medical journals, and a nationwide survey [10] revealed that 99% of obstetric departments give VK prophylaxis at birth (20% only to newborns at risk and 79% to all newborns). Routine VK prophylaxis is given in 53% i.m., in 17% s.c., and in 21% orally. Between 1986 and 1987 the number of cases fell from 27 to 11. Since 1988 we have learnt to five further cases. Of the 16 cases recorded by us since 1987: 12 did not receive VK prophylaxis at birth, 2 received oral, 1 subcutaneous, and 1 intramuscular VK prophylaxis. If we integrate our data into the survey data, the following conclusion can be drawn: (1) VK prophylaxis is effective in reducing the late form of VK deficiency as is indicated by the reduction in the number of cases after 1986. Since 1987 the risk for newborns who do not receive VK prophylaxis at birth is significantly higher than in newborns who do receive VK prophylaxis. (2) The parenteral route of administration seems to be more effective than the single oral dose in preventing the late form of VK-deficiency bleeding, however, this difference is statistically not significant. The data may change when more hospitals comply with the survey and when all recent cases have been included.

Note added in proof

After completing this study, 4 more patients with the late form of VK-deficiency bleeding between 1987 and 1989 came to our attention. The data is amended as follows: total patients, 20; no prophylaxis, 13; parenteral prophylaxis, 3; oral prophylaxis, 4. In addition, the British Paediatric Surveillance Unit informed us that: "Based on these preliminary data, the investigators concluded that intramuscular prophylaxis with vitamin K1, 1 mg protects against hemorrhagic disease of the newborn. The same dose of prophylaxis given orally is less effective, but probably better than no prophylaxis. If oral prophylaxis is to be used, regimens using larger or repeated doses, or different formulations, should be considered" (3rd Annual Report 1988–1989). Prof. Ekelund from Sweden informed us of 17 cases with the late form of VK deficiency bleeding, after he had evaluated a survey for the years 1987–89. In all cases which had informations about it, the babys were breastfed. All of them received an oral VK prophylaxis one time after delivery. All had an underlying disease, which may lead to a VK deficiency (secondary form). Nine were seriously ill, one died.

References

1. Künzer W (1971) Die Blutgerinnung bei Neugeborenen und ihre Störungen. Klin Wochenschr 49: 1–13
2. Göbel U, Sonnenschein-Kosenow S, Petrich C, Von Voss H (1977) Vitamin K deficiency in the newborn. Lancet II: 187–188
3. Sutor AH, Pancochar H, Niederhoff H, Pollmann H, Hilgenberg F, Palm D, Künzer W (1983) Vitamin-K-Mangelblutungen bei 4 vollgestillten Säuglingen im Alter von 4–6 Lebenswochen. Dtsch Med Wochenschr 108: 1635–1639
4. Sutor AH, Pollmann H, Von Kries R, Brückmann C, Jörres H, Künzer W (1988) Spätform der Vitamin-K-Mangelblutung. Bericht über 57 Fälle. Sozialpädiatrie 10: 557–560
5. McNinch AW, Upton C, Samuels M, Shearer MJ, McCarthy P, Tripp JH, Orme l'e R (1985) Plasma concentrations after oral or intramuscular vitamin K_1 in neonates. Arch Dis Child 60: 814–818
6. Verity CM, Carswell F, Scott GL (1983) Vitamin K deficiency causing infantile intracranial haemorrhage after the neonatal period. Lancet I: 1439
7. Sutor AH, Künzer W (1986) Physiologie und Pathophysiologie des Vitamins K. Roche, Basel Grenzach-Wyhlen
8. Künzer W (1986) Schlusswort. In: Sutor AH, Künzer W (eds) Physiologie und Pathophysiologie des Vitamin K. Roche, Basel Grenzach-Wyhlen, pp 243–244

9. Bergmann KH, Bremer HJ, Droese W, Grüttner R, Knübler W, Schmidt E, Schöch G; prepared for the Commission by Von Kries R, Göbel U (1986) Empfehlungen der Ernährungskommission der Deutschen Gesellachaft für Kinderheilkunde zur Vitamin K-Prophylaxe bei Neugeborenen. Monatschr Kinderheilk 134: 823–824; Kinderarzt 17: 1602; Sozialpädiatrie 8: 706–707; Dtsch Ärzteblatt 83: 3380–3383
10. Göbel U, Meier F, Von Kries R, Sutor AH (1989) Ergebnisse der Umfrage zur Vitamin-K-Prophylaxe in Deutschland. In: Sutor AH, Göbel U (eds) Gegenwärtiger Stand der Vitamin-K-Prophylaxe in Deutschland. Roche, Basel Grenzach-Wyhlen, pp 11–21
11. Scharbau O, Sutor AH (1989) Ergebnisse der Freiburger Auswertung. In: Sutor AH, Göbel U (eds) Gegenwärtiger Stand der Vitamin-K-Prophylaxe in Deutschland. Roche, Basel Grenzach-Wyhlen, pp 21
12. Hanawa Y, Maki M, Murata B, Matsuyama E, Yamamoto Y, Nagao T, Yamada K, Ikeda I, Terao I, Mikami S, Shiraki K, Komazawa M, Shirahata A, Tsuji Y, Motohara K, Tsukimoto I, Sawada K (1988) The second nationwide survey in Japan of vitamin K deficiency. Eur J Pediatr 147: 472–477
13. McNinch AW (1989) Haemorrhagic disease and vitamin K prophylaxis in Exeter UK. In: Sutor AH, Göbel U (eds) Gegenwärtiger Stand der Vitamin-K-Prophylaxe in Deutschland. Roche, Basel Grenzach-Wyhlen, pp 175–178
14. McCarthy PT, Shearer MJ, Gau G, Crampton OE, Barkhan P (1986) Vitamin K content of human liver at different ages. In: Sutor AH, Künzer W (1986) Physiologie und Pathophysiologie des Vitamins K. Roche, Basel Grenzach-Wyhlen, pp 95–104
15. Ekelund H (1989) Vitamin-K-Prophylaxe in Schweden. In: Sutor, Göbel U (eds) Gegenwärtiger Stand der Vitamin-K-Prophylaxe in Deutschland. Roche, Basel Grenzach-Wyhlen, pp 149
16. Tönz O, Schubiger G (1988) Neonatale Vitamin-K-Prophylaxe und Vitamin-K-Mangelblutungen in der Schweiz. Schweiz Med Wochenschr 118: 1747–1752
17. Von Kries R, Shearer M-J, Meier F, Göbel U (1989) Pharmakokinetiche Untersuchungen nach subkutaner Vitamin K-Gabe bei Neugeborenen. In: Sutor AH, Göbel U (eds) Gegenwärtiger Stand der Vitamin-K-Prophylaxe in Deutschland. Roche, Basel Grenzach-Wyhlen, pp 137–142
18. Shinzawa T, Mura T, Tsunei M, Shiraki K (1989) Vitamin K absorption capacity and its association with vitamin K deficiency. Am J Dis Child 143: 686–689
19. Motohara K, Endo F, Matsuda I (1986) Vitamin K deficiency in breast- fed infants at one month of age. J Pediatr Gastroenterol Nutr 5: 931–933
20. Sann L, Leclercq M, Guillaumont M, Bethenod M (1988) Faut-il supplémenter le nouveau-né en vitamine K? Arch Fr Pediatr 45: 775–777
21. Gädeke R (1989) Anmerkung zu dem bericht von A.H. Sutor et al. über den gegenwärtigen Stand der Vitamin-K-Prophylaxe. Padiatr Prax 38: 632
22. Mang K (1989) Intramuskuläre Vitamin-K-Prophylaxe bei Hämophilen. In: Sutor AH, Göbel U (eds) Gegenwärtiger Stand der Vitamin-K-Prophylaxe in Deutschland. Roche, Basel Grenzach-Wyhlen, pp 107–110
23. Müller-Vahl (1985) Schäden durch intramuskuläre Injektion. Dtsch Ärzteblatt 82: 2626–2633
24. Whitfield MF, Salfield SAW (1980) Accidental administration of Syntometrine in adulat dosage to the newborn. Arch Dis Child 55: 68–70
25. Tönz O (1989) Discussion remark. In: Sutor AH, Göbel U (eds) Gegenwärtiger Stand der Vitamin-K-Prophylaxe in Deutschland. Roche, Basel Grenzach-Wyhlen
26. Sutor AH, Suzuki S, Yoshioka H (1989) Vitamin-K-Prophylaxe in Japan. Pädiatr Prax 38: 629–631
27. Gädeke R (1989) Nebenwirkungen der Vitamin-K-Prophylaxe, deren haftungsrechtliche Beurteilung und deren Verhütung. In: Sutor, Göbel U (eds) Gegenwärtiger Stand der Vitamin-K-Prophylaxe in Deutschland. Roche, Basel Grenzach-Wyhlen, pp 115–122
28. Motohara K, Matsukane I, Endo F, Kijota Y, Matsuda, I (1989) Relationship of milk intake and vitamin K supplementation to vitamin K status in newborns. Pediatrics 84: 90–93

29. Künzer W, Niederhoff H (1988) Vitamin-K-Versorgung der Neugeborenen. Dtsch Med Wochenschr 113: 432–438
30. Allen AC (1988) for the Fetus and Newborn Committee of the Canadian Paediatric Society. The use of vitamin K in the perinatal period. Can Med Assoc J 139: 127–130
31. Von Kries R, Shearer M, Meier F, Göbel U (1989) Protrahierte orale Vitamin-K-Prophylaxe. In: Sutor AH, Göbel U (eds) Gegenwärtiger Stand der Vitamin-K-Prophylaxe in Deutschland. Roche, Basel Grenzach-Wyhlen, pp 201–209
32. Sutor AH, Göbel U, Von Kries R, Künzer W, Landbeck G (1989) Vitamin-K-Prophylaxe. Stellungnahme der Teilnehmer am 2. Freiburger Vitamin-K-Symposion und der GTH-Arbeitsgruppe Hämostaseologie im Kindes- und Jugendalter. Pädiatr Prax 38: 625–628

3.9 Antithrombin III Administration in Premature Infants with Intracranial Hemorrhage

Tsuyomu Ikenoue, Satoshi Ibara, Takahiro Hirano, and Yuko Ninomiya[1]

Introduction

Intracranial hemorrhage (ICH) is a significant cause of mortality and morbidity in the neonatal intensive care unit. Abnormalities of coagulation have been implicated as one of the important causes of intracranial hemorrhage in premature infants. Recent advances in the technique of ultrasound diagnosis of ICH in premature infants have made it possible for us to determine the presence of ICH even in the early stages of the disease. This study was conducted to ascertain whether antithrombin III (AT III) inhibits the progress of ICH in prematurely born infants.

Patients and Methods

Thirty-five premature infants of 24–31 weeks gestation were enrolled in this study immediately after documentation of ICH by real-time ultrasound (Aloka SSD 250) examinations, which were performed on admission and repeated intermittently at intervals of at least eight hours thereafter. When ICH was documented by ultrasound examination, the first blood samples for coagulation study were obtained from indwelling umbilical or radial arterial lines through which heparinized saline was continuously infused at the rate of 0.5 unit per h. After carefully clearing the line of any infusion fluid, a total of 1.0 ml of citrated whole blood was withdrawn. The citrated sample was immediately centrifuged at 2500 g for 20 min and the citrated plasma was immediately frozen and stored at −80 °C until tests were performed. Subsequent blood samples were obtained in the same fashion on day 1, 2, 3, and 7 when patient condition allowed. The progression of ICH was observed for seven days following documentation by

[1]Perinatal Medical Center, Kagoshima Municipal Hospital, Kajiya-cho 20–17, Kagoshima, Japan

ultrasound examination and was expressed using the criteria of Papile et al [1], based on the ultrasound examination findings.

Results

Immediately after diagnosis of ICH 18 infants received AT III concentrate (Behringwerke AG) 60 units/kg twice a day; this regimen continued for three days subsequently. Seventeen infants who did not receive AT III concentrate were chosen as a control group. This control group consisted of the infants who were treated in our neonatal intensive care unit before the AT III concentrate became available. Throughout the total observation period of 2 years and 3 months, there were no essential changes in the treatment protocols for ICH in premature infants except for the use of AT III concentrate. The patients' backgrounds are listed in Table 1.

Table 1. Background of 35 infants with ICH

		AT III (+) ($n = 18$)	AT III (−) ($n = 17$)	
Gestational age		27.7 ± 2.3 wks	27.5 ± 1.7 wks	N.S.
Birth weight		1062 ± 343 g	1014 ± 284 g	N.S.
Apgar score (1 min)		5.9 ± 2.7	4.7 ± 2.8	N.S.
Blood gas pH (adm.)		7.26 ± 0.11	7.26 ± 0.13	N.S.
RDS	(+)	13	14	N.S.
	(−)	5	3	
Infection	(+)	8	4	N.S.
	(−)	10	13	
Hypotension	(+)	12	11	N.S.
	(−)	6	6	
FFP or fresh	(+)	9	8	N.S.
Whole blood	(−)	9	9	
Exchanged blood	(+)	8	5	N.S.
trans.	(−)	10	12	

ICH, intracranial hemorrhage; AT III, Antithrombin III

The mean gestational week of the AT III treated group was 27.7 ± 2.3 weeks and that of the AT III non-treated group was 27.5 ± 1.7 weeks. The mean birth weight of the AT III treated group was 1062 ± 343 g and that of the non-treated group was 1014 ± 284 g. The mean Apgar score one min in the treated group was 5.9 ± 2.7 and in the non-treated group the mean was 4.7 ± 2.8. The blood pH on admission was 7.26 ± 0.11 and 7.26 ± 0.13 respectively. The incidence of mechanical ventilation to support respiratory distress was 13/18 and 14/17. The incidence of clinical evidence of infection was 5/18 and 4/17. The incidence of hypotension which required catecholamine administration to keep the systolic

Table 2. Change of ICH hemorrhagic grade

ICH	AT III (+)	AT III (−)
No change	14	4
Advanced	4	13
Total	18	17

P<0.01
ICH, intracranial hemorrhage; AT III, Antithrombin III

pressure above 40 mmHg was 12/18 and 11/17. The incidence of fresh frozen plasma or fresh whole blood infusion was 9/18 and 8/17. The incidence of exchange blood transfusions for various reasons was 8/18 and 5/12. None of these background factors differed significantly between the two groups.

The effect of AT III infusion on the progression of intracranial hemorrhage in premature infants is listed in Table 2. Antithrombin III was given in 18 cases, and among them only 4 cases developed further hemorrhage and worsened disease states, while all of the rest stayed in the same grade, without any further progression of ICH. On the other hand, out of 17 cases who did not receive AT III concentrate, only 4 cases stayed in the same grade of ICH; the others showed further progression. These differences were significant ($\beta < 0.01$).

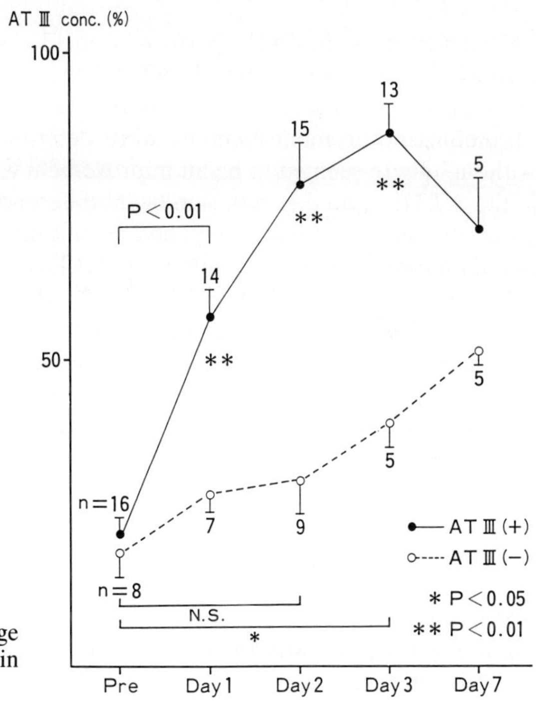

Fig. 1. Intracranial hemorrhage cases, changes of Antithrombin (AT) III conc. (%)

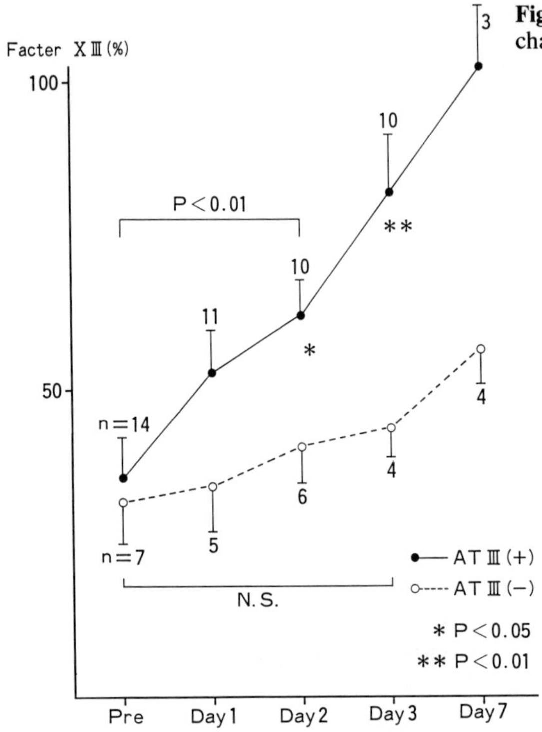

Fig. 2. Intracranial hemorrhage cases, changes of factor XIII (%)

Coagulation studies were performed in 13 cases of the AT III group and in 7 cases of the group to which AT III was not given. Factor XIII, AT III, Fibrinogen, Fibrin Degradation Product (FDP)-D dimer, platelet counts, and Thrombin-antithrombin complex were determined for each group of infants. Although there seemed to be an improvement tendency in the coagulation data in the AT III treated group, significant differences in AT III were found in this group on days 1, 2, and 3 only; and significant differences in Factor XIII were found on days 2 and 3 after initiation of AT III treatment (Figs. 1, 2).

We examined Factor XIII in the patients who did not have intracranial hemorrhage. The number observed is still scanty at present; we could not see significant differences between the two groups—AT III treated and non-treated—patients (Fig. 3). It is, therefore, likely that the consumption of Factor XIII associated with the occurrence of intracranial hemorrhage is inhibited by the administration of AT III.

Conclusion

We studied the effects of AT III administration on the clinical course of intracranial hemorrhage in premature infants. When AT III concentrate was given after documentation of the presence of hemorrhage, progression of the disease

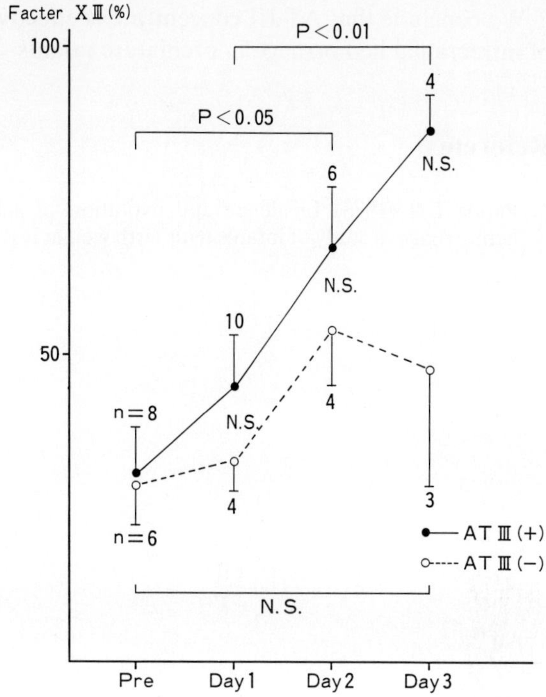

Fig. 3. Non-intracranial hemorrhage cases, changes of factor XIII (%)

occurred in only 22.2% of the patients while in the AT III non-treated control group clinical progression occurred in 76% of the patients. We conclude that AT III concentrate is effective in inhibiting the progression of intracranial hemorrhage.

Summary. Intracranial hemorrhage (ICH) in premature infants is a significant cause of mortality of morbidity in the neonatal intensive care unit.

After ICH was documented by ultrasound examination, AT III concentrate (Behringewrke AG) 60 unit/kg, was given twice a day and continued for three days subsequently. The progression of ICH, based on Papille's classification, was observed for 7 days.

Eighteen infants (mean: 27.6 weeks, 1069 g) received AT III concentrates while a control group of seventeen infants (mean: 27.9 weeks, 1027 g) did not. Gestational age, birth weight, Apgar scores, pH on admission, incidence of respirator care, episodes of hypotension, fresh frozen plasma administration, blood transfusion, exchange blood transfusion and infection did not differ significantly between the two groups.

Of 18 infants who received AT III concentrate, only 4 infants developed a worsened hemorrhagic grade. On the other hand, 13 of the 17 infants who did not receive AT III concentrate developed progression of the hemorrhage after initial documentation of ICH. Coagulative study revealed the increase of Factor XIII and the elevation of AT III in the AT III treated group.

We conclude that AT III concentrate is effective in inhibiting the progression of intracranial hemorrhage in premature infants.

Reference

1. Papile LA (1978) Incidence and evolution of subependymal and intraventricular hemorrhage: a study of infants with birth weight less than 1,500 grm. J Pediatr 902: 529

3.10 Six Cases of Alpha-1-Antitrypsin Deficiency Presenting as a Bleeding Diathesis with Intracranial Hemorrhage in the Newborn

GÜNTER AUERSWALD[1] and ANTON H. SUTOR[2]

Introduction

Alpha-1-antitrypsin (alpha-1-AT), or alpha-1-protease inhibitor is a glycoprotein with a molecular weight of about 52. 000 daltons. More than 90% of it is synthesized by the liver. The concentration in serum in healthy children is 2.0–3.3 g/l. Alpha-1-AT constitutes about 90% of the whole alpha-1-globulin fraction. The gene responsible for the production of alpha-1-AT is situated on the long arm of chromosome 14.

Alpha-1-AT exists in more than 50 different biochemical variants known collectively as the Pi-system, the abbreviation standing for "protease inhibitor". The variants are designated by a capital letter corresponding to their mobility in isoelectric focusing. The common variant is known as type M, whose frequency in most populations is between 0.866 and 0.994. Other important variants are known as S and Z. The six possible phenotypes derived from M, S, and Z are shown in Table 1. Type Z homozygous persons have about 10%–15% of the normal serum alpha-1-AT concentration.

Homozygotes of type Z have been most commonly implicated in the pathogenesis of emphysema and hepatocellular damage. Disabling shortness of breath can occur as early as 30 years of age, or later. The effect on the liver, however, begins much earlier. This complication afflicts only a minority of infants with this phenotype, but those affected may experience serious long-term consequences. In some of these infants hepatitis seems to develop. They usually present in the first few weeks of life with hepatocellular damage and obstructive jaundice.

The outcome of 67 type Z infants (Table 2) who presented with hepatitis was assessed in a study carried out in the United Kingdom [1]. The maximal duration

[1] Professor Hess-Kinderklinik, ZKH St.-Jürgen-Straße D-2800 Bremen 1, Federal Republic of Germany

[2] Universitäts-Kinderklinik, D-7800 Freiburg i.Br., Federal Republic of Germany

Table 1. Serum α_1-AT concentrations associated with the commoner phenotypes. (From [6])

Phenotype	Serum α_1-AT concentration (g/l)		Mean percentage contribution (%)
	Mean	SD	
MM	2.86	0.73	100
MS	2.15	0.47	75
MZ	1.64	0.44	57
SS	1.49	0.23	52
SZ	1.06	0.34	37
ZZ	0.45	0.08	16

Table 2. The outcome of 67 type Z infants. (From [1])

Death from liver disease	28%
Cirrhosis	28%
Persisting clinical or biochemical abnormalities (without cirrhosis)	21%
Completely normal	22%

Table 3. Special findings

1. The bleeding disorders did not begin without early signs
2. In all six children a severe bleeding diathesis with intracranial haemorrhage was found
3. The infants (two female and four male) became ill between the 3rd and 6th week of age
4. None of the children had received vitamin K after birth
5. All children were fully breast-fed
6. In all six children vitamin K, fresh frozen plasma or PCC returned the prothrombin time and partial thromboplastin time to normal values
7. All six children had a homozygous (pi-type ZZ [PiZZ]) α_1-antitrypsin deficiency

of follow-up was 17 years. Twenty-eight percent of the patients died of liver disease, 28% had established cirrhosis, and 21% had persisting clinical or biochemical abnormalities (without cirrhosis). Only 22% appeared to be completely normal. Bleeding disorders due to alpha-1-AT deficiency and liver disease in early childhood are often reported in the literature. We found only a few reports of severe intracranial hemorrhage as the first important symptom of alpha-1-AT deficiency due to lack of vitamin K dependent coagulation factors [2,3,4,5]. This is probably explained by the decreased intestinal absorption of vitamin K resulting from the cholestatic liver disease.

Results

The case reports of six infants with homozygous Pi ZZ-type alpha-1-AT deficiency who were born between 1982 and 1986 are described. Specific findings for these children are shown in Table 3. Of special interest is the fact that in all cases

Table 4. Details of the six infants (all children were breast-fed and had not received vitamin K at birth)

	Case 1	Case 2	Case 3	Case 4	Case 5	Case 6
Serum α_1-antitrypsin level [g/l]	0.86	0.48	0.32	0.36	0.82	0.47
Pi phenotype	ZZ	ZZ	ZZ	ZZ	ZZ	ZZ
Neonatal jaundice	+ (Phototherapy)	+	+ (Phototherapy)	+	+	–
Direct bilirubin	↑	↑	↑	↑	↑	n.i.*
First clinical symptoms	3rd week: increased bleeding from venepuncture site	From 2nd week: vomiting, failure to thrive	From 3rd week: flatulency, failure to thrive	From 2nd week: failure to thrive faeces with blood	From 3rd week: restlessness, vomiting	In the 3rd week: bleeding from the navel ground and nose
Intracranial haemorrhage at age (weeks)	6	5	4	3	4	4
Current clinical status	Hydrocephalus, developmental delay	Hydrocephalus, severe spastic syndrome (see figs. 1 + 2)	Hydrocephalus, severe developmental delay, epilepsy, exitus letalis at age of 35 months	Hydrocephalus, developmental delay	Moderate ventricular enlargement, mild developmental delay	Exitus letalis after 6 days

*Not investigated

the diagnosis of alpha-1-AT deficiency was made after the intracranial hemorrhage occurred. It should be emphasized that in all six cases, intracranial hemorrhage was the first serious complication of alpha-1-AT deficiency. As a result, hydrocephalus was seen in 4 cases and serious neurological damage was seen in all cases (Table 4).

Computed tomography (CT) findings for child 2 (Figs. 1, 2) show the beginning of enlarged ventricles and blood in the subarachnoid space above the tentorium as well as a small amount of bleeding frontoparietally in the right hemisphere. Fig. 2 shows the CT of the same child 3 years later; now with multicystic encephalomalacia and nearly complete destruction of the cerebral hemispheres. One child (case 6) died six days after intracranial hemorrhage was diagnosed. Another child (case 3) died after 35 months with clinical signs of severe liver cirrhosis, extreme developmental delay, and convulsions which did not respond to treatment. In one child (case 5) the hemorrhage caused mild hemiplegia of the left side and only moderate ventricular enlargement without elevated intracra-

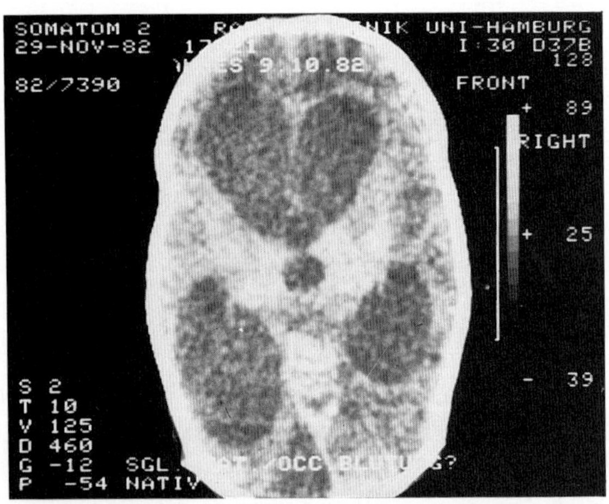

Fig. 1. Computed tomography (CT) findings for child 2

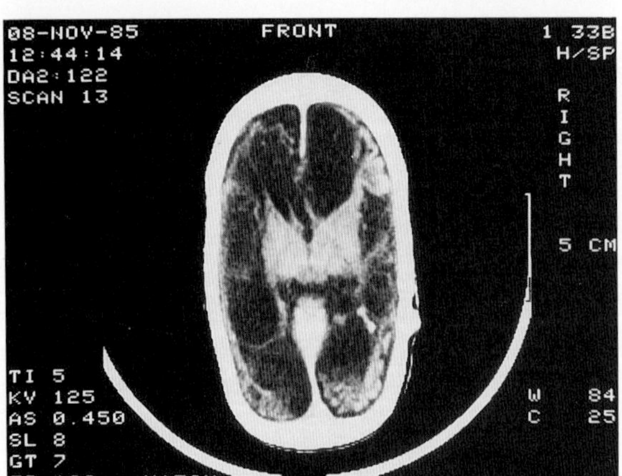

Fig. 2. Computed tomography (CT) findings for child 2 three years later

Table 5. Coagulation at clinical presentation

		Case 1	Case 2	Case 3	Case 4	Case 5	Case 6
PT (Quick's test)	[%]	10	2	<1	4,2	<1	<1
PTT	[sec]	120	160	180	180	200	200
Factor II	[%]	10	n.i.	1.3	10	n.i.	10
Factor VII	[%]	10	11	<1	10	n.i.	10
Factor IX	[%]	n.i.	<1	<1	<1	n.i.	<1

n.i., not investigated

nial pressure. The other 3 children (cases 1, 2, and 4) developed hydrocephalus with psychomotor retardation and developmental delay.

In all cases studied the coagulation tests (Table 5) showed the expected prolongation of prothrombin time and partial thromboplastin time. The levels of vitamin K dependent factors II, VII and IX, when investigated, were greatly reduced. We did not find any signs of disseminated intravascular coagulation (DIC). Treatment with either vitamin K, fresh frozen plasma or Prothrombin complex concentrate returned the prothrombin time and partial thromboplastin time to normal values within a few hours. All the children had only borderline elevation of liver enzymes and had normal platelet counts. Five children had hyperbilirubinaemia in the neonatal period and two needed phototherapy for not more than 48 hours.

An important finding is that all the children had histories of problems during the second or third week of life (Table 4). Three children (1, 4, and 6) had mild bleeding problems. This was possibly the first indication of vitamin K deficiency. Mild hyperbilirubinaemia, failure to thrive, and vomiting may provide clues to the existense of cholestatic liver disease and homozygous alpha-1-AT deficiency. Intracranial hemorrhage occurred between the third and sixth week of age. There was no subsequent evidence of bacterial or viral infections in any of the children. None of the children had received vitamin K prophylaxis after birth and all were fully breast-fed.

Discussion

This report concerns six fully breast fed infants with homozygous alpha-1-AT deficiency, who did not receive vitamin K prophylaxis after birth, and who suddenly became ill between the third and sixth week of life with signs of acute

Table 6. Risk factors

1. Decreased intestinal absorption of vitamin K due to the cholestatic liver disease caused by α-1-AT deficiency
2. Diet consisting solely of breast milk, which is known to contain little vitamin K
3. Failure to administer prophylactic vitamin K at birth

deterioration of the CNS. In the computed tomography all showed the signs of intracranial hemorrhage. The coagulation studies (Table 5) confirm vitamin K deficiency. The final diagnostic confirmation was the rapid therapeutic response to vitamin K administration.

The cause of vitamin K deficiency could be decreased intestinal absorption of vitamin K, due to cholestatic liver disease induced by alpha-1-AT deficiency (Table 6). Another cause could be the diet which consisted solely of breast milk, which is known to contain low concentrations of vitamin K.

A striking similarity between previously reported patients with late-onset hemorrhagic disease and our 6 patients was the failure to administer prophylactic vitamin K at birth. Not all neonates with homozygous alpha-1-AT deficiency have severe jaundice or other obvious signs of hepatic dysfunction. Accordingly, it seems important to obtain at least one measurement of total and direct bilirubin in any jaundiced newborn to screen for direct hyperbilirubinaemia associated with cholestasis. Even mild liver enzyme abnormalities deserve attention and evaluation. Any hint of a bleeding diathesis needs coagulation tests.

Conclusion

Our experience should remind clinicians of the potentially serious consequences of failing to administer vitamin K at birth and of failing to give supplementary vitamin K to all solely breast-fed infants who have conditions such as alpha-1-AT deficiency with the consequent decreased absorption of fat soluble vitamins.

Summary. Six cases of alpha-1-antitrypsin deficiency are reported. Each infant who presented with intracranial hemorrhage responded to vitamion K. All children were fully breast-fed and did not receive vitamin K at birth. Although it was subsequently proved that five of the six infants had conjugated hyperbilirubinaemia, their presentation was with severe hemorrhagic phenomena rather than with prolonged jaundice. The levels of alpha-1-AT in all infants were below 90 mg/100 ml with a phenotype PIZZ. They all presented between the second and sixth week of life. Bleeding disorders due to alpha-1-AT deficiency and liver disease in childhood are often reported in the literature but there are only a few reports of severe intracranial hemorrhage as the first important symptom of homozygote alpha-1-AT deficiency due to the lack of vitamin K dependent factors.

References

1. Psacharopoulos HT, Mowat AP, Cook PJL, Carlile PA, Portmann B, Rodeck CH (1983) Outcome of liver disease associated with alpha-1-antitrypsin deficiency (Pi Z). Arch Dis Child 58: 882–887
2. Payne NR, Hasegawa DK (1984) Vitamin K deficiency in newborns: a case report in α-1-antitrypsin deficiency and a review of factors predisposing to hemorrhage. J Pediatr 73: 712–716

3. Fidalgo I, Vazquez C, Rodriguez-Soriano J (1982) Intracranial hemorrhage due to vitamin K deficiency associated with alpha-1-antitrypsin deficiency type Pi Z. Arch Dis Child 57: 722
4. Jenkins HR, Leonard JV, Kay JDS (1982) Alpha-1-antitrypsin deficiency, bleeding diathesis, and intracranial hemorrhage. Arch Dis Child 57: 722–723
5. Hope PL, Hall MA, Millward-Sadler GH, Normand ICS (1982) Alpha-1-antitrypsin deficiency presenting as a bleeding diathesis in the newborn. Arch Dis Child 57: 68–70
6. Hutchison DCS (1988) Natural history of alpha-1-protease inhibitor deficiency (Suppl. 6A). Am J Med 84: 3–12

Index